RECONSTRUCTION OF THE HEAD AND NECK

RECONSTRUCTION OF THE HEAD AND NECK

Edited by

Malcolm A. Lesavoy M.D., F.A.C.S.

Assistant Professor of Surgery
Division of Plastic Surgery
U.C.L.A. School of Medicine
Los Angeles, California

Chief, Plastic and Reconstructive Surgery
Harbor General Hospital
Torrance, California

Chief, Plastic and Reconstructive Surgery
Long Beach General Hospital
Long Beach, California

SANS TACHE

WILLIAMS & WILKINS
Baltimore/London

Made in the United States of America

Library of Congress Cataloging in Publication Data

Main entry under title:

Reconstruction of the head and neck.

Includes index.
1. Head—Surgery. 2. Neck—Surgery. 3. Surgery, Plastic. I. Lesavoy, Malcolm A.
RD521.R42 617'51 79-24352
ISBN 0-683-04949-6

Composed and printed at the
Waverly Press, Inc.
Mt. Royal and Guilford Aves.
Baltimore, Md. 21202, U.S.A.

DEDICATION

To my wife, Jeannie, and my children, Brian, Jordan, and Nikki
for their love, devotion, patience and support.

Malcolm A. Lesavoy, M.D., F.A.C.S.

PREFACE

This book is designed to elucidate the basic principles and techniques of reconstruction of the head and neck region. It is not meant to be a "how to do it" textbook. It is meant to scratch the surface and illustrate to the reader a number of ways of attacking a particular problem. It is by no means a definitive and "only way" textbook. It is meant to pique and stimulate the readers' imagination toward newer and better ways of reconstruction.

Any textbook on plastic and reconstructive surgery can never be definitive. Various other textbooks already published deal with similar problems. This textbook attempts to deal with construction of parts of the human anatomy above the clavicles in a segmental fashion. One has to constantly keep in mind, however, that although various parts of our body are segmental in nature, everything is connected. One cannot contemplate plastic and reconstructive procedures on the "head bone" without considering the "neck bone" to which it is connected.

Reconstructive surgery is a constantly changing field. Newer techniques of microvascular reconstruction and recent advances in the repair and reconstruction of craniofacial anomalies have given plastic and reconstructive surgeons new outlooks for tackling functional and cosmetic parts of our anatomy.

It is with utmost humility that the editor and contributing authors offer this book for use by practicing physicians, residents, interns and medical students interested in imagination in reconstructive surgery.

CONTRIBUTORS

Thomas C. Calcaterra, M.D., F.A.C.S.
Professor of Surgery
Division of Head and Neck Surgery
U.C.L.A. School of Medicine
Los Angeles, California

Andrew E. Choy, M.D.
Clinical Instructor
Department of Ophthalmology
U.C.L.A. School of Medicine
Los Angeles, California

Rollin K. Daniel, M.D., F.R.C.S.(C)
Chief, Division of Plastic Surgery
Royal Victoria Hospital
Montreal, Canada
Associate Professor of Surgery
McGill University School of Medicine
Montreal, Canada

Frederick R. Eilber, M.D., F.A.C.S.
Professor of Surgery
Division of Oncology
U.C.L.A. School of Medicine
Los Angeles, California

Henry K. Kawamoto, Jr., M.D., D.D.S.
Acting Chief
Division of Plastic Surgery
Sepulveda Veteran's Administration Hospital
Sepulveda, California
Assistant Clinical Professor
Division of Plastic Surgery
U.C.L.A. School of Medicine
Los Angeles, California

Malcolm A. Lesavoy, M.D., F.A.C.S.
Assistant Professor of Surgery
Division of Plastic Surgery
U.C.L.A. School of Medicine
Los Angeles, California
Chief, Plastic and Reconstructive Surgery
Harbor General Hospital
Torrance, California
Chief, Plastic and Reconstructive Surgery
Long Beach General Hospital
Long Beach, California

John William Little III, M.D.
Assistant Professor of Surgery (Plastic)
and Director,
Division of Plastic and Reconstructive Surgery,
Georgetown University Medical School
Consultant in Plastic Surgery,
the National Cancer Institute,
National Institutes of Health,
Washington, D.C.

Timothy A. Miller, M.D., F.A.C.S.
Chief, Plastic and Reconstructive Surgery
Wadsworth Veteran's Administration Hospital
Los Angeles, California
Associate Professor of Surgery
Division of Plastic Surgery
U.C.L.A. School of Medicine
Los Angeles, California

Walter R. Mullin, M.D.
Clinical Assistant Professor
Division of Plastic Surgery
University of Miami School of Medicine
Miami, Florida

Jon A. Perlman, M.D.
Chief Resident in Plastic Surgery
U.C.L.A. School of Medicine
Los Angeles, California

F. Kristian Storm III, M.D., F.A.C.S.
Assistant Professor of Surgery
U.C.L.A. School of Medicine
Los Angeles, California

S. Anthony Wolfe, M.D., F.A.C.S.
Clinical Associate Professor
Division of Plastic Surgery
University of Miami School of Medicine
Miami, Florida

Harvey A. Zarem, M.D., F.A.C.S.
Professor and Chief
Division of Plastic Surgery
U.C.L.A. School of Medicine
Los Angeles, California

ACKNOWLEDGMENTS

No medical textbook can be written alone. Aside from the numerous contributing authors that appear in print, many extremely important people behind the scenes carry out the tasks that make the completion of a book successful. It is here that the editor and contributing authors would like to acknowledge secretaries, medical illustrators, patients, medical students and residents, and family that have enabled thought and hard work to come to fruition.

I would personally like to acknowledge the long hours and tremendous work contributed by Mrs. Patty Lindsly, Mrs. Juanita Navarette, and Mrs. Janet Lewis. Their collation, typing, efficiency, and patience contributed greatly to the successful completion of this book. I would also like to thank Mrs. Hermina Kavanah for her excellent medical illustrations and her professional expertise in being able to put on paper what is in one's mind.

I would like to thank our residents and medical students who constantly stimulate our minds to deeper thought, our patients who allow us to care for them tenderly, but efficiently, for relief of disease, pain, and disfigurement and who allow us to continue to learn.

Gratitude and acknowledgment must be given to Mrs. Susan Vitalle and Mr. George Stamathis of Williams & Wilkins. Their cooperation, professional expertise, and consistent patience have made the publishing of this book a true cooperative venture.

Finally, I would like to thank my parents, Harry and Rae Lesavoy, who stimulated and supported my early medical education.

Malcolm A. Lesavoy, M.D., F.A.C.S.

CONTENTS

CHAPTER 1

Evaluation and Examination

Malcolm A. Lesavoy, M.D., F.A.C.S.

In any reconstructive problem, evaluation of the deformity by taking the history and doing a physical examination is of utmost importance. One's evaluation is made up of many factors. The reconstructive surgeon must always keep in mind that beauty is definitely not in the eye of the beholder, but in the "beholdee." The patient's needs and desires should be foremost in the surgeon's mind, not the reverse. Many an experienced plastic and reconstructive surgeon has entered the examining room for initial consultation with a patient and is confronted with the visual impact of a large nose. The first words out of his mouth are, "Mrs. Jones, I am Doctor Smith, and I'll be glad to take care of you and correct your nasal deformity." Mrs. Jones then replies, "Doctor Smith, what is wrong with my nose? I think it is quite nice, as does my husband. It is the small mole that I have behind my ear that I would like removed." This principle is then re-enforced to the surgeon that beauty is not in the eye of the beholder, but in the eye of the "beholdee." The constructive surgeon should spend large portions of time conversing with his patient so that information can be gained about his patient's wants, desires, and expectations. This is the appropriate time for elucidating a patient's possible unrealistic wants on how he or she will look after the "magic restorative surgery."

It is important to stress to the patient differences between function and cosmesis. There has to be a marriage between these two factors in any discussion of facial reconstruction. The patient must understand that a surgeon should never jeopardize function for cosmesis. A sunken and enophthalmic globe can be improved and better symmetry attained with the contralateral normal globe, but the procedures are limited by good functioning extrinsic muscles and a somewhat chronically contracted and fibrosed optic nerve of the affected eye. The patient must completely understand the anatomical limitations and become an active and participating member in the restorative process.

The discussion with the patient preoperatively will save heartaches on both sides of the operative scalpel postoperatively. If patients are fully aware of their particular deformity and taking an active role in planning and understanding of the staged reconstructive procedures, they will then have realistic and satisfied results. The day of the doctor saying, "Don't worry Mrs. Jones, I understand the problem, so leave everything in my hands and I'll take care of it," is long gone. The patient should be considered sophisticated, intelligent, and should be given the opportunity to take an active part in their own care.

PRINCIPLES

As in anything in life, there are certain rules and regulations one must live by. In this relatively new field of plastic and reconstructive surgery, some principles of care have been elucidated by the father of modern plastic surgery, Sir Harold Gillies. These principles have subsequently been documented, expanded, and flourished by one of his disciples, D. Ralph Millard, Jr., one of the most prolific and imaginitive surgeons in the last few decades. A recounting of these principles as described by Gillies and Millard in their book, *The Principles and Art of Plastic Surgery* should be read and applied by all who cherish plastic surgery. Overemphasis of these principles cannot be done and a recapitulation is definitely in order. The first principle and most basic is "observation is the basis of surgical diagnosis." The surgeon must observe and look, not just with his eyes, but with his mind. He must observe, not just his patients, but patients of other surgeons, and learn from past and present mistakes. Another part of this "observation principle" is to "know the normal."

To "know the normal" is not an easy task. All human faces have two eyes, two ears, one nose, two nostrils, one mouth, etc. Understanding the relationship of these structures to one another and to themselves is something that requires great study. Once the normal is known, the next principle can then be delineated.

The second principle of Gillies and Millard is "diagnose before you treat." This can have many ramifications, however, basically one must determine what the true defect is. Looks are definitely deceiving, and an apparent small defect can be converted into a much larger, truer defect when this principle is appreciated.

Once the true defect is found, the third principle of "making a plan and a pattern for this plan" can apply. To exercise one's gray matter and to mentate to make a plan is one of the greatest intellectual challenges and stimulations one has in reconstructive surgery.

The fourth and fifth principles are "documentation," and "the life boat." Obviously, without good record-keeping, preoperative photographs, appropriate sketches and diagrams, one's fantastic ideas, and moments of genius will be past and forgotten once the flap settles. We must learn by successes as well as failures, therefore, documentation is of utmost importance. Most importantly, one plan is not enough, one must have a number of plans preoperatively, so that various "life boats" can be used if so needed. The sixth principle of "good style" can only be appreciated if one pays attention to details, applies principles of surgery to the gentleness and dexterity of handling tissue.

Seventh, and high in priority in this order of principles is, "replace what is normal in normal position and retain it there." Healthy wounds heal by scar contracture and normal structures can be shifted and transposed by the mighty myofibroblast. In time, this action can be used to the patient's benefit, but after severe traumatic deformities, normal tissue can be displaced from their normal anatomic positions, and the true defect subsequently masked prior to soft tissue or bony reconstruction. The visions of one's plan should be made to retain the new transposed normal tissue in its normal position, otherwise, this tissue will migrate back to its abnormal home.

The next principles laid down by Gillies, and enumerated by Millard, were to "treat the primary defect first," and to "borrow from Peter to pay Paul, only when Peter can afford it." One should not be unnecessarily concerned with a secondary defect, but keep in mind the main goal and mission of the reconstructive exercise. The patient is in need of reconstruction of a particular organ, and if the secondary defect is acceptable after transposition of tissue to the primary site, go for it. Add to this the ninth principle of "losses must be replaced in kind." An example is that thin ruberous skin should be replaced with similar skin. Obviously, to the contrary, thin ruberous skin should not be used to reconstruct thick pale skin. The principle of "never throwing anything away," is an extremely important one and emphasizes that every little bit counts and can be used at sometime during any particular reconstruction. There always is a piece of tissue that had been excised and thrown away, but later on was needed and could have been used as the final piece of the puzzle. A plastic surgeon's mind must always remain young and "never let routine methods become your master": a rule we should all keep in mind. One should never "always" do a particular procedure one way or the other. Being stuck in a rut is when the imaginative mind falters. Having the constant stimulation of new tracks or new procedures, is limited only by one's imagination. It does not mean, however, that if a particular procedure has worked satisfactorily in a similar case, that it should not be tried again. The second time it is done, efforts should be made to improve that same procedure.

"Consulting other specialists," as suggested by Gillies and Millard, can be most helpful. Discussing procedures and problems with colleagues can pique interest and stimulate further imagination. Using a colleague's mind as a sounding board can be most productive. Finally, "never do today what can honorably be put off till tommorow": scars in need of revising, flaps in need of thinning, and defects to be reconstructed. Tincture of time will heal and soften many wounds, and the more of this tincture, the better the stage is set for further reconstruction. The surgeon who is interested and compulsive, always striving for perfection, and who pays great attention to detail, will never be finished with any particular reconstructive case. That surgeon will always be wanting to "thin this" or "defat that" and eventually will come close to the ideal.

PHYSICAL EXAMINATION

Once a historical recounting of the particular problem by the patient has been accomplished and the principles of plastic and reconstructive surgery understood, one must then lose all abandon and examine the patient. In the examination of the face, one should concentrate on the particular defect at hand after all other normal structures are inspected and examined. Underlying bony structures of the neck, face, and skull can be easily palpated. Almost the entire inferior border of the mandible can be felt for deformity. Intraoral examination for masses and abnormalities is extremely important and bimanual palpation can easily be done. Occlusal relationships of the mandibular to the maxillary teeth are important to document and understand. The relationship between the two jaws is the key to the underlying facial bony contour. For that reason, an understanding of dental occlusion should be accomplished. Functional movement of the mandible should be examined in all six positions: opened, closed, right and left lateral movement, anterior projection, and posterior projection.

Observation and palpation of symmetry of both malar bones and their confluent zygomatic arches should be made. Similar palpation of the infraorbital rim under the thin lower eyelid skin should also be done as well as the lateral and superior orbital margins, visual acuity, and extraocular movements of both eyes. Palpation of the nasal bones along with their cartilaginous extensions should also be made. Intranasal examination for septal deviations, nasal polyps, tubinate hypertrophies, or assymmetries should be noted.

Examinations of the soft tissue of the face and neck are relatively self-explanatory. Knowledge of "knowing the normal" comes from experience and close observation. Basic courses in sculpturing or line drawing are most helpful to a surgeon's powers of true meaningful observation.

If the particular reconstructive problem involves underlying bony structures, x-rays can add to one's basic information. It is not the purpose of this chapter to elucidate the 15 or 20 various types of facial and skull x-rays. These can be gathered from any number of other textbooks, however a few selected x-rays are most often used. A posterior, anterior, and lateral

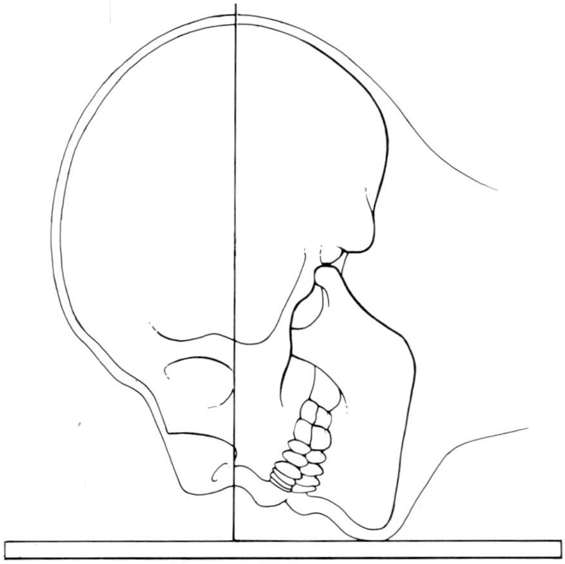

Figure 1.1 Waters' view—the face is placed on the x-ray plate so that the mastoid process and mandibular condyles are shifted out of the x-ray path; thus, the maxillary sinus and inferior orbital rim can easily be seen.

view of the face, along with a Waters' view (Fig. 1.1) are ostensibly the main x-rays from which one gleans the most basic information. One should constantly keep in mind that the facial bones are membranous in structure and heal by fibrous union. Previous osteotomies or prior fractures can be seen on x-rays for many years. Facial bones do not heal by callus formation as do the long bones of our anatomy. This is quite fortunate, because it would be difficult to imagine a large callus forming in an orbital floor fracture. A large callus in this region would not only hamper the extrinsic muscles of the eye, but may increase the intraorbital pressure by decreasing the intraorbital volume and cause severe functional impairment on the globe. Aside from this near disastrous sequela on the eye, a terrible cosmetic deformity would result. Teleologically the good Lord figured this out quite well. For functional weight bearing the long bone fractures produce bulky calluses contrary to a lack of bulk in the fibrous union of the much more delicate facial bones.

The recent use of computerized axial tomography (CAT) scans has also been helpful in evaluation of various congenital and traumatic bony deformities. The use of CAT scans and cephalometrograms can be extremely helpful in the annual monitoring and documentation of growth in congenital deformities of the skull and face. The results from Panorex x-rays for mandibular deformities is unparalleled, but these have limitation at the temporomandibular joint areas, which can be separately viewed if so desired on special projections.

PLAN

Once appropriate history, physical examination and x-rays are accomplished, a diagnosis of the defect has to be made. This is not always easily done. One has to determine whether there is an underlying bony defect, and overlying soft tissue defect, or both. It is not always necessary or desirable to return normal bony tissue to its normal position if the functional occlusion is satisfactory. There are, therefore, exceptions to the rules and principles of Gillies and Millard. An example is a patient who had a traumatic LeFort III fracture (suffered by being stepped on by a bull) and has had two or three reconstructive procedures at outside hospitals to

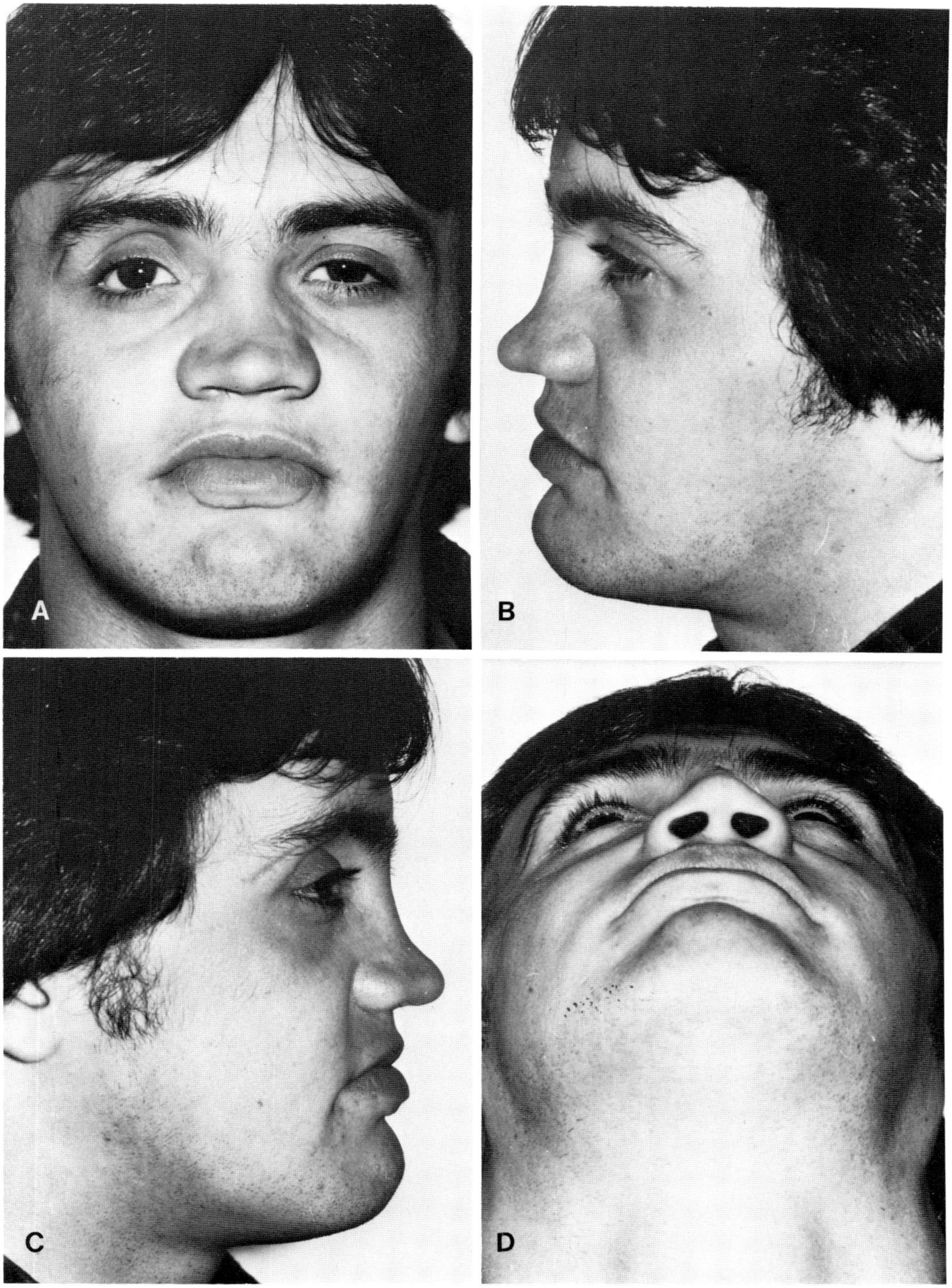

Figure 1.2 (*A*) Adequate postoperative occlusion status post-traumatic LeFort III fracture with unsatisfactory facial contour—frontal view, (*B*) left lateral, (*C*) right lateral, and (*D*) mental view.

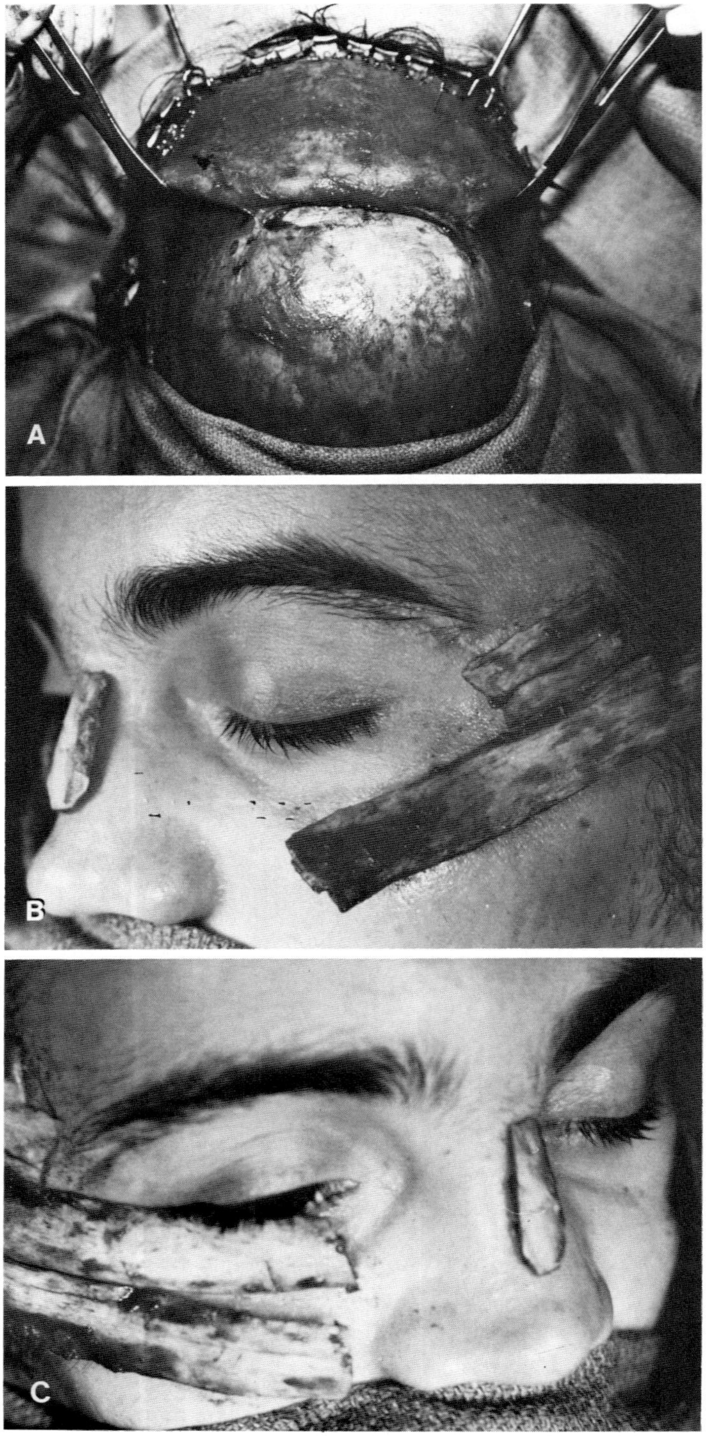

Figure 1.3 (*A*) Bicoronal flap is elevated for easy access. (*B*) Split autogenous rib grafts on left lateral. (*C*) right lateral views.

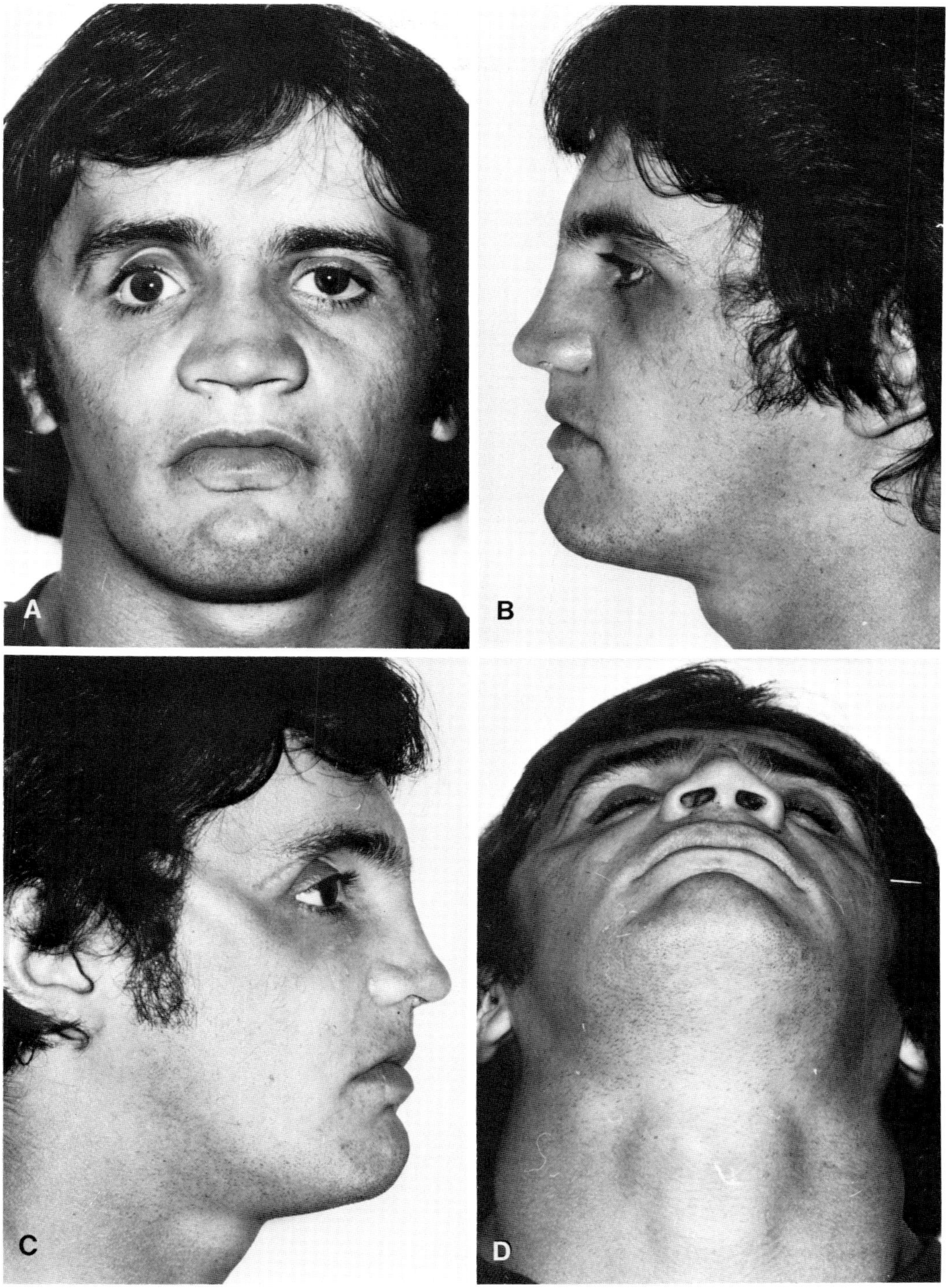

Figure 1.4 (*A*) Status post autogenous rib grafts through bicoronal approach—frontal view. Revision of right anophthalmic-enophthalmic global prosthesis is planned. (*B*) Left lateral, (*C*) right lateral, and (*D*) mental view.

reconstruct the satisfactory occlusion. After this was accomplished, the patient was still left with a "dishpan" facial deformity (Fig. 1.2). A LeFort III osteotomy and maxillary advancement of the midface might have been the theoretical plan of attack, but the more straightforward and easier approach (and depending on the patient's desires) was relatively simple augmentation of the malar and nasal bones with autogenous bone grafts (Fig. 1.3) to achieve satisfactory contour (Fig. 1.4). Here we are taking "extra" normal tissue and placing it in a normal position, and again getting back to principles.

Once the original defect is defined and a number of technical plans are formulated, one should not be forced to adhere to these plans once manipulation of the tissue has been accomplished intraoperatively. One should be flexible enough to "wing it," assuming that there is a solid reason for bending the original plans. Keeping general principles in mind, one should be able to serially improve any dire situation.

References

1. Bonanno, P. C., and Converse, J. M.: Primary bone grafting in management of facial fractures. *N. Y. State J. Med.*, *75:*710, 1975.
2. Braunstein, P. W.: Medical aspects of automotive crash injury research. *J.A.M.A.*, *163:*249, 1957.
3. Brown, J. B., Fryer, M. P., and McDowell, F.: Internal wire-pin immobilization of jaw fractures. *Plastic Reconstr. Surg.*, *4:*30, 1949.
4. Converse, J. M.: Fractures of the maxilla, in *Kazanjian and Converse's Surgical Treatment of Facial Injuries*, Ed. 3, Williams & Wilkins, Baltimore, 1974.
5. Dingman, R. O., and Alling, C. C.: Open reduction and internal wire fixation of maxillofacial fractures. *J. Oral Surg.*, *12:*140, 1954.
6. Dingman, R. O., and Natvig, P.: *Surgery of Facial Fractures*, W. B. Saunders, Philadelphia, 1964.
7. Georgiade, N., and Nash, T.: An external cranial fixation apparatus for severe maxillofacial injuries. *Plastic. Reconstr. Surg.*, *38:*142, 1966.
8. Gillies, H. D., and Millard, D. R.: *The Principles and Art of Plastic Surgery*. Little Brown, Boston, 1957.
9. Kazanjian, V. H., and Converse, J. M.: *The Surgical Treatment of Facial Injuries*, Ed. 2, Williams & Wilkins, Baltimore, 1959.
10. Knorr, N. J., Hoopes, J. E., and Edgerton, M. T.: Psychiatric-surgical approach to adolescent disturbance in self-image *Plast. Reconstr. Surg.*, *41:*248, 1968.
11. LeFort, R.: Etude expérimentale sur les fractures de la machoire supérieure. *Rev. Chir.*, *23:*208, 360, 479, 1901.
12. Macgregor, F. C.: Symposium on cosmetic surgery. *Surg. Clin. North Am.*, *51:*289, 1971.
13. Rowe, N. L., and Kiley, H. C.: *Fracture of the Facial Skeleton*, Ed. 3, Williams & Wilkins, Baltimore, 1968.
14. Schultz, R. C.: *Facial Injuries*, Year Book, Chicago, 1970.

CHAPTER 2

Surgery of the Scalp and Skull

Malcolm A. Lesavoy, M.D., F.A.C.S.

ANATOMY

The scalp is an extremely vascular part of the human anatomy, and has readily dissectable cleavage planes. Anatomically, the scalp is composed of the cranium, galea aponeurotica, occipitofrontalis muscle, subcutaneous tissue, and skin. The cleavage plane between the galea aponeurotica and the pericranium is relatively avascular, as there are no major perforating vessels in this plane, and fairly rapid finger dissection can be accomplished. The other side, however, of the double edge sword is that infection beneath the galea can spread rapidly without significant mechanical barrier, and a subgaleal abscess can be most devastating.

Vascular arterial inflow is supplied by the temporal, supraorbital, supratrochlear, posterior auricular, and occipital arteries. Venous outflow follows these named arteries, although there are many other various unnamed channels.

Reconstruction of the scalp may be necessary under varied circumstances. Deformities of the scalp result from massive trauma, neoplastic extirpation, and congenital malformation. Reconstruction of the tissue overlying the skull may be necessary for both functional and cosmetic reasons.

TRAUMA

Traumatic deformities of the scalp can run the gamut of minor scalp lacerations from an unexpected fall or from a falling object, to massive and total avulsion. All that is required for the former is relatively simple debridement and primary closure where the latter requires extremely sophisticated miscrovascular techniques for the successful replanation of the avulsed scalp.

Lacerations of the scalp usually result from the sequelae of blunt trauma and occasionally are caused by contact with sharp instrumentation. In the usual emergency room case following a blow to the scalp and skull from a blunt object or the results of an unexpected fall, extreme care must first be taken to ascertain underlying structural damage. An accurate and detailed history must be documented in order to rule out possible medical reasons for the fall that should be prevented in the future. Seizure disorder, transient ischemic attacks, alcoholism, and vestibular malfunction all can contribute to possible answers for the reason for the fall. Investigation of the underlying problem should always be carried out as early as possible. Subsequently, physical examinations at times will reveal bone fractures visible through the scalp laceration and obviously this would lead one toward the x-ray suite. A complete and thorough neurologic examination is of the utmost importance and should give clues to some underlying problems.

Assuming all the aforementioned factors are negative, evaluation of the actual scalp laceration should then be accomplished. Because of the usual type of contused laceration of the scalp, copious irrigation and excision of the bruised and damaged wound edges should be carried out. It is a easy task to infiltrate with a local anesthetic within the wound margins itself to effect fairly rapid and complete anesthesia over the area in question. Once this has been accomplished and irrigation and debridement has been done, closure of these wounds can be accomplished with relatively large gauge nylon hemostatic sutures (3-0 or 4-0 locking sutures).

It is relatively futile and impossible to try to obtain electrocautery hemostasis, and one should not waste time (and blood) in the emergency room for this task. The main obstacle to hurdle in hemostasis in scalp lacerations is vessel retraction. A number of factors contribute to this: first, the scalp, itself, is quite rigid and has little retractile force, whereas arteries and veins are quite retractile and hide under the nongiving scalp skin. Secondly, the galea aponeurotica inhibits full vascular retraction and maintains luminal patency so continuous bleeding occurs. Hemostatic and tight (but not strangulating) sutures of the scalp are the best and quickest remedy. Once the wound is closed, a relatively watertight dressing can be applied with liquid collodion. Sutures can then be removed at the surgeon's discretion approximately 10 days to 2 weeks later.

Occasionally, one will be called to the emergency department by the junior house officer to deal with a scalp wound that is "missing." If the laceration is through the galea and perpendicular to the muscular fibers, by mere inspection, lack of muscular continuity will present a gaping soft tissue defect. These gaping wounds can be fairly easily approximated with stout sutures under moderate tension.

If, however, there has been a tangential defect, or if there is such massive contusion that debridement leaves an area of the skull devoid of soft tissue covering, local flaps can be employed. It should be remembered that the scalp, itself, has very little inherent elasticity. The lack of elasticity is contributed, too, by its vertical thickness and anatomic relationship of the underlying galea which splints the scalp. Simple undermining of the scalp will gain very little advancement. One may be able to gain a slight advantage in length by serial incisions within the galea perpendicular to the access of desired advancement (Fig. 2.1). However, even if one undermines the entire scalp and serially incises the galea, only approximately 1–2 cm of advanced length will be gained. It should, therefore, be concluded that if there are significant scalp defects to be covered, advancement and closure under tension will not suffice and the formation of local scalp flaps will become a necessity.

Is a scalp flap necessary? Depending on the situation, and depending on the known anatomic defect, in most cases, simple split thickness skin grafting of the scalp defect may suffice (Fig. 2.2). If the pericranium is intact, split thickness skin grafts will cover the defect beautifully and allow one to return at a later date to re-evaluate what once was an untidy wound. The advantages of thin split thickness skin grafts is that they will allow the wound to contract a certain degree and work in the patient's favor—so that, 6–8 months later, repeated serial excisions of this skin graft can convert a once untidy primary wound to a simple scar. Even if the pericranium is not intact, and bare cortical bone of the calvarium is exposed, one can produce granulation tissue over this cortical bone with multiple drill holes through the outer cortex and into the diploe. (It should be noted that small drill bits, although well meaning,

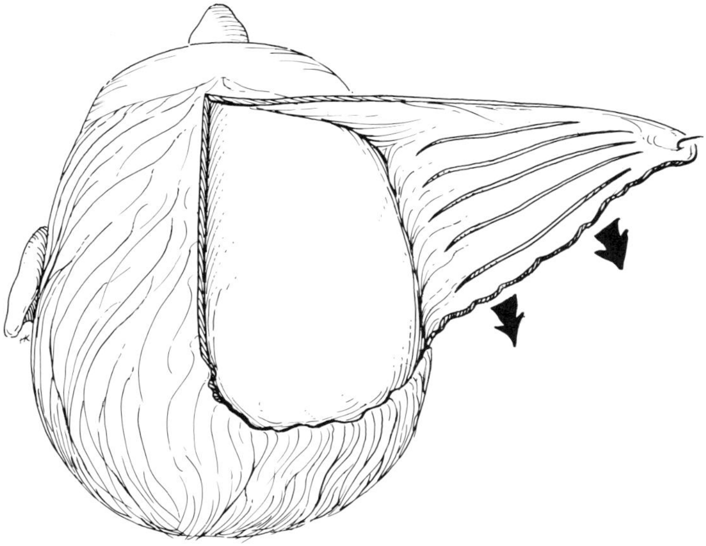

Figure 2.1 Parallel incisions in the undersurface of the galea for minimal expansion.

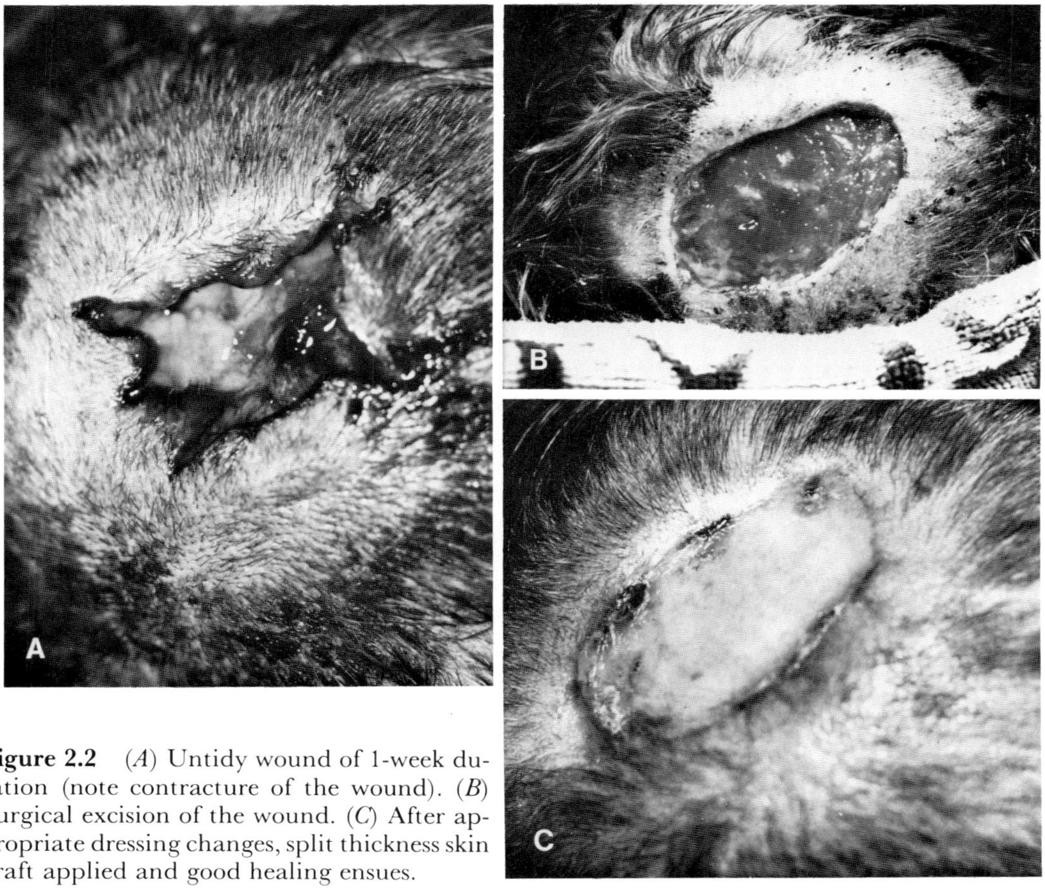

Figure 2.2 (*A*) Untidy wound of 1-week duration (note contracture of the wound). (*B*) Surgical excision of the wound. (*C*) After appropriate dressing changes, split thickness skin graft applied and good healing ensues.

will cause clots to form within their bony diameter and not allow granulation to exude through their openings.) One may even remove the cortex of the skull and place split thickness skin grafts on a medullary exposed diploe portion of the cranium. If absolutely necessary, it is even possible to skin graft exposed dura mater (Fig. 2.3). Obviously, a skin graft does not have the inherent structures that scalp tissue itself has, and for that reason will always be maintained as a "bald spot" in a hair-bearing area. It will also not provide sufficient support for continued use and may break down with frequent abrasions from head gear and/or wigs, etc. However, skin grafts should always be considered the first line of reconstruction in these type of scalp defects and further reconstruction can be carried out at a later date. If, for many reasons, the split thickness skin graft seems not to be the procedure of choice, and a significant scalp defect is present, local flap coverage is the next choice for coverage. One can start with a simple incision parallel to the scalp defect and create a bipedicle flap that can be transposed into the defect while the donor area is covered with a split thickness skin graft. If the original scalp defect is large enough, a bilateral bipedicle transpositon may be needed. Bipedicle flaps in the scalp if possible should be oriented in the anterior-posterior direction through well known vascular channels. It is possible to have horizontal bipedicle flaps if these are based on the anterior or posterior branch of the superficial temporal artery. Essentially, bipedicle flaps work mechanically as a relaxing incision would in the groin for repair of an inguinal hernia.

Rotation flaps are frequently used in the scalp for closing irregular central defects. Because the scalp has little elasticity, there is small room for error in the basic design of rotation flaps. One must constantly keep in mind the basic principles of Gillies and Millard, and remember that the small cutback at the end of the flap is most important to relieve tension on rotation flaps. (Fig. 2.4). Without this cutback, the rotational flap loses its geometric advantage. Occasionally, multiple rotation flaps can be employed to cover one central defect.

Large scalp and scalping flaps should be considered arterialized flaps and, for this reason, virtually the entire skull can be pared of its overlying scalp by two or three large axial flaps. The ability to totally replant an entire avulsed scalp by one or two microvascular arterial anastomoses has proven the anatomic presence of arterialized scalp flaps. Orticochea in 1971 graphically described the use of large arterialized scalp flaps analogous to that of a boy peeling a banana.

Scalp flap transpositions and rotations can be demonstrated for the restoration of hairline

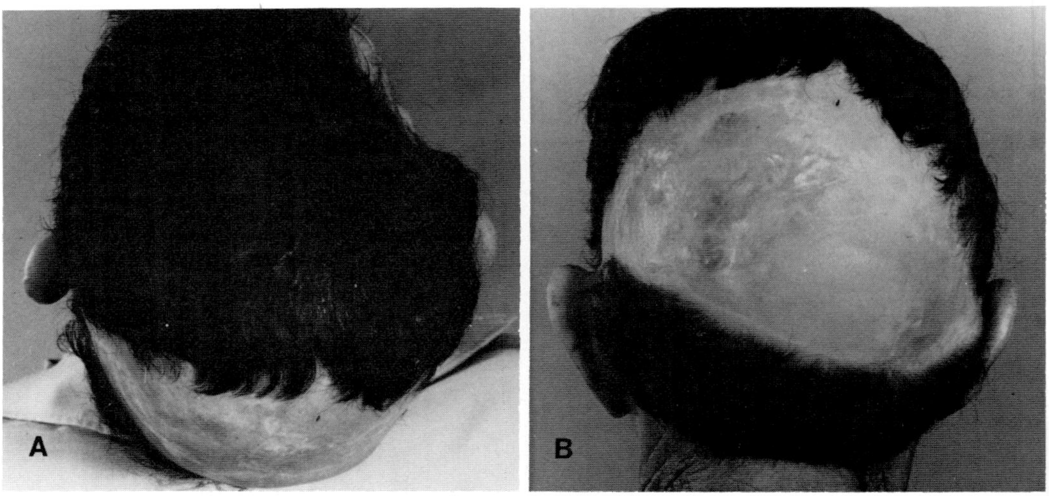

Figure 2.3 Scalp and cranial defect following wide and agressive excision of basal cell carcinoma. Wounds are totally healed with split thickness skin graft coverage.

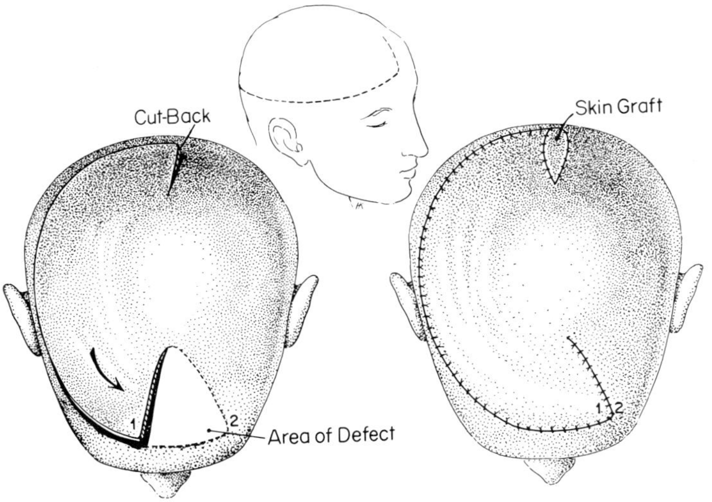

Figure 2.4 Hemiscalp rotation flap (this particular flap is random and demonstrates excellent vascularity of the scalp.

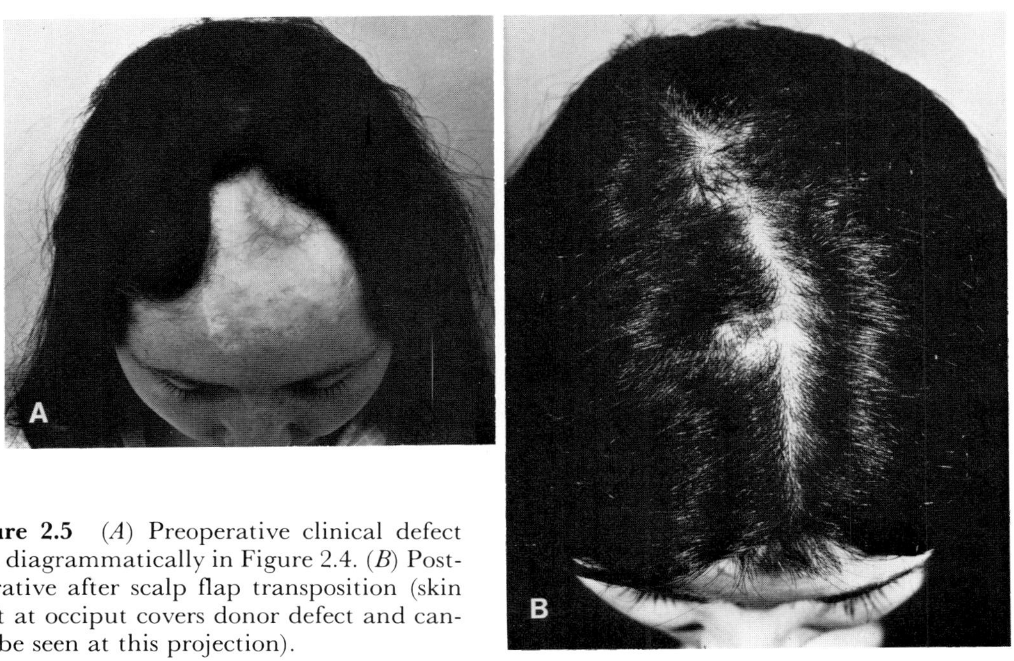

Figure 2.5 (*A*) Preoperative clinical defect seen diagrammatically in Figure 2.4. (*B*) Postoperative after scalp flap transposition (skin graft at occiput covers donor defect and cannot be seen at this projection).

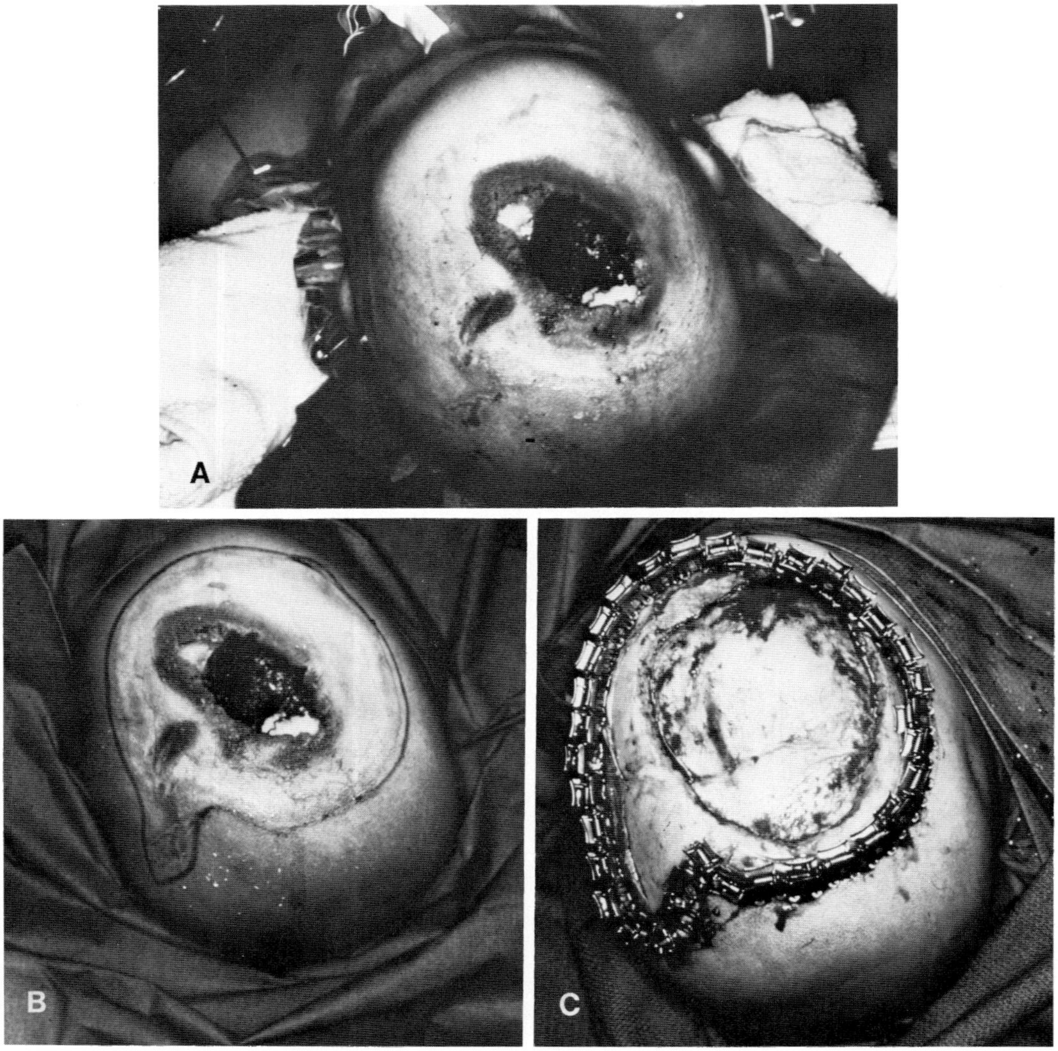

Figure 2.6 (*A*) Severe penetrating electrical burn of scalp, skull, and brain. (*B*, *C*) Debridement marked and carried out with scarred dura seen at the depth of the wound.

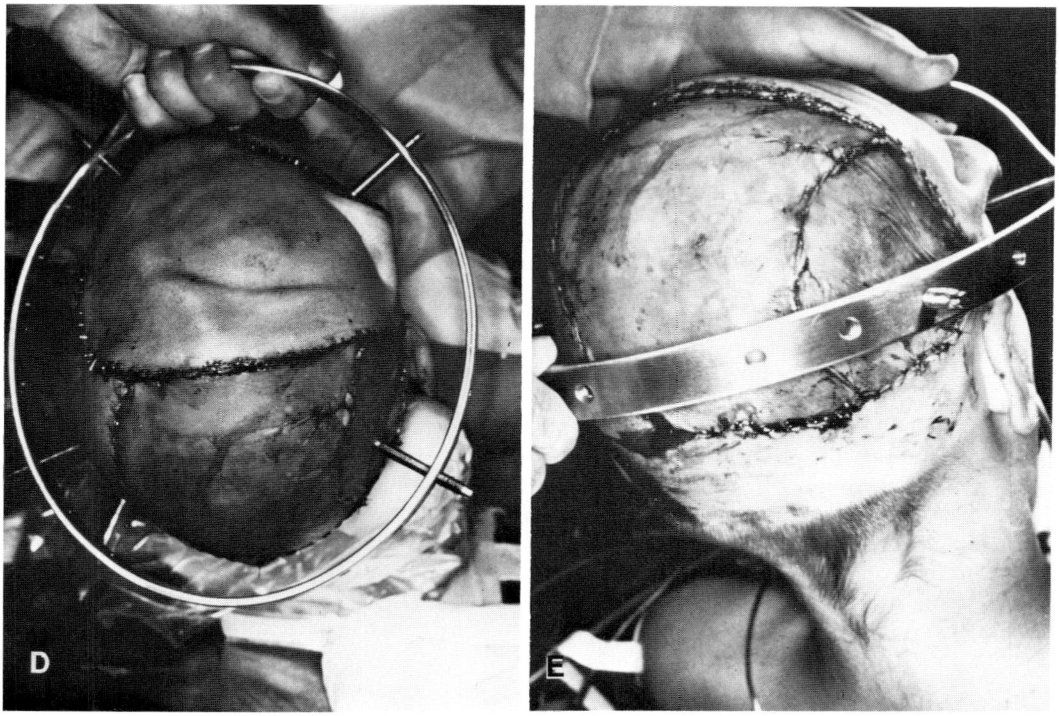

Figure 2.6 (*D*) Scalp flap transposition based on right superficial temporal artery. (*E*) Split thickness skin graft placed on posterior donor site and application of halo for protection of wound. (Courtesy of Michael McGuire, M.D.)

continuity in dermal burns, where simple movement of a posterior unburned area to an anterior scarred and allopecic area is advantageous. Similarly, a case is demonstrable of a young woman who underwent traumatic scalp loss from an automobile accident. Considerable embarrassment ensued while riding in open cars or swimming. A right scalp flap rotation was carried out to allow for continuity of the important forehead hairline (Fig. 2.5). In contrast, a lifesaving large scalp flap transpositon was carried out to cover a severely traumatized scalp, skull, and brain injury from a high energy electrical source (Fig. 2.6 *A*). After adequate debridement of the scalp and skull (Fig. 2.6, *B* and *C*), coverage of the thrombosed sagittal sinus and burned dura was accomplished with a large occipital scalp flap based on the superficial temporal artery (Fig. 2.6 *D*). The donor defect is then grafted with split thickness skin. This case also illustrates the excellent use of the halo device for isolation and protection of the wound (Fig. 2.6 *E*). (Unfortunately, this young boy died 6 days later from severe intracranial hemorrhage, however, the flap remained viable to the end.)

Scalp flap transpositions and rotations have come from the thoughts of imaginative surgeons dealing with severe burns or traumatic injuries of the scalp. These same principles have allowed reconstructive surgeons to deal with the problem of male pattern baldness where temporal and occipital flaps are transposed into non-hair-bearing scalp. Gillies and Millard described this years ago and, recently, Juri has popularized the use of parieto-occipital scalp flaps with prior delay procedures (Fig. 2.7). This is based on the presumption that the parieto-occipital portion of the male scalp will maintain its hair follicles and not become subsequently bald (Fig. 2.8 *A*). After one or two delay procedures, this parieto-occipital flap can be raised and transposed into the allopecic area (Fig. 2.8, *B* and *C*). Two months later, a similar flap on the contralateral side can be raised and transposed if necessary (Fig. 2.8 *D*). The bald areas between can then be feathered and filled in with hair plug transplantation from the posterior scalp (Fig. 2.8 *E*).

Many authors have described the use of hair plugs from the parietal or occipital regions of the scalp for hair transplantation. Recently, Devine has produced an innovative square punch knife to make use of more hair follicles. Hair plug transplantation is time consuming, expensive, and many times unaesthetic. It has been faster, more inexpensive, and more aesthetic to employ scalp flap transposition in cases that require large amounts of hair.

An interesting and demonstrative case employing the point of thinking ahead is that of a patient who sustained traumatic loss of his eyebrow. This was reconstructed with a hair-bearing arterial flap based on the anterior branch of the superficial temporal artery. It was not

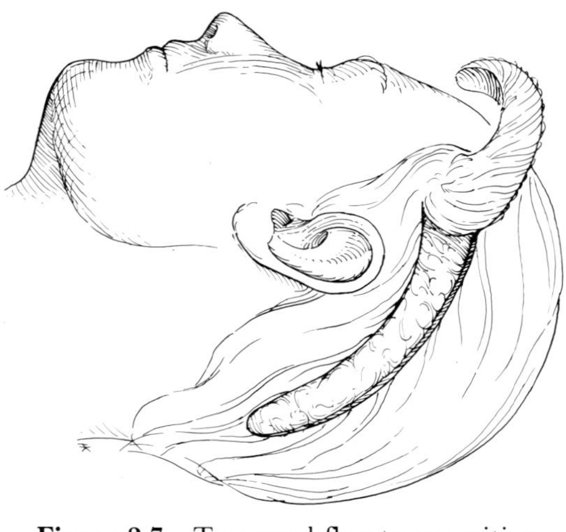

Figure 2.7 Temporal flap transposition.

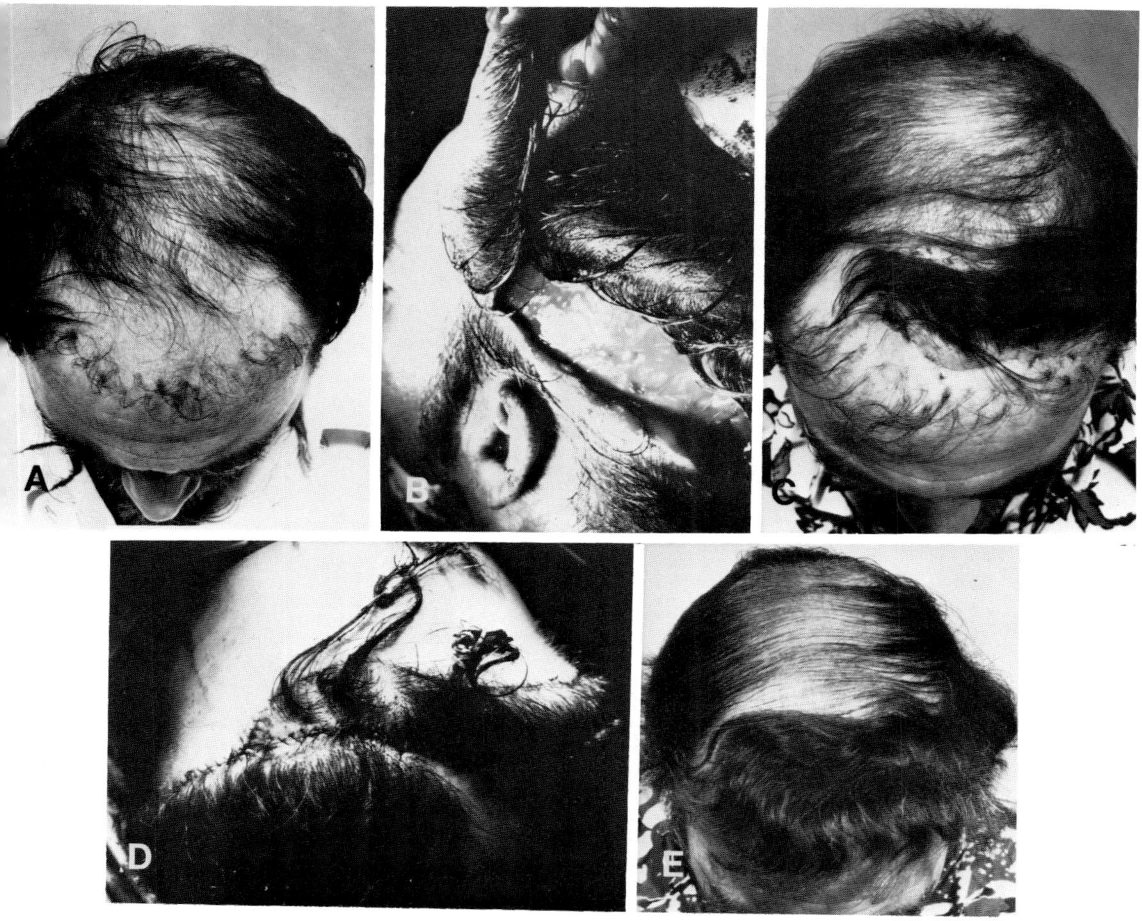

Figure 2.8 (*A*) Preoperative male pattern baldness (anterior hair plugs placed by outside physician prior to patient's self-referral). (*B*) After two previous delays, scalp flap is raised and based on the branch of the superficial temporal artery (only the proximal third of this flap is actually arterial, the distal two-thirds are random). (*C*) Left temporal parietal flap in place. (*D*) Right temporal parietal flap transposed anterior to left flap 6 weeks later. (Courtesy of Howard (Sam) Seider, M.D.) (*E*) Postoperative result.

anticipated by the surgeon, that, as years passed, this patient's hereditary and/or genetic disposition would render his temporal area bald and subsequently he would lose the hair in his reconstructed eyebrow (Fig. 2.9, *A* and *B*).

A small technical but important point should be made that, whenever incisions are made in the scalp for cosmetic reasons, the knife blade should be beveled parallel to hair follicles. If one holds the knife blade perpendicular to the skin edge and incises at 90°, a few hair follicles will be damaged in the path of the knife blade and a bald scar will result. This can be avoided by cutting parallel to the hair follicles and subsequently hair will not be damaged close to the acutal suture line. It should also be mentioned that, when relaxing incisions are made within the galea aponeurotica to take advantage of whatever small advancement one might achieve in the scalp, one has to take great care not to damage the subdermal vessels superficial to

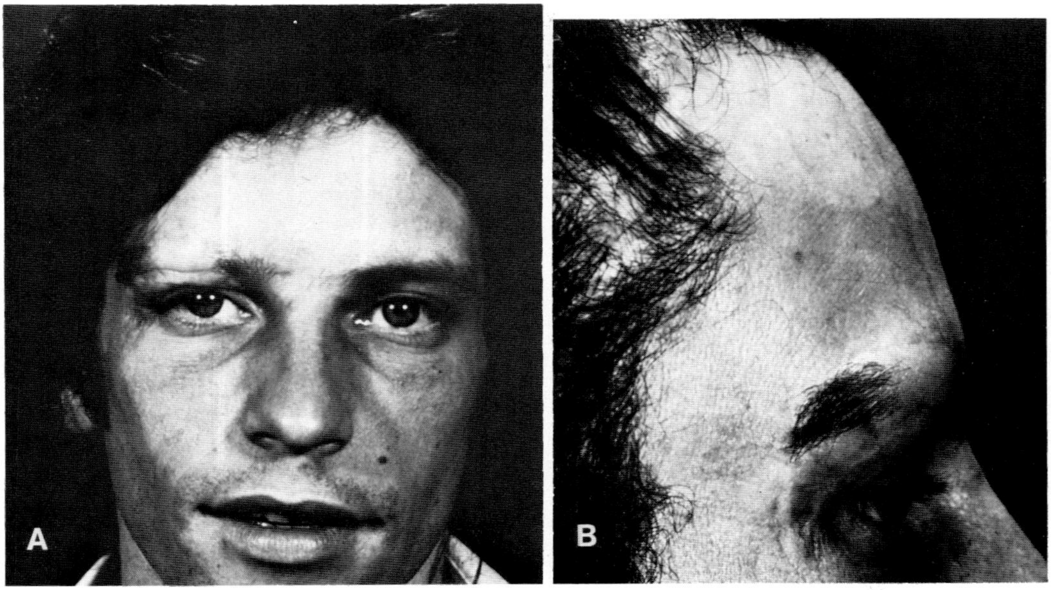

Figure 2.9 (*A*) "Balding" reconstructed right eyebrow. (*B*) Second case. Courtesy of Henry K. Kawamoto, Jr., M.D., D.D.S.)

galea. If one is using an axial flap, it is usually better to make parallel incisions rather than perpendicular incisions to the flap so that one has less chance of injuring the parallel axial vessels.

NEOPLASM

Neoplastic invasion of the scalp is not uncommon and frequently seen in large practices. Differentiation between basal cell carcinoma and squamous cell carcinoma is often very difficult to make; however, basal cell carcinomas are more frequently seen in the scalp. These lesions are usually seen late after their onset because of the patient's lack of awareness of the lesion that he cannot see, and because of the surrounding hair about these lesions. Only if these lesions become traumatized by hair utensils such as combs and brushes, will they be brought to the attention of the physician. If the tumors are large and necessitate wide defects, similar principles of reconstructive scalp surgery are applied (Fig. 2.10). A tumor of rarity of the scalp, hemangiopericytoma (Fig. 2.11), is shown after one recurrence in a scalp flap transposition. This patient has remained free of disease to date after extensive wide excision.

Underlying cerebral intracranial tumors that have been irradiated can have overlying skin and soft tissue breakdown. It is very difficult in these situations to reconstruct and cover exposed calvarium, etc., with the adjacent radiated tissue. The scalp is not immune to the ravaging excesses of radiation therapy, and progressive endarteritis will take its toll. When bone is exposed, skin grafts will not suffice, and scalp flap transposition may be necessary. Ian McGregor has advocated leaving these exposed areas of calvarium to their own devices, because this area is relatively avascular, it is not prone to infection and therefore manipulations sometimes will be to the patient's detriment. This is one man's opinion, and most plastic surgeons would employ previous principles of scalp reconstruction to cover exposed skull.

CONGENITAL

Congenital problems of the sc; lp are rare (Figs. 2.12 and 2.13), though there are a number of reported cases of cutis aplasia in this area. This has been described by a number of authors, the first of which was Campbell in 1826. This defect is variable in its extent; however, most cases involve simply the scalp and underlying skull. There may be a recessive genetic factor involved, but it is the author's impression that the defect may be a result of intrauterine pressure on the affected parts.

Treatment can be nonoperative or aggressively operative. In our particular case, (Fig. 2.14 *A*), we elected to treat these lesions the same as a burn with silver sulfadiazine. Remarkably in time, the areas gain in thickness, texture, and epithelial elements (Fig. 2.14 *B*).

Industry has become more and more aware of scalping injuries in women affecting long hair styles. Safety measures force women working around geared machinery to wear protective hair coverings. Recently, there have been a number of reports in the literature of total scalping avulsions that have been microvascularly replanted successfully. This is obviously the ultimate in scalp reconstruction, described as employing one or two arterial anastomoses and four or five venous anastomoses.

Since the recent advent of microvascular surgery, a sophisticated method of soft tissue coverage can be accomplished by the use of a free vascularized omental flap. This can be accomplished after harvesting the greater omentum and revascularizing this tissue with anastomoses of either the right or left gastroepiploic artery and vein to a recipient artery and vein in the scalp (usually the superficial temporal artery and vein) (Fig. 2.15, *A* and *B*).

Once the vacularized omental flap is in place, split thickness skin grafts can be placed on this vascular bed and excellent coverage will be obtained (Fig. 2.15 *C*). A difficulty arises in these types of cases when the donor omentum is very thin and membranous-like. Obviously, not much bulk will be obtained and there may be subsequent breakdown after adequate healing has occurred. A thicker and more durable one-stage microvascular free flap transposition can be accomplished with a groin flap. (Newer and more recently described free flaps such as the latissimus dorsi and tensor fascia lata flaps could also be used).

Obviously, microvascular free flap transposition for covering large scalp soft tissue and bony defects are usually a surgeon's last choice. However, with the explosion of microsurgery and improvement of techniques in recent years, if flap coverage is needed, free flaps may be the quickest avenue toward success. The need for multistaged delayed and pedicle flaps will be relegated to history. It should emphasize, however, that, if local scalp flaps are available, they should definitely be used before microvascular free flap transfer.

CONTOUR

For many reasons, it is possible to have a bony skull contour deformity without associated overlying soft tissue defects. These can be either congenital or aquired. The most frequently

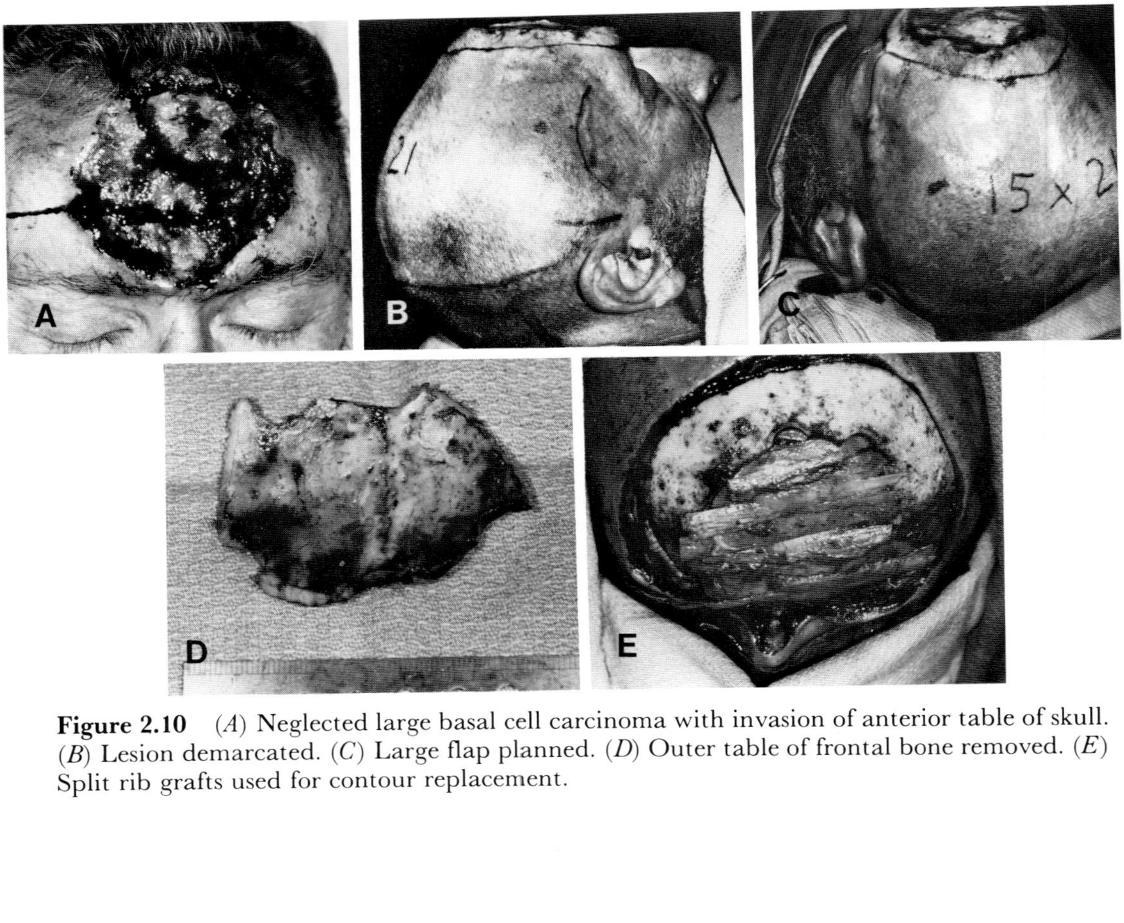

Figure 2.10 (*A*) Neglected large basal cell carcinoma with invasion of anterior table of skull. (*B*) Lesion demarcated. (*C*) Large flap planned. (*D*) Outer table of frontal bone removed. (*E*) Split rib grafts used for contour replacement.

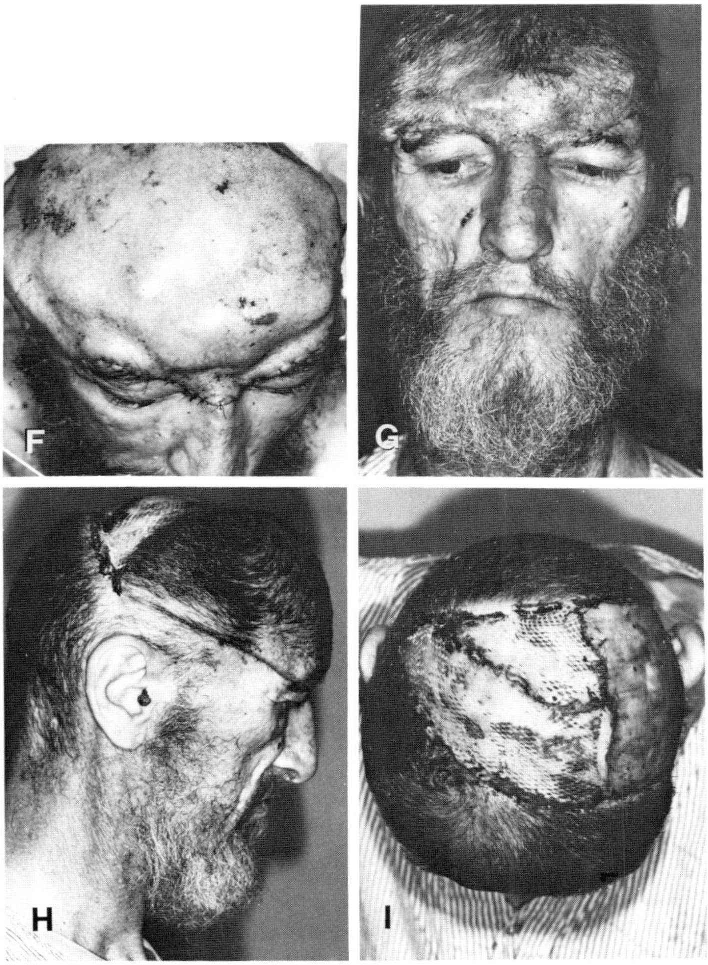

Figure 2.10 (*F*) Scalp flap in transposed position. (*G*) Postoperative frontal view. (*H*) Postoperative right lateral view. (*I*) Donor defect at top of scalp. (Courtesy of James K. Wright, M.D.)

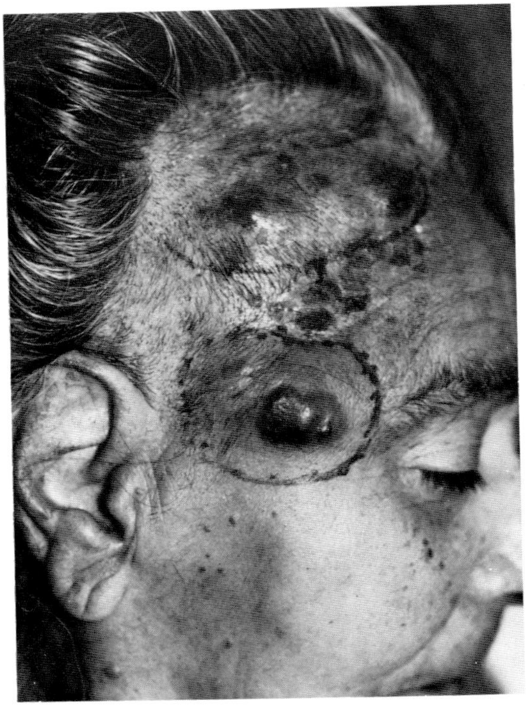

Figure 2.11 Recurrent scalp hemangiopericytoma.

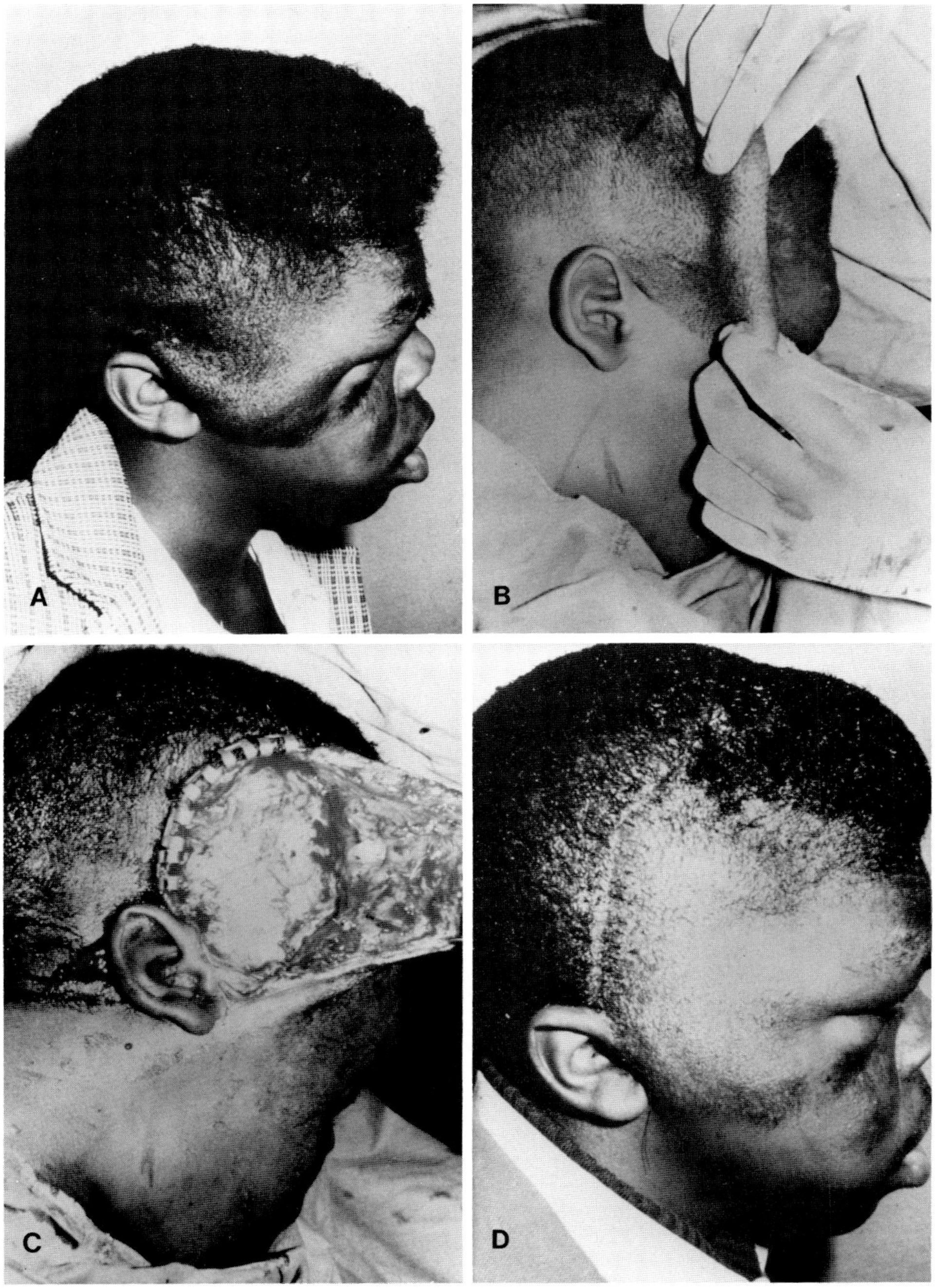

Figure 2.12 (*A*) Severely involved scalp neurofibromas (*B*) Excess scalp tissue. (*C*) Excision. (*D*) Postoperative result.

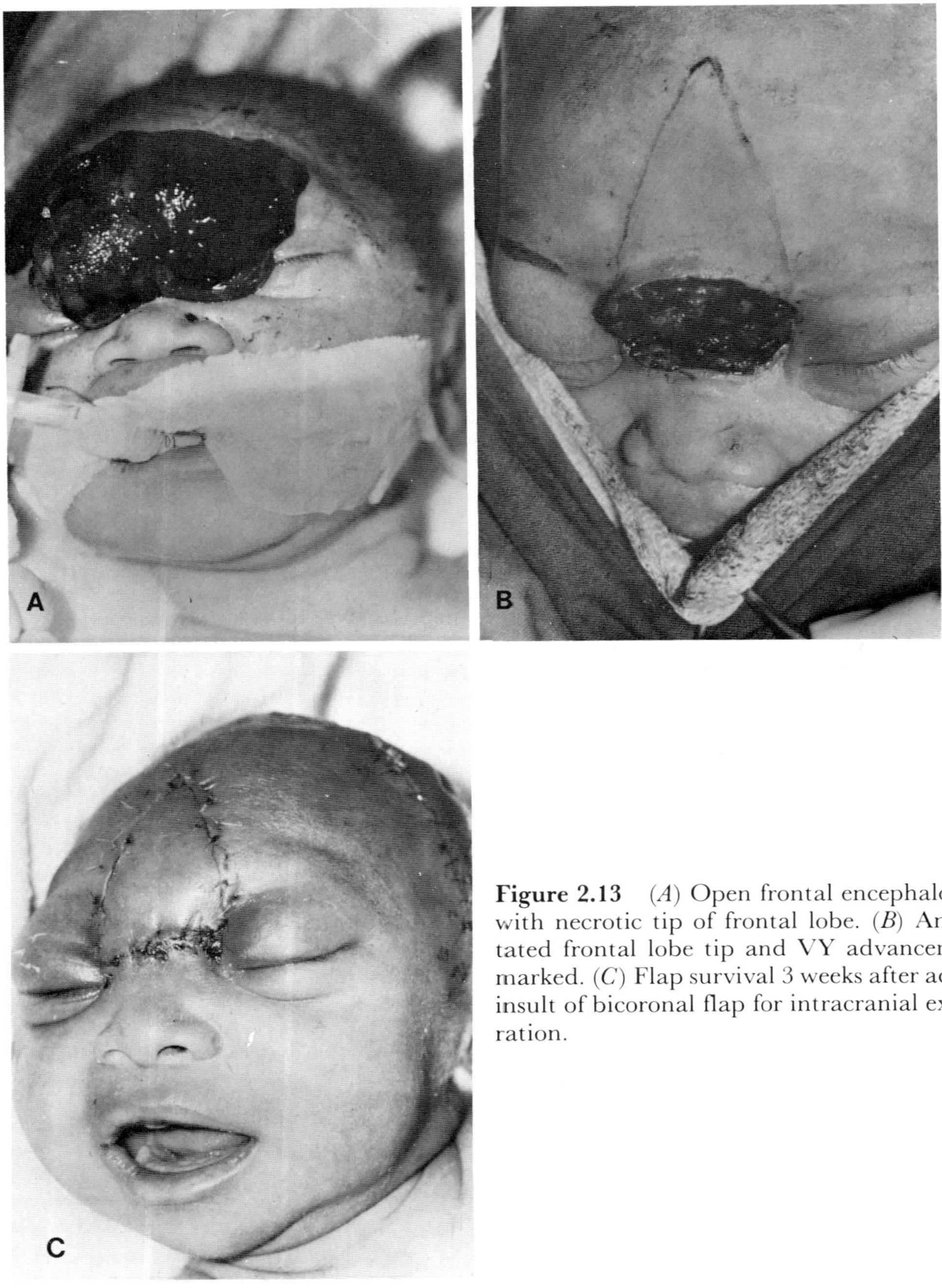

Figure 2.13 (*A*) Open frontal encephalocele with necrotic tip of frontal lobe. (*B*) Amputated frontal lobe tip and VY advancement marked. (*C*) Flap survival 3 weeks after added insult of bicoronal flap for intracranial exploration.

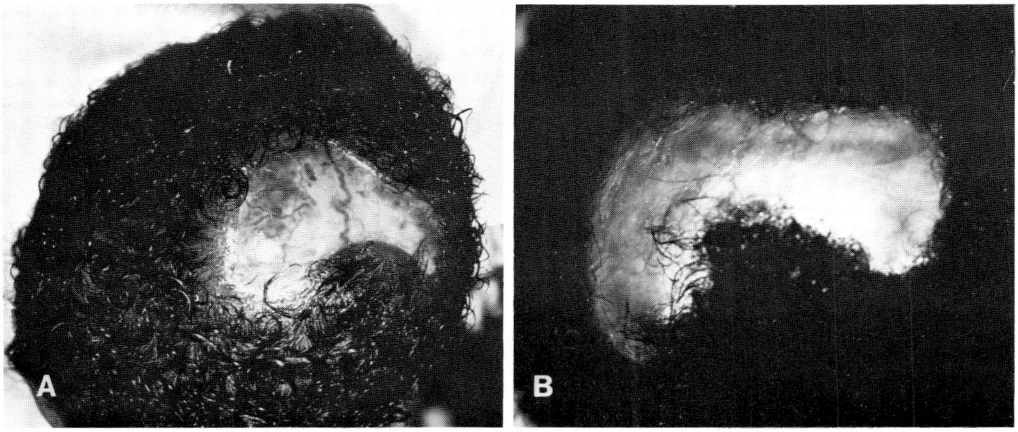

Figure 2.14 (*A*) Two days of age with translucent dura (?). Brain can be seen. (*B*) After conservative therapy re-epithelialization was ensued.

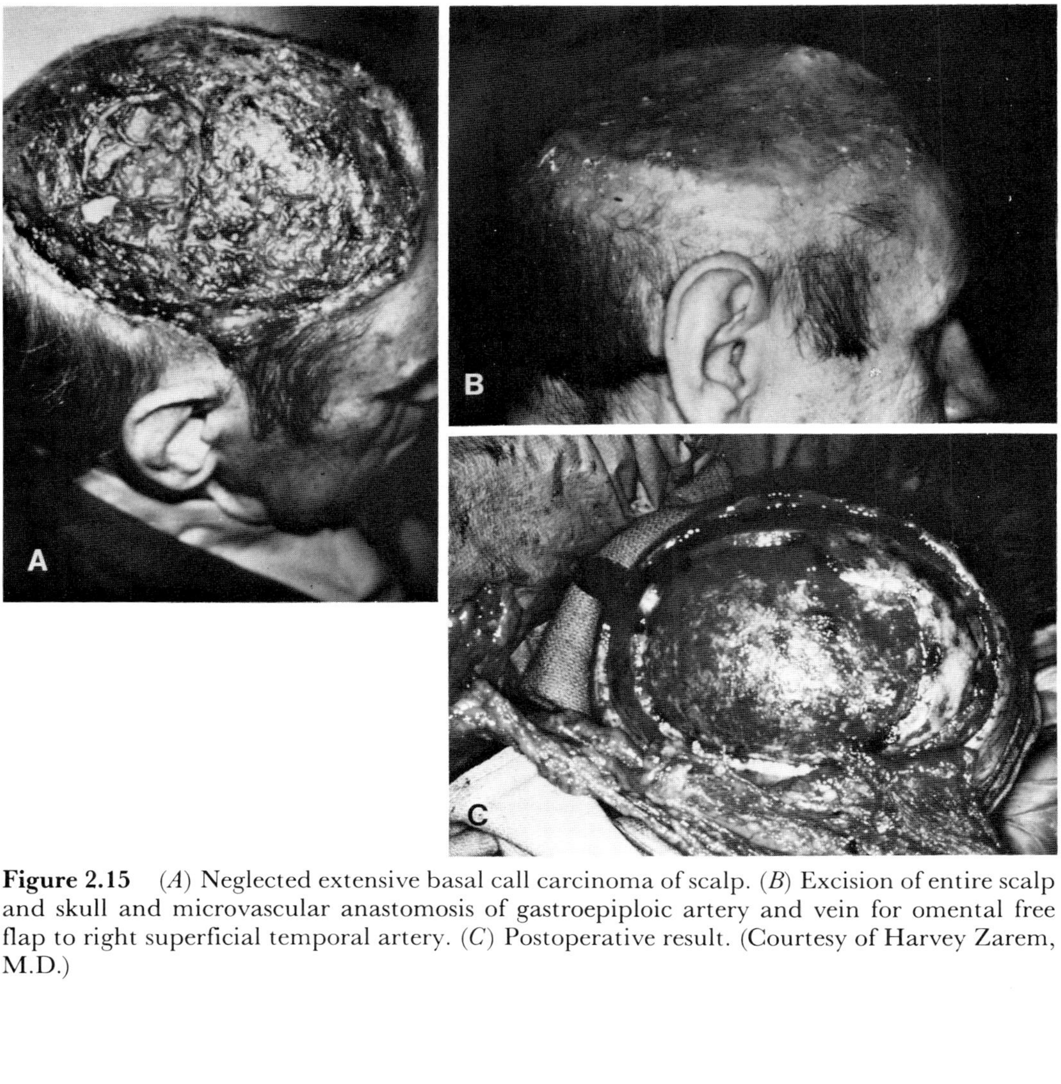

Figure 2.15 (*A*) Neglected extensive basal call carcinoma of scalp. (*B*) Excision of entire scalp and skull and microvascular anastomosis of gastroepiploic artery and vein for omental free flap to right superficial temporal artery. (*C*) Postoperative result. (Courtesy of Harvey Zarem, M.D.)

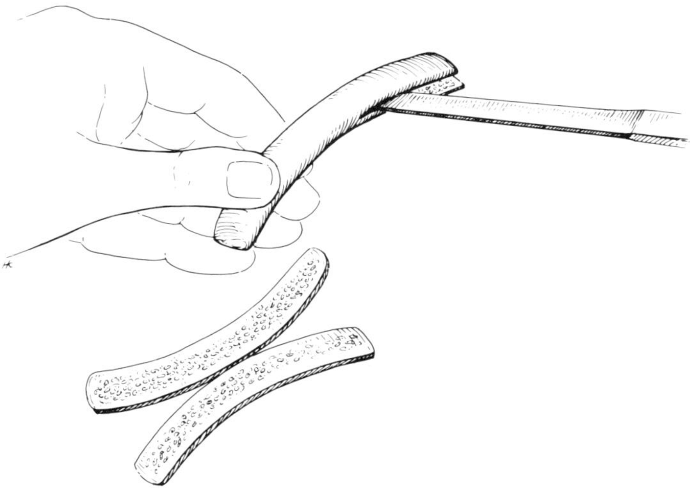

Figure 2.16 Osteotome used for horizontal splitting of rib grafts.

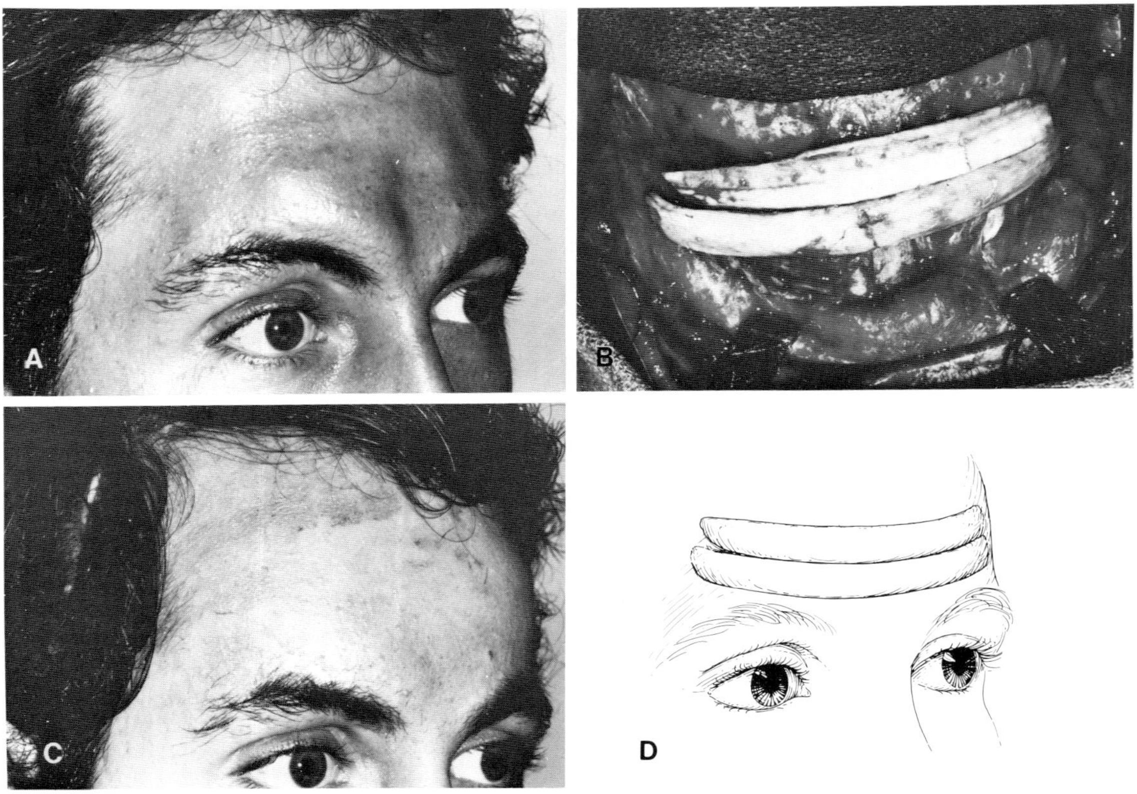

Figure 2.17 (*A*) Preoperative deformity. (*B*) Split rib grafts applied through bicoronal approach. (*C*, *D*) Excellent contour results.

seen is that of acquired skull deformity; after trauma or necessary resection of neoplasm (Fig. 2.3 *A*). Before deciding on the methods for reconstruction, one has to decide whether or not reconstruction is necessary. Many times, a bony skull defect can be masked within the hair-bearing scalp by the hair itself. Unless this bony defect is massive and brain injury is eminent because of lack of protection, reconstruction may not be necessary. If, however, the bony contour is obvious and is psychologically distressing to the patient, recontouring can be beneficial. The latter occurs most frequently in frontal sinus and frontal bone fractures.

Reconstruction of the bony calvarium can be accomplished with various methods. Techniques include the use of either alloplastic materials, autogenous tissue, or both. Occasionally, if large bony defects of the scalp are missing, the use of formed methyl methacrylate can be employed (see Chapter 11). This has the disadvantage of being a foreign body and occasionally is a nidus for infection. Although these methyl methacrylate plates can be wired into place beautifully to correct contour and brain coverage deformities, the perimeter never truly "heals" and for that reason there is constant motion.

It is the author's feeling that autogenous split grafts offer advantages that alloplastic materials cannot have. Once ribs are harvested, they can be split in a horizontal fashion (Fig. 2.16) so that their length and width are doubled. Split ribs can then be shaped to fit any contour desired, and have the advantage of being autogenous tissue (Fig. 2.17). The perimeter of bone graft and calvarium "heals," however, the disadvantage is that of the donor-chest scar.

Combinations of alloplastic and autogenous bone "mush" have recently been popularized by several authors and combined advantage (but still maintain disadvantages) of each technique.

References

1. Ballin, J.: A method of cranioplasty. *Surg. Gynecol. Obstet.*, *33:*79, 1921.
2. Barlett, S. C.: Removal of entire scalp: wound healed by skin grafting. *Am. J. Med. Sci.*, *63:*573, 1872.
3. Brookes, W. L.: A case of complete avulsion of the scalp. *Indian Med. Gazette*, *61:*128, 1926.
4. Converse, J. M.: Techniques of bone grafting for contour restoration of the face. *Plast. Reconst. Surg.*, *14:*332, 1954.
5. Crockford, D. A., and Converse, J. M.: The ilium as a source of bone grafts in children. *Plast. Reconstr. Surg.*, *50:*270, 1972.
6. Delack, Z.: Successful replacement of the completely avulsed scalp. *Br. J. Plast. Surg.*, *8:*55, 1955.
7. Devine, J. W.: Square scalp grafts combined with strip grafts for treatment of male pattern baldness. *Plast. Reconstr. Surg.*, *62:*716, 1978.
8. Holmstrand, K., Longacre, J. J., and de Stefano, G. A.: Biophysical studies of split-rib grafts in the repair of the cranium. *Plast. Reconstr. Surg.*, *26:*286, 1960.
9. Juri, J.: Use of parieto-occipital flaps in surgical treatment of baldness. *Plast. Reconstr. Sugr.*, *55:*456, 1975.
10. Kazanjian, V. H., and Converse, J. M.: *The Surgical Treatment of Facial Injuries*, Ed. 2, Williams & Wilkins, Baltimore, 1959.
11. Kazanjian, V. H., and Webster, R. C.: The treatment of extensive losses of the scalp. *Plast. Reconstr. Surg.*, *1:* 360, 1946.
12. Kirhn, C. L., and Grino, A: Iliac bone grafts replacing tantalum plates for gunshot wounds of the skull. *Am. J. Surg.*, *85:*395, 1953.
13. Korlof, B., Nylen, H., and Kietz, K.: Bone grafting of skull defects. *Plast. Reconstr. Surg.*, *52:*378, 1973.
14. Koss, N., Robson, M. C., and Krizek, T. J.: Scalping injury. *Plast. Reconstr. Surg.*, *55:*439, 1975.
15. Law, A. A.: Avulsion of the scalp. *Surg. Gynecol. Obstet.*, *19:*229, 1914.
16. Longacre, J. J.: Surgical correction of extensive defects of scalp and skull with autogenous tissue, in *Transactions of First International Congress of Plastic Surgeons, Stockholm, 1955*, p. 346.
17. Longacre, J. J., and de Stefano, G. S.: Reconstruction of extensive defects of the skull with split-rib grafts. *Plast. Reconstr. Surg.*, *19:*186, 1957.
18. Longacre, J. J., and de Stefano, G. S.: Further observation of the behavior of autogenous split-rib grafts in reconstruction of extensive defects of the calvarium and facial skeleton, in *Transactions of Second International Congress of the Plastic Surgeons*, London, 1959, pp. 290.
19. Lu, M. M.: Successful replacement of avulsed scalp. *Plast. Reconstr. Surg.*, *43:*231, 1969.
20. Macomber, D. W.: Cancellous iliac bone in depression of forehead, nose and chin. *Plast. Reconstr. Surg.*, *4:*157, 1949.
21. McClintock, H. G., and Dingman, R. O.: The repair

of cranial defects with iliac bone. *Surgery, 30:*955, 1951.

22. McLean, D. H., and Buncke, H. J.: Autotransplant of omentum to a large scalp defect with microsurgical revascularization. *Plast. Reconstr. Surg., 49:*268, 1972.
23. Miller, G. D. G., Anstee, E. J., and Snell, J. A.: Successful replantation of an avulsed scalp by microvascular anastomoses. *Plast. Reconstr. Surg., 58:*133, 1976.
24. Nowlem, R.: Cancellous chip bone grafts; report on 75 cases. *Lancet, 2:*746, 1944.
25. O'Brien, B., and Drake, J.: Congenital defects of the skull and scalp. *Br. J. Plast. Surg., 24:*184, 1971.
26. Orticohea, M.: Four flap scalp reconstruction techniques. *Br. J. Plast. Surg., 20:*172, 1967.
27. Orticohea, M.: New three-flap scalp reconstruction technique *Br. J. Plast. Surg., 24:*184, 1971.
28. Phemister, D. B.: The fate of transplanted bone and regeneration of its various consituents. *Surg. Gynecol. Obstet., 19:*303, 1914.
29. Scott, M., and Wyeis, H. T.: Experimental observations on the use of stainless steel for cranioplasty. *J. Neurosurg., 3:*310, 1946.
30. Small, J. M., and Graham, M. P.: Acrylic resin for the closure of skull defects. *Br. J. Surg., 33:*106, 1945.
31. Sutliff, F. B.: Prolonged survival after avulsion of the entire scalp. *Occidental Med. Times, 4:*129–131, 1890.
32. White, J. C.: Late complications following cranioplasty with alloplastic plates. *Ann. Surg., 128:*743, 1948.

CHAPTER 3

Surgery of the Forehead and Cheek Regions

Walter R. Mullin, M.D.

As a surgeon who is involved with the removal of lesions or the repairing of defects of the face, one should strive to arm himself with as many of the basic surgical skills, techniques and philosophies that lend themselves to this special area of the body. To lay a foundation for this, more than casual knowledge of the detailed anatomy of the area should be mastered. If accomplished, this knowledge will add confidence to the decision-making process, when one is faced with any of the many different situations that each unique surgical challenge in this area offers.

Considering the cheek and forehead separately is valid since they are so similar topographically. They offer the largest smooth surface of the face. Also, they are in themselves aesthetic units and irregularities that are present in these specific areas are often more noticeable than a similar defect would be in a junction point of an aesthetic unit, i.e., nasolabial fold, etc. Furthermore, in considering the areas of the face separately, one is encouraged to focus in more detail on the specific characteristics of the area more thoroughly. Therefore, one will be confident in dealing with different structures in the area that may be violated either by trauma or surgery. Injuries to structures, contained in these areas, demand that they be recognized, evaluated and treated appropriately, so that the end result will be optimal.

ANATOMY

Superiorly the forehead is bound by the hair-bearing scalp area or, in bald individuals, the junction of the area which had previously been hair-bearing. Its boundary laterally and inferiorly is the hair-bearing area of the temporal region continuing to a line from the lateral aspect of the eyebrow to the temporal area parallel to the zygoma, then across the superior edge of the eyebrow joining the other side by crossing the bridge of the nose. Many wrinkled individuals have a transverse wrinkle in this area of the nasal root that follows this joining line (Figs. 3.1 and 3.2).

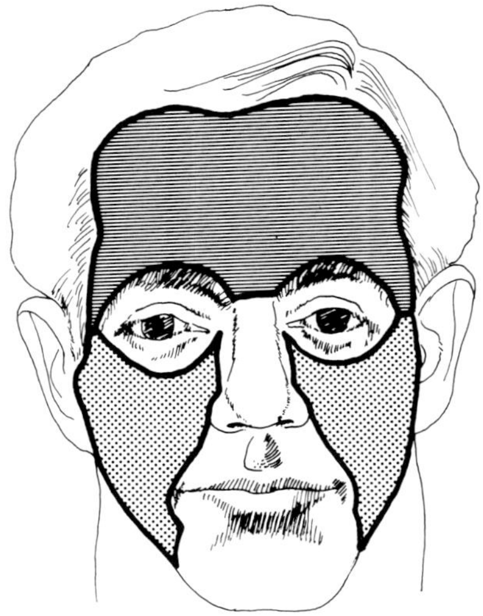

Figure 3.1 Boundary of forehead.

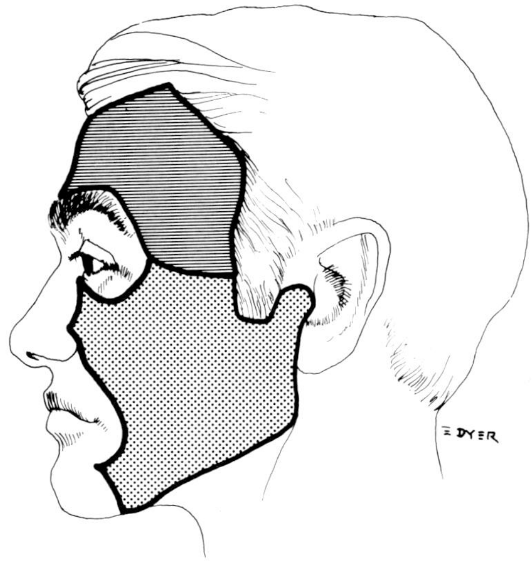

Figure 3.2 Boundary of the cheeks.

The limits of the cheek are as follows: (1) superiorly the area of junction is with the thin, pliable lower eyelid skin; (2) laterally the junction is with the lower aspect of the line from the lateral aspect of the eyebrow to the sideburn hair. It becomes academic whether or not to consider the sideburn area cheek or scalp (true sideburn being defined as the location of the hair-bearing area in the preauricular area in females of all ages and in preadolescent males). It seems it should be included in the consideration of the cheek, continuing the lateral brow line to the junction area of the ear helix root to the temporal area.

The lateral limit includes the preauricular skin, which follows a line from the junction area of the ear helix root inferiorly and splits the tragus vertically, then down to the preauricular skin fold to the junction point of the lobule to the face. From this point, the line parallels the lower edge of the mandible to a point where the labiomental line meets the lower edge of the mandible. This line then goes superiomedially up to and across to joint the more definite nasolabial fold, which is followed to the lower part of the alar groove. From here, an imaginary line crosses to the most medial aspect of the aforementioned infraorbital line at the junction of thin lower eyelid skin and the cheek skin.

Next, the concept of resting skin tension lines (RSTL)[1] (Fig. 3.3) should be understood to the degree that one is able to visualize them on any specific location of the face, even on a child's unwrinkled face. These lines most often parallel wrinkle lines and are usually at right angles to the direction of pull of the facial muscles. It becomes obvious that any elective surgical incision should be parallel to the RSTL in that specific area. The corollary, i.e., any incision that is at angles to the RSTL, requires special consideration.

It is of some interest to note the unusual area in the glabella area and perioral area where the wrinkles meet at right angles. Other somewhat unusual wrinkles to be aware of that are found in some individuals are wrinkles that come out of the temporal bay area to a point in the general area of the arch of the eyebrow. Another unusual wrinkle can sometimes be found in the malar area going at right angles to the normal RSTL (Fig. 3.3).

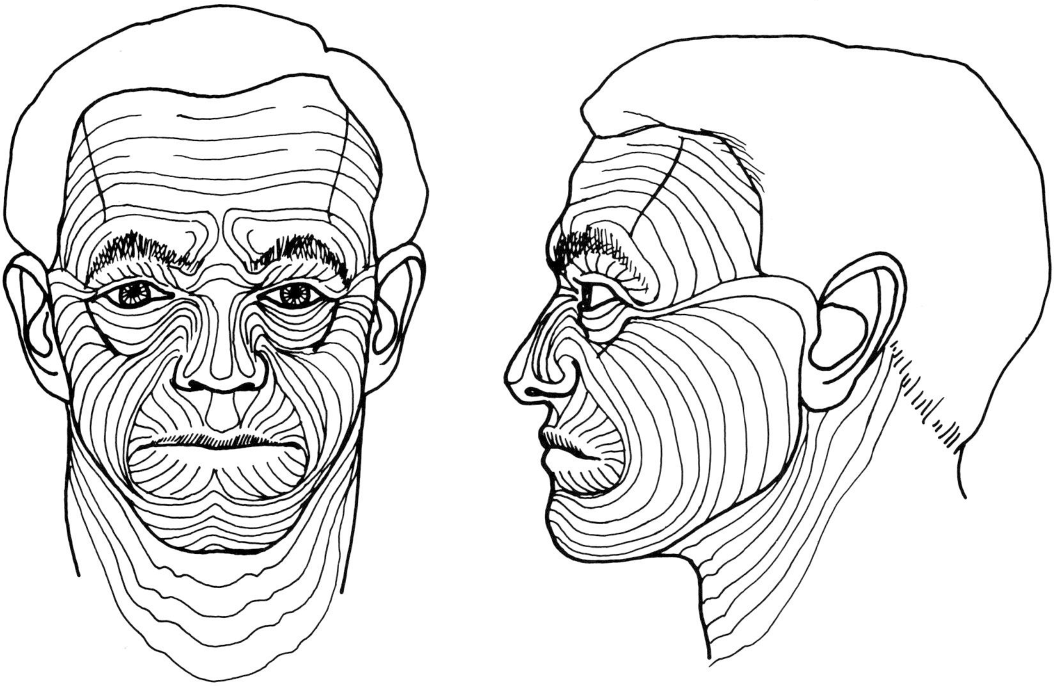

Figure 3.3 Face wrinkle lines.

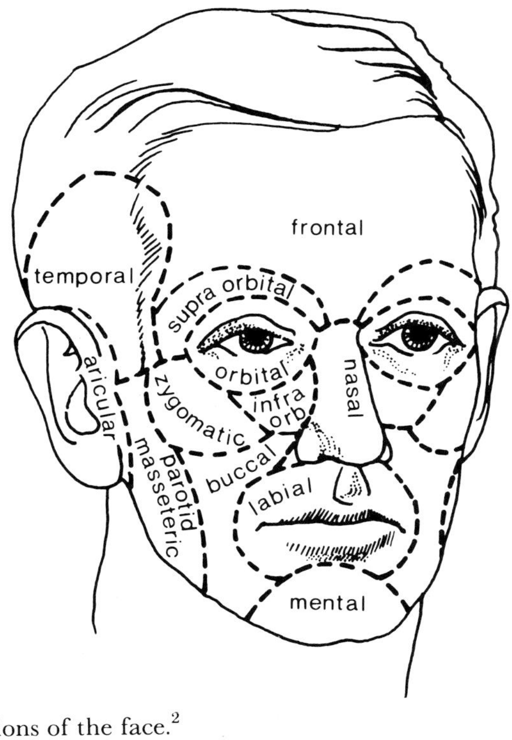

Figure 3.4 Named regions of the face.[2]

Factors which have been incriminated in the development of wrinkles are: the genetic makeup of each unique individual, activity of facial expression, sun exposure, sleeping face down against the bed, and smoking. Incisions that take advantage of these wrinkles, both for sheer camouflage and reduction of stress across the closure, and that are meticulously closed with a competent plastic closure, have the best chance of leaving the least noticeable scar.

Another very important point should be made. Namely, one should make every effort to avoid an elective incision that crosses the border of the mandible, even if the incision follows the RSTL. When these scars contract even with normal healing they invariably form a depression at the lower edge of the mandible and are usually unsightly. This potential for a poor outcome should be recognized and the patient clearly informed in both trauma cases that present this situation and in mandatory elective incision of this area.

Incision in the hair-bearing cheek area should be carefully placed so that no follicle will be transected. If an incision is closed over such transected follicles, then cyst formation and chronic irritation of the scar in that area are likely.

Next one should be aware of the mobility of the skin in the area of concern. This can best be judged on an individual basis, simply by placing one's index finger on the area being evaluated and moving it in different directions. This is a most important maneuver prior to any surgical intervention of any area.

Another special consideration involves the central butterfly area of the face as it goes out onto the cheeks. This skin is very different, especially with respect to its texture and type of pores. Some individuals have very thick, oily skin with prominent depression at each pore in this area. Even carefully closed incision under optimal conditions in this particular area have a tendency to remain red longer and tend toward a final scar that may be wide and depressed.

Next, more specific anatomic detail of the areas involved will be considered. The facial nerves must always be kept in mind when dealing with any problem concerning the face. Transection or damage by scalpel or electrocautery is tragic to both the patient and the surgeon. In traumatic wounds, when the nerve gap is not great, primary microsurgical funicular repair should be carried out (see Chapter 16). The nerve stimulator will be helpful in locating the distal end up to 72 hours after transection. Delayed repair usually results in retraction of the ends. The neuroma and glioma resection required is such that most often a nerve graft is required to bridge the gap. Due to the extensive arborization medial to a vertical line dropped from the lateral canthus of the eye, a transection medial to this line will, in many cases, result in a return of functioning after passage of time. Frey's syndrome (gustatory sweating) is another bothersome complication of injury to the facial nerve. The surgeon should be aware of this complication and be prepared to discuss it with his patients. One quickly becomes aware of the importance of these nerves, and a fresh cadaver dissection of them in their entirety by anyone who is involved with surgery of the face would be time well spent. The reconstruction of the paralyzed face is a book in itself and will not be covered in this chapter.

The next specific structure is the parotid system. The parotid duct is located approximately one finger breadth below the zygomatic arch and runs horizontally to cross the medial edge of the masseter muscle to exit in the buccal mucosa opposite the second upper molar tooth.

The duct can be easily palpated by clenching one's teeth, thus flexing the masseter, whereby one can roll the duct beneath the tip of the index finger. Its location becomes important so that transections are recognized and treated appropriately. If repair is possible, then careful microsurgical technique should be utilized. Stinting the repair with a Silastic tube of appropriate size for 3–6 weeks is thought to aid in the patiency rate after closure. If the transection is such that repair is not possible, then ligation of the duct may be the treatment of choice, but this usually results in transitory edema and tenderness of the gland. Direct injury to the gland parenchyma may result in cystic collection at the site of injury after closure of the skin. The size will increase and drainage will usually occur with increased salivation. Most often these symptoms will resolve with time. However, in persistent cases, frequent

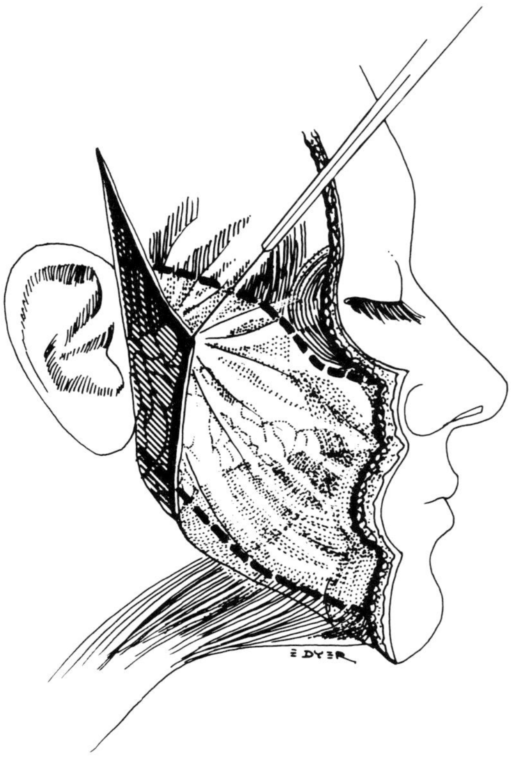

Figure 3.5 The superficial musculo-aponeurotic system (SMAS).[3]

needle aspiration may be required and, if unsuccessful, low dose radiation to the area may become necessary.

The next anatomic areas for consideration are the facial muscles and fascia. The system of muscles, fascia and dermis becomes important for lack of approximation at a deep level may result in an unsatisfactory depression in that area (Fig. 3.5). This results in an unsightly scar since shadows catch in the depths of such scars and are very noticeable.

TECHNIQUE OF REPAIR

Other general considerations in repairing traumatic or surgical defects of the face are sutures and drains. A minimal number of sutures should be used to obtain the desired result and they should be removed from the skin as early as 3 days to prevent the objectionable hatch marks. In the face, if the sutures are in longer than 5 or 6 days, then these unsightly marks usually remain. After suture removal, special adhesive tapes should be placed for longer support. Sutures to approximate deep structures should be buried as deeply as possible with their knots inverted (Fig. 3.6). The material used varies, but most often it is absorbable in nature. The newer synthetic materials of polyglycolic acid seem to be less reactive than catgut. If one encounters a stitch abcess which is sometimes seen after using nonabsorbable material deeply or even absorbable sutures placed too close to the surface, the use of a small crochet hook to

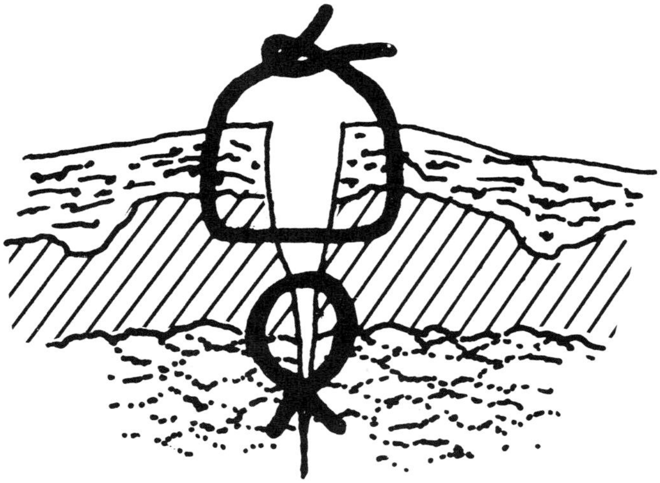

Figure 3.6 Relationship of sutures in two-layer closure.

"fish" these buried sutures out of the draining sinus is a handy method of removal of the irritating "foreign body."

Another often discussed topic is the use of drains in the face. It should be rare for one to use a drain of any sort, for great care should be spent to obtain meticulous hemostasis. If a drain is felt necessary, then the ones fashioned from a No. 19 butterfly scalp vein set connected to a Vacutaner tube is a good choice. The tube should exit the skin in an inconspicuous spot. This is especially useful beneath larger flaps and in areas of parotid gland injury. Closure of extremely contaminated injuries of the face of puncture wounds, such as from dog fangs, should be avoided if at all possible. The reliance on a drain to prevent infection is both wishful thinking and hazardous. A great deal of one's own individual judgment, coupled with his own and the experience of others, becomes paramount in optimally managing some of these difficult problems. Needless to say, any drain should be removed as soon as its intended job is finished and before it becomes a source of irritation to the wound or an avenue for infection.

PLANNING

Following the preceding generalizations, a more specific consideration of the thought process leading to choice of a reconstructive technique will be of interest. First, if one feels he is dealing with a malignant process, then, of course, no compromise should ever be considered so as to fit the excision into a pre-chosen method of convenient reconstruction. This concept cannot be stressed enough. The opposite of this is the ablative surgeon who purports the philosophy of cutting everyone "high, wide and handsome," thus, unnecessarily ruining some choice method of reconstruction. Hence, even if the reconstructive surgeon is not the ablative surgeon, he should be consulted with the intent of avoiding unnecessary damage to needed reconstructive sources. The most simple choice of reconstruction should first be considered, and the use of a method simply because the surgeon is fascinated by it from a textbook drawing often results in a disastrous result. The stepwise progression of choices should be as follows: (1) simple excision and closure, (2) closure with undermining, (3) skin grafts, (4) local flaps, and (5) distant flaps.

It is appropriate to mention here that other methods of therapy enter in the discussion. It is not within the scope of this chapter to discuss radiation, electrocautery and cryosurgery of lesions. There is an obvious lack of micropathologic control of the limits of removal. Mohs' chemosurgery is aimed at this problem in the ultimate sense. Mohs' chemosurgery, done expertly, has enjoyed a very good success rate for tumor removal, especially in dealing with morphea-type basal cell carcinoma and recurrent tumors. It also provides some interesting reconstructive challenges after the wounds have "healed" by contracture.

Another important pitfall is sometimes seen when a patient is sent to a surgeon for excision of a lesion that has recurred several times. The complimented surgeon sometimes may feel he will be able to cure this patient by re-excising the lesions, for he feels himself a much better surgeon. Bad mistake! At this point, one would be wise to slow down and consider other possibilities and obtain other studies in an attempt to determine the cause of the prior failures. A case in point was a patient who had a "recurrent" squamous cell carcinoma over the malar area which had been excised three times. Sinus films revealed it to be an "iceberg" type lesion arising from the maxillary sinus.

RECONSTRUCTION

The following is a compilation of diagrams of useful techniques in managing surgical defects of the cheek and forehead. The diagrams are not intended to be used in a cookbook fashion in that they may not represent the best method of closure for all patients with a defect in the same location of the diagram. They are intended only to demonstrate the particular surgical exercise in a stylized fashion. One must keep in mind that the only thing that the forehead-cheek areas and the paper these techniques are depicted on have in common is that they are both relatively flat. The plasticity of skin offers an advantage in that it can be adjusted to fit by careful suture technique, so that the standing cones (dog ears) are less severe due to the flow and stacking of skin. These advantages are diminished by the fact that one must be ever mindful of blood supply, tension, hematoma and infection. Also, these methods must be used so that the majority of the suture closure lines lie in the most optimal direction with respect to RSTL, units, and camouflage areas. The ultimate artistic and economic use of tissue will then be accomplished.

Fusiform Excision with Primary Closure

These methods are usually best suited for removal of relatively small lesions which are in an area where the resulting edges are easily approximated. Significant facial landmarks must be considered and not distorted by the closure. Use of the crown excision as shown (Fig. 3.7*B*) may be helpful in accomplishing this end by having the patient demonstrate exaggerated facial expressions that involve the area of concern. By checking the mobility of the local tissue with one's index finger, the surgeon can most often precisely locate the most suitable alignment of the long axis. These maneuvers obviously must be carried out prior to distorting or paralyzing the area with anesthesia. Also, one must carry an exact mental picture of the locations of the RSTLs so that he may apply this knowledge to the very young face or to the patient under general anesthesia.

In excising the fusiform, one must take care to make vertical cuts and to cleanly incise the two corners. The length to width ratio of the excision will be approximately 4:1 to allow for a smooth closure at the ends. The local tissue will also determine to some extent the amount of standing cone or "dog ear" that will occur. Although it is often thought that these settle with time, one should not rely on this too heavily.

Next, the edges should be undermined enough to allow for eversion of the closure. This

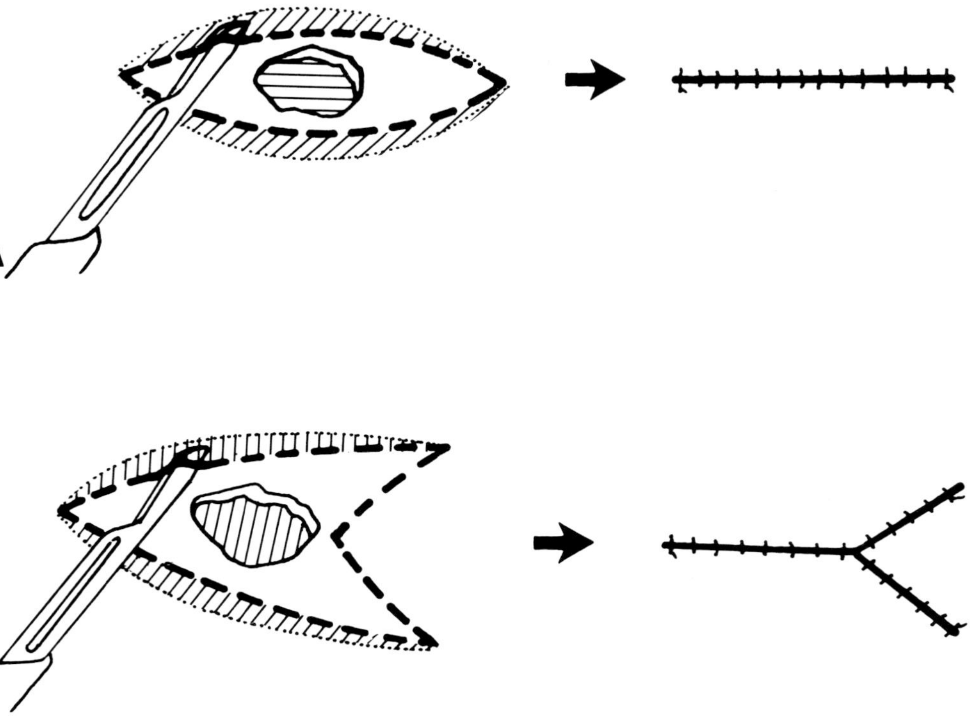

Figure 3.7 (*A*) Fusiform excision with primary closure. (*B*) Crown excision.[4]

undermining should be at the dermal-subdermal level and followed by careful pinpoint electrocautery hemostatis prior to careful two-layer closure. This method will be very adequate for the majority of small lesions of the forehead and cheeks, and should be reconsidered when one finds himself wanting to use one of the more "fancy flaps" depicted later.

More Extensive Undermining

The next method of closure is the same as the fusiform and closure, but advantage may be taken of the fact some areas may be undermined in the cheek and forehead area at the dermal-subdermal level to allow closure of larger defects. The undermining should be carried out in an area away from any landmarks of the face so that distortion is minimal (Fig. 3.8).

Local Flaps

There are a multitude of local flaps and modifications of modifications of local flaps. A few more basic and applicable flaps will be illustrated along with a few brief comments. First, one must be convinced that a flap is needed, and that a more simple method would not give the same or better result. When used correctly, flaps offer an excellent method of repair, for they repair the defect with tissue that is most similar to that which is missing and they avoid the central depression of the linear scar which has real or relative dog ears at each end as is

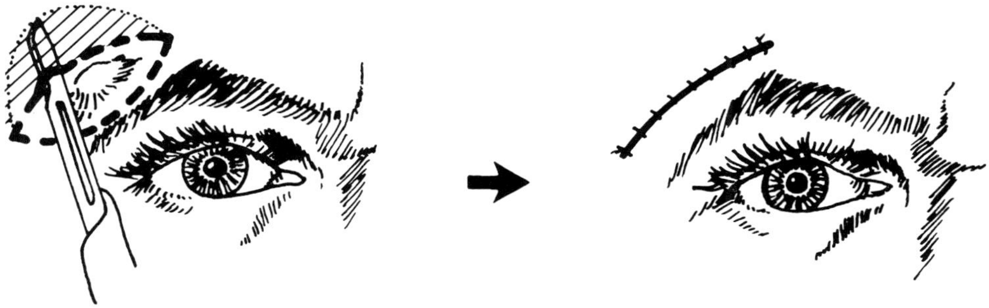

Figure 3.8 Demonstration of undermining away from facial landmarks.

sometimes seen with fusion excisions. Careful planning is a must in using any method of flap reconstruction. Using a reverse pattern, i.e. walking backward mentally through each step and considering the consequences with respect to donor defects, distortion at closure, the defect that would result if the flap is lost, and the question: "Will more than one step be necessary?" are all very important to visualize and discuss with the patient.

Other considerations such as the local mobility, texture, thickness and blood supply of the area, along with alternate plans, all should precede any well thought out flap. Most flaps of the forehead and cheek area do not require delays unless the surgeon has some reason to suspect the local blood supply in the area is compromised, i.e., old scar, radiation or previous surgery. The most common types of local flaps will be illustrated (Fig. 3.9–3.16). Less attention should be paid to the ratios and numbers often associated with these flaps and more attention should be focused on the use of common sense with respect to the direction of alignment of the vessels in the local area, size of the base of the flap, awareness of old scars, and avoiding hematoma, kinking and tension, all of which are so important to the success of these flaps.

DERMAL ISLANDS

See Figure 3.17.

SUBCUTANEOUS ISLANDS

See Figure 3.18.

VASCULAR ISLANDS

See Figure 3.19.

Other Special Flaps to Cover Larger Areas

The deltopectoral flap (Fig. 3.20) will cover defects up to the zygoma and is especially good to provide cover to the cheek and mandible area. It is sturdy and fairly reliable even without delay.

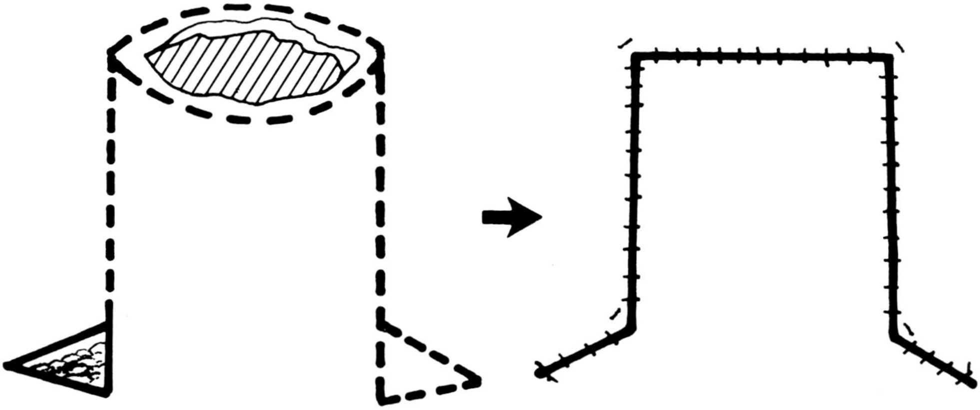

Figure 3.9 Local advancement flap[6] is seldom used as such since resultant scars are usually unsightly; more often serial excision may be used to close an area that has been previously grafted or a lesion such as a hairy nevus.

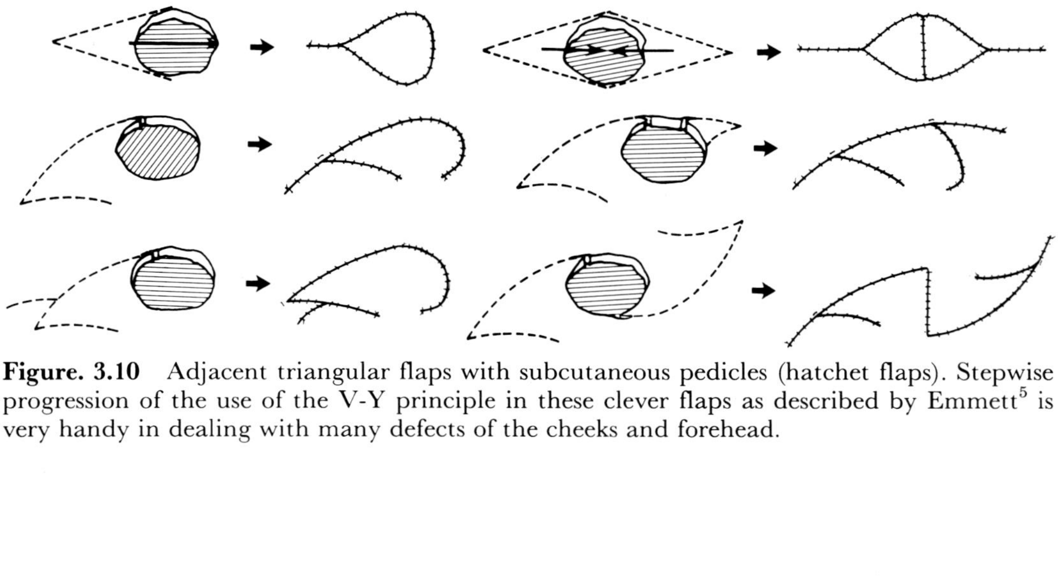

Figure. 3.10 Adjacent triangular flaps with subcutaneous pedicles (hatchet flaps). Stepwise progression of the use of the V-Y principle in these clever flaps as described by Emmett[5] is very handy in dealing with many defects of the cheeks and forehead.

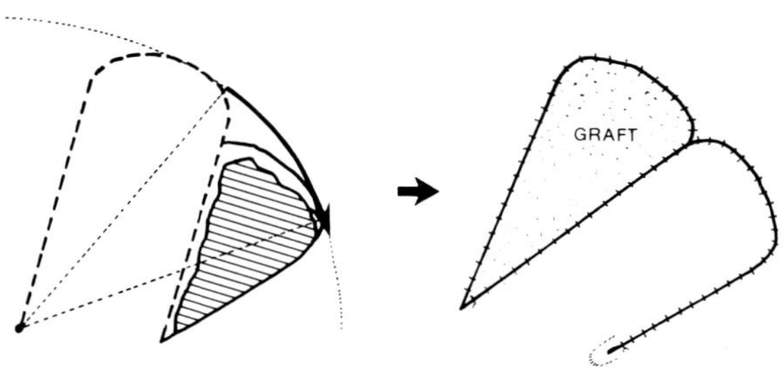

Figure 3.11 Local transposition flap.[6] Major point to consider is making sure donor area can afford to give the flap. Make the flap long enough to fit the defect without tension.

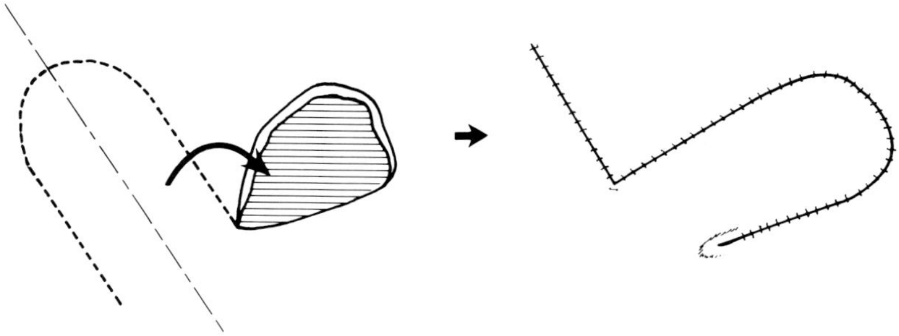

Figure 3.12 Interpolation flap simply jumps over intact tissue; usually used when the most desired donor area is more remote.

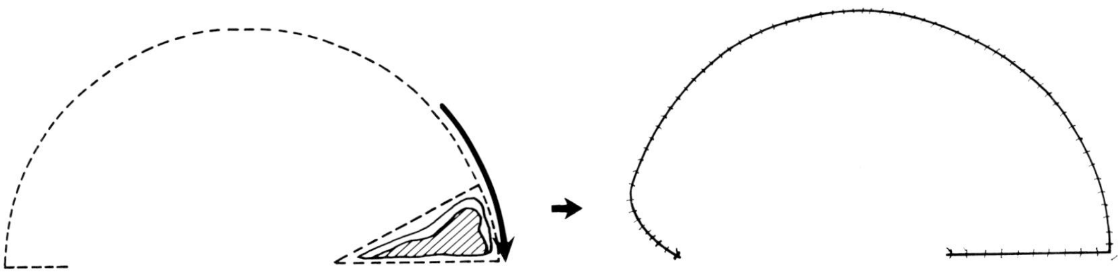

Figure 3.13 Rotation flap[7, 9] seldom used in the strict design as shown in more application in the larger areas of the scalp. The flap must be large enough to allow rotation.

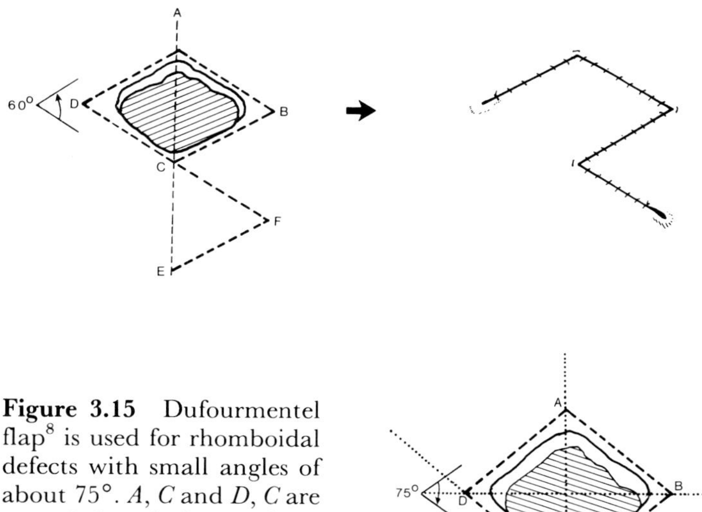

Figure 3.14 Lemberg flap[8] designed for use in a rhomboidal defect with a small angle of about 60°. *A, C* is extended to *E* and *D, C* is extended to *F* so that *C, F* = *A, B* and *E, F* = *C, B*. Mobility of the local area is a must.

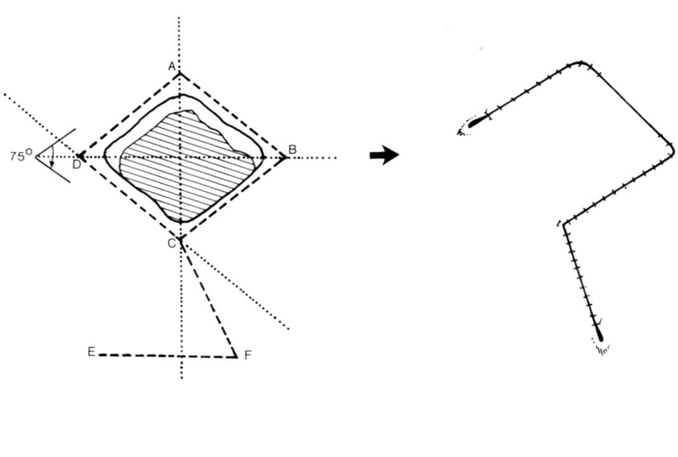

Figure 3.15 Dufourmentel flap[8] is used for rhomboidal defects with small angles of about 75°. *A, C* and *D, C* are extended and the resulting angle bisected so that *C, F* = *A, B* and *E, F* = C, *B*. *E, F* is horizontal to *D, B*. Once again, local mobility is a must.

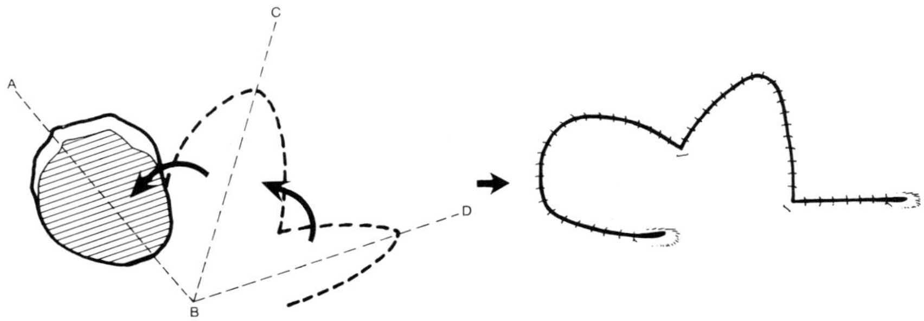

Figure 3.16 Bilobe flap[12] is a very useful flap and it avoids the need for a skin graft to a donor area that is too large to close primarily. The axis point *B* is located and then *A*, *B* is drawn. The primary flap required is bisected by *B*, *C* is outlined next usually slightly smaller in total area of the primary defect. Next, the secondary flap is outlined so that its area is smaller than the defect of the primary flap, and its donor area may be closed primarily. Angle *A*, *B*, *C*, should equal *C*, *B*, *D*. Obviously, the larger the angle *A*, *B*, *D*, the more kinking and tension of the flap.

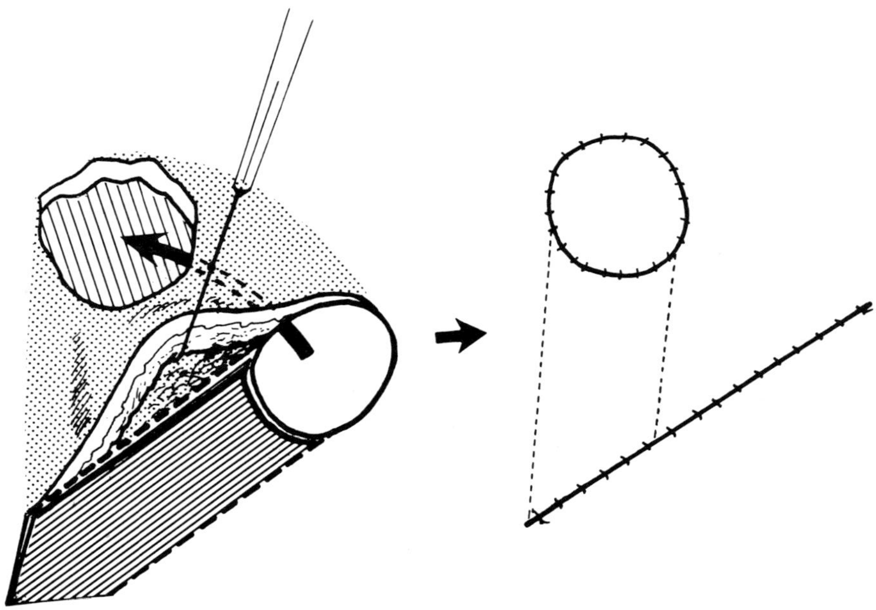

Figure 3.17 The epithelium on the pedicle that is to be buried is removed as a split thickness graft. The flap is then elevated in the dermal-subcutaneous fat plane leaving the subdermal plexus of vessels intact. The cover tissue is then tunneled into position at the defect site. These flaps are of limited value since they leave depressions and bulges in their wake. These depressions may be filled with local fat flaps or buried depithelized dermis that is excised at the end of the donor area for closure. Another disadvantage is the blood supply is often tenuous. Edema or hematoma easily necrose this flap since the pedicle is trapped below an intact bridge of tissue. If this flap is used, great care must be taken to make the pedicle long enough to reach the defect without a kink.

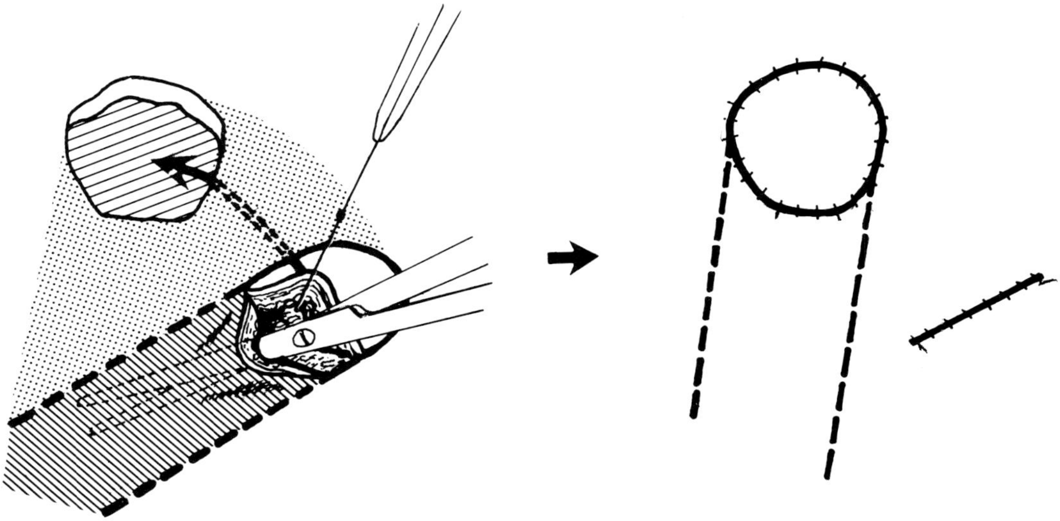

Figure 3.18 The difference in this flap and the dermal island flap is that these flaps receive their blood supply from a pedicle of subcutaneous tissue and not the dermis. Most of the negative comments with respect to the dermal flap pertain to this flap also.

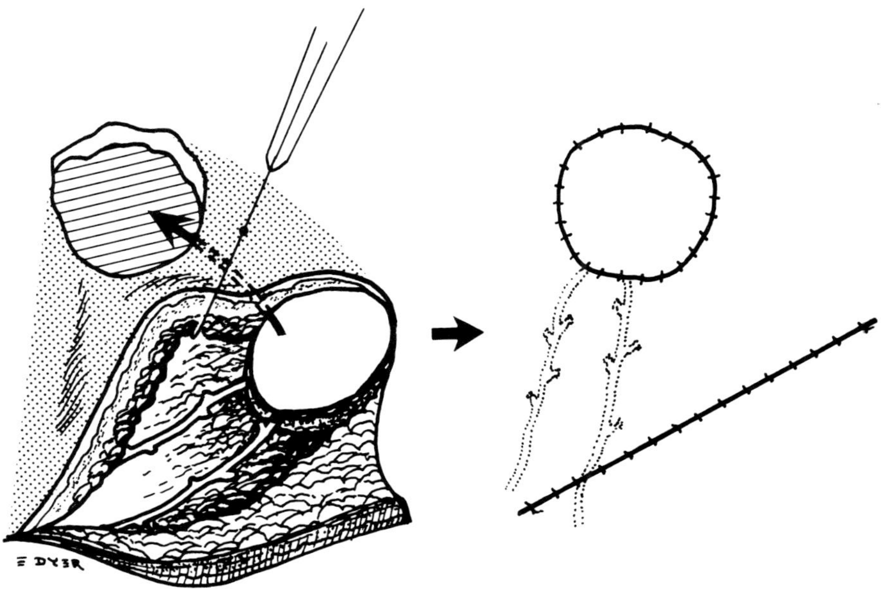

Figure 3.19 A very specialized flap that requires very special circumstances to be used. The vessels must be large enough to allow dissection and the surgical technique used must be exacting. The failure rate of this flap is due to many of the problems mentioned with respect to subcutaneous and dermal island flaps.

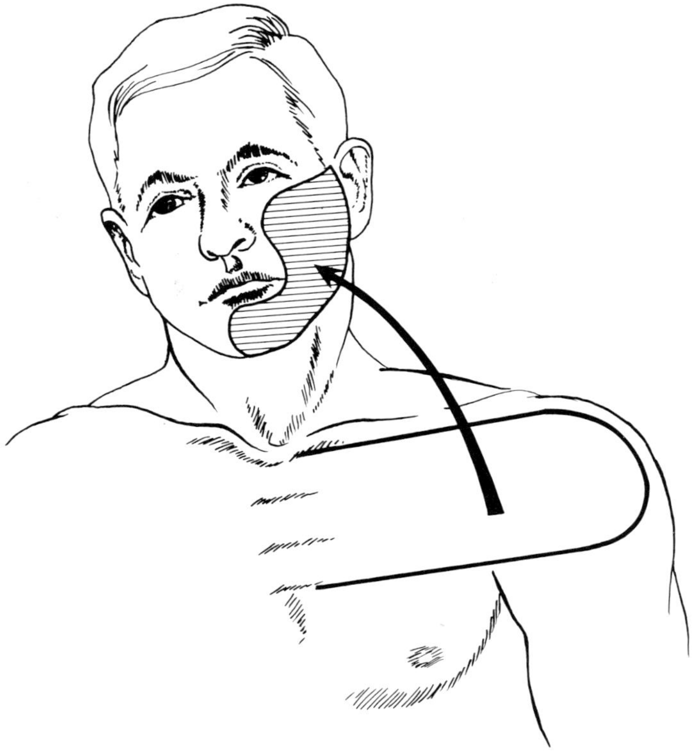

Figure 3.20 Deltopectoral[10] flap.

The Zovickian-Owens neck shoulder flap (Fig. 3.21) is another flap that may be considered to cover much the same area mentioned. It may be delayed; it may be used as a myocutaneous flap. The longitudinal scars on the neck and the potential of contracture is a drawback to this flap and it is usually used after the deltopectoral area has been used.[10]

FOREHEAD FLAPS

Total forehead flaps (Fig. 3.22) are (a) based on temporal and auricular vessels. (b) When taken as one entire unit and the border is at the exact edge of the hair and brow line, the resulting defect is least noticeable. (c) Usually no delay is necessary (except in cases where vessels have been damaged after head and neck surgery or radiation. (d) In planning, the thickness and kinking of the flap must be allowed for. (e) Intact periosteum must be left behind for graft to take. (f) The graft should be uniform and in one piece. However, McCurdy[15] feels meshing the graft with very little expansion offers good camouflage and prevents the unattractive shiny look. (g) Will cover most areas of cheek externally or internally.

In smaller central forehead flaps (Fig. 3.23), (a) it should be possible for the defect to be closed primarily. The laxity of the skin must be assessed preoperatively. (b) Isolated forehead grafts should be avoided and, if possible, they should be excised at a later date. (c) Larger defects can be closed by wide undermining and closure with more than usual tension. The transverse scoring beneath such flaps to gain length is often not helpful and may even

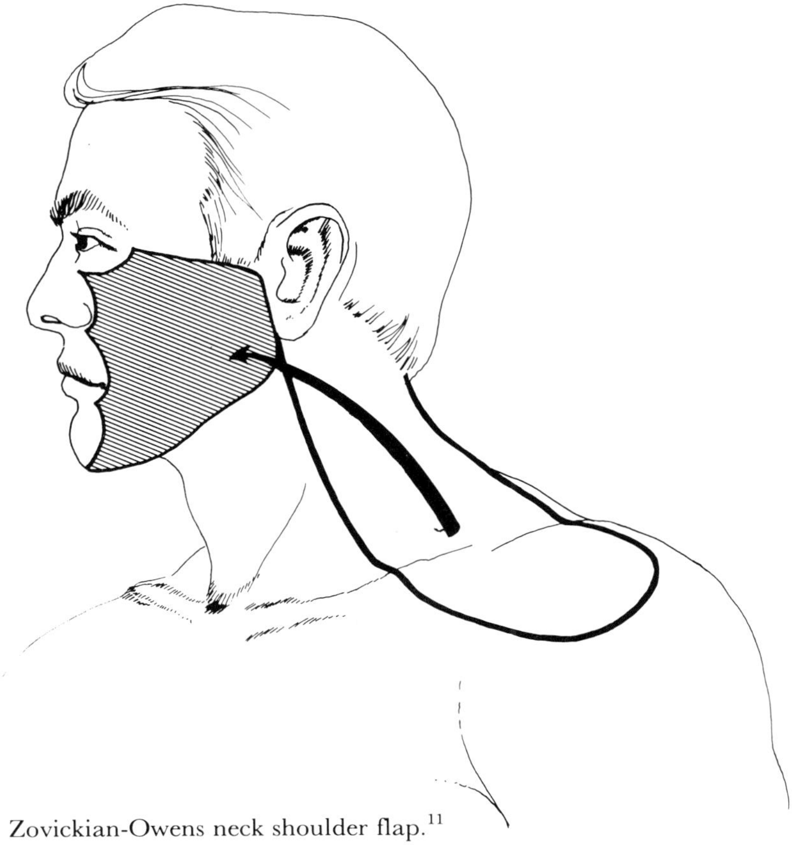

Figure 3.21 Zovickian-Owens neck shoulder flap.[11]

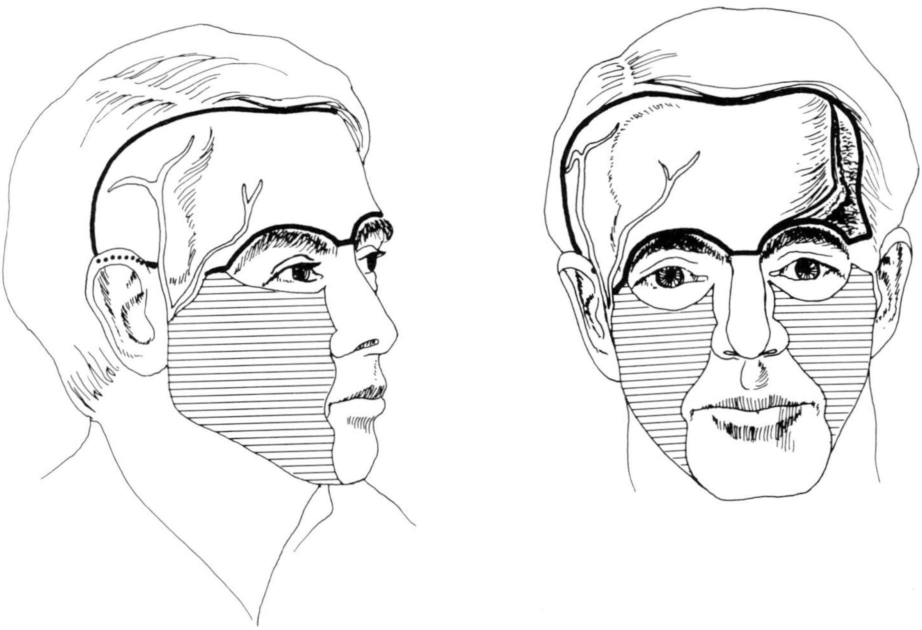

Figure 3.22 Total forehead flaps.

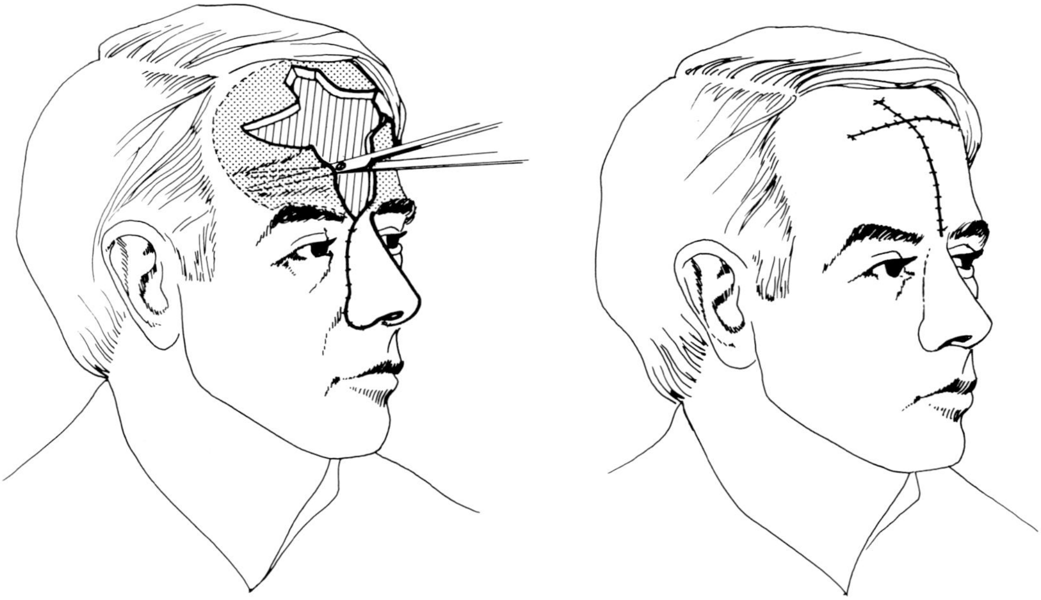

Figure 3.23 Smaller central forehead flaps based on the supratrochlea vessels.

jeopardize the flap's circulation. (d) Larger central defects may be closed by a larger sliding type V-Y flap along the temporoparietal occipital area based on the temporal vessels, if necessary.

CHEEK FLAPS

The largest cheek flaps are found in the meloplasty. This demonstrates the viability of flaps elevated at that level receiving blood supply medially.

If a cheek flap is chosen to fill a defect of the lower eyelid, malar or maxillary area, then the modification of the Mustarde cheek flap by McGregor is nice to consider for the surgery is less extensive and the lateral canthus of the eye has less chance of being pulled inferiorly.

Points to consider in using the McGregor modification flap (Fig. 3.24) are: (a) Attention must be directed at not forming a step deformity in the sideburn area. (b) Pay close attention to the marked change in thickness of the eyelid and cheek skin.

POSTAURICULAR FLAPS (INTERPOLATION)

See Figures 3.25 and 3.26.

NECK FLAPS[10]

See Figure 3.27.

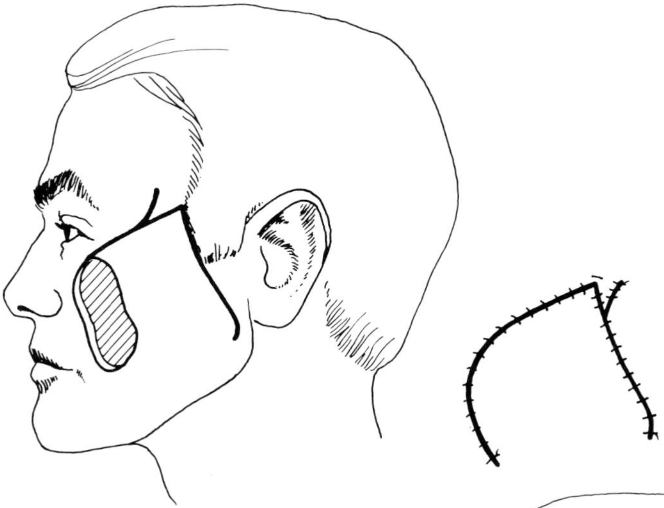

Figure 3.24 McGregor modification of cheek flap.

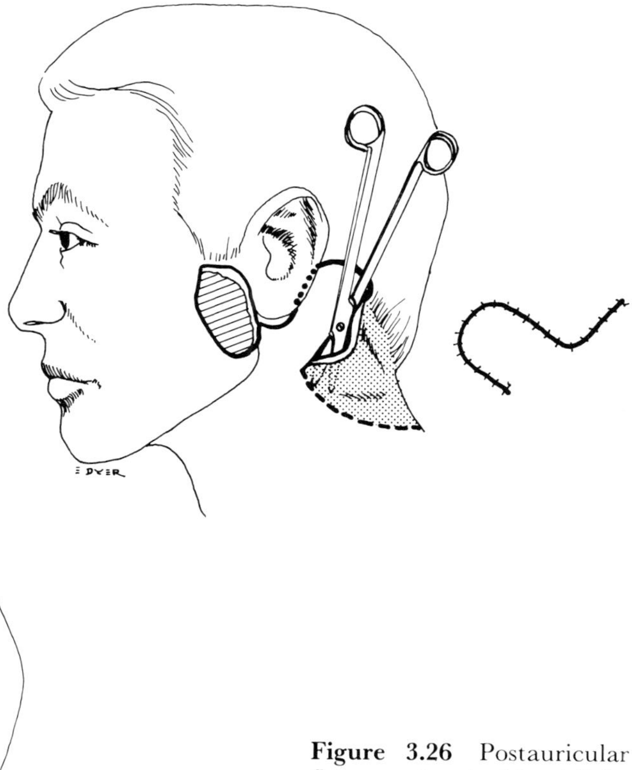

Figure 3.25 Primary postauricular flap with graft to retroauricular defect or advancement of neck skin to gain closure.

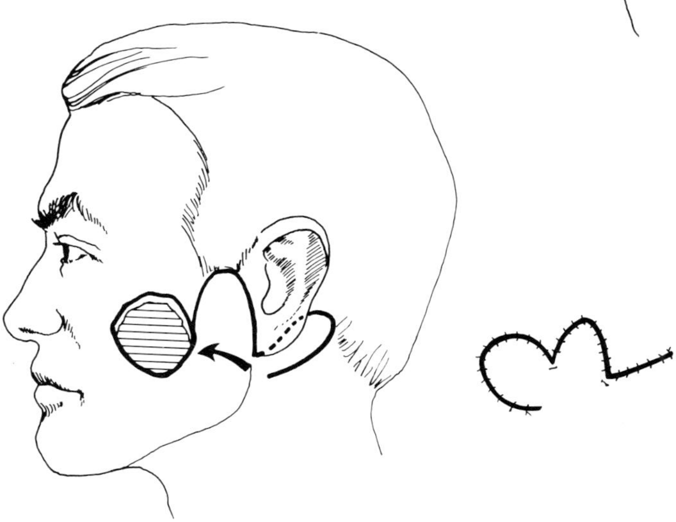

Figure 3.26 Postauricular flap associated with a bilobe flap.

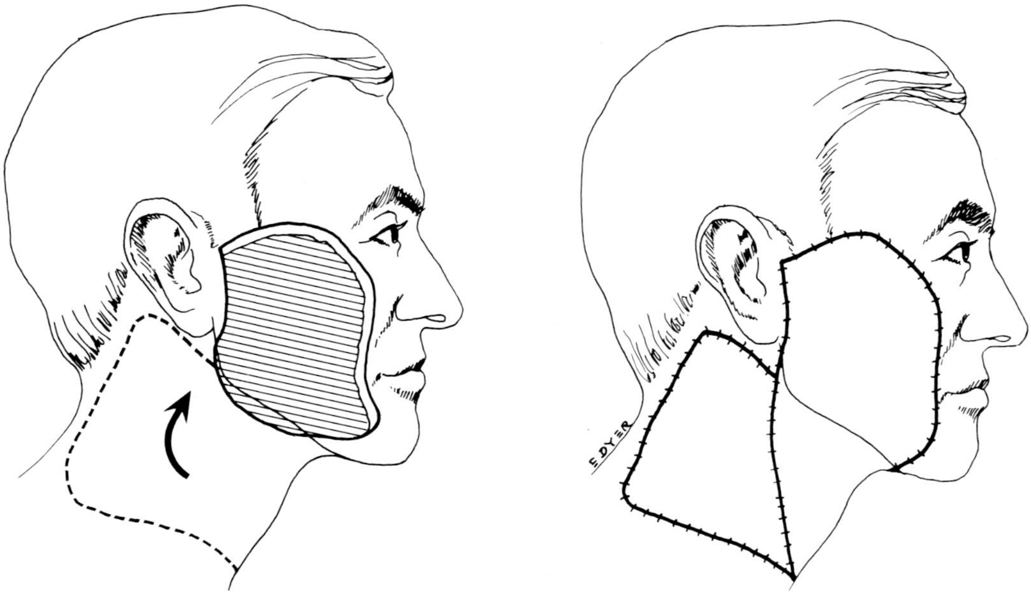

Figure 3.27 Transposition flap with STG to defect of neck.

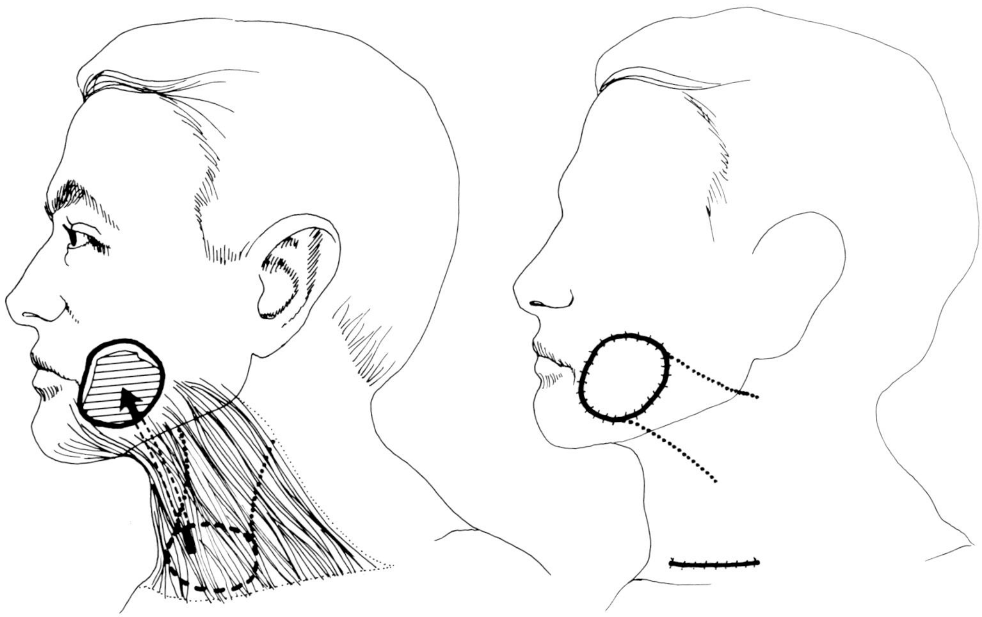

Figure 3.28 This flap has the advantage of leaving a small defect in donor area and providing good color match to cheek skin. Its tenuous blood supply must be guarded with the most careful surgical technique.[11]

MYOCUTANEOUS BASED ON PLATYSMA MUSCLE

See Figure 3.28.

Other more distal sources of cover are tubed pedicle flaps carried on a wrist carrier. This is a last resort, but sometimes becomes necessary, especially if the local donor areas are not available. The disadvantages are the multiple stages involved in the surgery. The tissue, when in place, is often bulky and has a poor color match.

Microsurgery has all but made the tubed flap method obsolete in many cases and will be discussed in Chapter 16. In modern reconstructive surgery, the tubed pedicle flap is relegated to history.

The use of skin grafts for defects with satisfactory beds on the cheek and forehead often provide a simple and satisfactory result. If the skin is taken from the blush area, i.e. above the clavicles, it will usually have a more satisfactory color match. Technically, this may be done by "ballooning out" the supraclavicular area with saline injections and using a drum dermatome to harvest the graft. Of course, the thicker the graft, the less secondary contracture of the graft and the better cosmetic result. In some cases, a thinner skin graft may be utilized to cover an area so that time is allowed to settle or make the defect smaller and possibly more satisfactory for flap reconstruction at a later date.

One should not forget the possibility of using a combination of the techniques outlined above in affecting a closure of more complicated defects.

Synthetic prostheses should be considered for patients who, for one reason or another, are not candidates for reconstruction. The advantages, along with the disadvantages, should be explained. Also, one should be aware of the individual facilities in one's own medical community so that the referring surgeon has a clear understanding of what the patient can expect from such a referral.

SUMMARY

This chapter is intended to offer a surgeon, who finds himself dealing with lesions of the forehead and cheek, a better familiarity with the basic philosophies of treating such lesions, along with an outline of some of the basic methods available to provide tissue for reconstruction. This is the point when the artistic ability of the individual plastic surgeon is called into action in an attempt to leave the patient with the best result possible today.

References

1. Boreges, A. F.: *Elective Incisions and Scar Revisions*, p. 1, Little Brown, Boston, 1973.
2. Converse, J. M.: *Reconstructive Plastic Surgery*, p. 26, W. B. Saunders, Philadelphia, 1964.
3. Mitz, V., and Peyronie, M.: The superficial musculo-aponeurotic system (SMAS) in the parotid cheek area. *Plast. Reconstr. Surg., 58*:80, 1976.
4. Robbins, T. H.: The "crown" excision of facial skin lesions. *Plast. Reconstr. Surg., 57*:251, 1976.
5. Emmet, A. J.: Adjacent triangular flaps with subcutaneous pedicles. *Plast. Reconstr. Surg., 59*:45, 1977.
6. McGregor, I. A.: *Fundamental Techniques in Plastic Surgery*, Ed. 6, Churchill Livingston, New York, 1975.
7. Worthen, E. F.: Repair of forehead defects by rotation of local flaps. *Plast. Reconstr. Surg., 57*:204, 1976.
8. Jeris, W., Salyer, K., Busquets, M., and Atkins, R.: Further application of Lemberg and Dufourmental flaps. *Plast. Reconstr. Surg., 54*:335, 1974.
9. Crow, M. L., and Crow, J. F.: Resurfacing large cheek defects with rotation flaps from the neck. *Plast. Reconstr. Surg., 58*:196, 1976.
10. Bakamjian, V. Y.: The delto-pectoral flap, in *Skin Flaps*, edited by W. C. Grabb and M. B. Myers, Ch. 16, Little Brown, Boston, 1975.
11. Wang, M. K. H.: The shoulder flap, in *Skin Flaps*, edited by W. C. Grabb and M. B. Myers, Ch. 17, Little Brown, Boston, 1975.
12. Barron, J. N.: Subcutaneous pedicle flaps, in *Skin Flaps*, edited by W. C. Grabb and M. B. Myers, Ch. 18, Little Brown, Boston, 1975.

13. Dean, R. K., Kelleher, J. C., Sullivan, J. G., and Baibak, G. J.: Bilobed flaps, in *Skin Flaps*, edited by W. C. Grabb and M. B. Myers, Ch. 20, Little Brown, Boston, 1975.
14. Littlewood, M.: Compound flaps, in *Skin Flaps*, edited by W. C. Grabb and M. B. Myers, Ch. 21, Little Brown, Boston, 1975.
15. McCurdy, J. A.: The secondary deformity of forehead flaps: improved appearance with meshed skin grafts. *Br. J. Plast. Surg., 30:*177, 1977.
16. Gillies, S. H., and Millard, D. R.: *The Principles and Art of Plastic Surgery*, Little Brown, Boston, 1957.

CHAPTER 4

Eyelid Reconstruction

Timothy A. Miller, M.D., F.A.C.S.

ANATOMY

The skin of the eyelid is thin and loosely connected to the pretarsal fibers of the orbicularis oculi muscle. These loose attachments allow for significant accumulation of periorbital edema following facial injury, surgery or infection. They also allow for significant movement of adjacent tissue to repair skin defects by primary approximation. The eyelids close by contraction of the orbicularis oculi muscle, which is innervated by the facial (VII) nerve. The cornea is covered and protected by the upper lid. The periodic closing of the upper lid, as in reflex blinking, serves to moisten the keratinized epithelium of the cornea and prevent desiccation. The cornea can thus be exposed as a result of an injury that prevents the full excursion of the upper eyelid or damages the nerve supply to the orbicularis muscle, such as facial nerve palsy.

Functionally, therefore, the upper eyelid is more important than the lower. The upper lid tarsal plate, which provides structured support, is considerably larger and thicker. This condensation of fibrous connective tissue measures approximately 10 mm in height and 20 mm in width. It is the site of the primary insertion of the levator muscle aponeurosis. This flexible support provides convex integrity to the eyelid as it makes its excursion from the closed to the open position. Eyelid opening is innervated by the oculomotor (IV) cranial nerve. When it is incomplete, ptosis results, usually due to an abnormality of the levator muscle of the upper lid. The lower eyelid, in contrast to the upper lid, is completely stationary.

The tarsal plates are connected to the orbital septum which in turn attaches to the periosteum of the orbital rim and canthal ligaments medially and laterally. These structures form the anterior support for the contents of the bony orbit: the globe, extraocular muscles and nerves, periorbital fat, retinal artery and optic nerve. The orbit is a cone-shaped cavity formed by the sphenoid bone posteriorly, and the frontal and ethmoid bones superiorly. The floor, formed by the zygomatic and palatine bones, is particularly thin in the area medial to the narrow canal containing the infraorbital nerve. It is in this medial area that the floor can be ruptured by an anterior blow that herniates orbital contents into the maxillary antrum: the orbital "blow-out" fracture.

This publication was supported by VA Surgical Research Funds.

The globe is suspended within the cone-shaped bony orbit by a series of ligamentous structures resembling a hammock. At either end, the fusion of this connective tissue forms the medial and lateral canthal ligaments inserting on the nasal process of the maxilla and tubercle of the frontal process of the zygoma. It is the integrity of these supporting structures that holds the individual globes in position and then stability allows binocular vision.

Superior to the lateral canthus and beneath the lateral orbital rim, the lacrimal gland provides tears to moisten the cornea. These tears are collected by the lacrimal apparatus, which is anatomically associated closely with the medial canthus. Tears travel by capillary action along the eyelid rim and drain into puncta in the medial margin of each eyelid. The lower punctum collects approximately 90% of the total tear secretion. Each puncta drains into a superior and inferior canaliculus, both of which communicate with the lacrimal sac, an epithelium-lined pouch partially protected within the lacrimal bone. Tear drainage is emptied from the sac into the nose in the region of the inferior turbinate bone. This process is assisted by a negative pressure in the lacrimal sac which results from the contraction of the orbicularis oculi muscle.

MALIGNANT TUMORS OF THE EYELID

The most common malignant tumor of the eyelid is the basal cell carcinoma. In most large series of patients this tumor accounts for 90% of all malignant neoplasms. Squamous cell epitheliomas and malignant melanoma are comparatively rare.

Basal cell carcinoma is characteristically a slow growing, well defined, modular tumor which invades surrounding tissue by direct extension. In its early course, the tumor involves only the skin. Excision is relatively easy, and the defect can usually be closed by primary approximation. The clinical appearance and gross characteristics of the tumor are important. The classical nodular form presents as a pearly, almost translucent mass that is usually well demarcated from the surrounding normal tissue. Other forms of basal cell epitheliomas have less distinct borders. In some ulcerating tumors, and particularly those of the morpheic or sclerosing variety, ill defined borders make it difficult to determine the tumor margin and extent of peripheral invasion. It is important to emphasize that such carcinomas require a wider margin of resection to ensure the clearance of subepithelial tumor extensions. Although arbitrary limits cannot always be achieved, clear borders of 2 to 3 mm are usually appropriate. In the eyelid, acceptable borders of resection obviously depend on the anatomic location. Regardless of the defect created, however, the surgeon must be certain that the tumor has been completely removed. Examination by a pathologist, using frozen sections at the time of excision to confirm the absence of tumor in the margin, is extremely important. If possible, preoperative examination of the patient by the pathologist will enhance the accuracy of interpretation of these results.

Basal cell carcinoma has a greater tendency to involve the lower eyelid. Although the reason for this consistent finding is not entirely clear, it is possible that such factors as the relatively greater sunlight exposure, tear drainage and chronic environment irritants are important etiological aspects. Because these tumors generally develop slowly, the patient is often unconcerned. However, even though metastasis is extraordinarily rare in basal cell epitheliomas, these tumors pose grave danger to the eye and even to the patients survival. Once the tumor reaches the conjunctiva, extension can be quite rapid. This situation must be recognized promptly and managed aggressively despite the natural timidity often shared by both physician and patient when the area around the eye is involved. The fact that this type of malignant tumor does not usually metastasize should be regarded as an additional reason for even more aggressive management to achieve its complete eradication. Lesions around the bulbar conjunctiva and canalicular apparatus, in particular, require careful evaluation inasmuch as tumor involvement may be extensive and frequently requires radical surgical therapy and, at times, orbital exenteration. Preoperative facial and sinus roentgenograms and tomography, as well as orbital venography, may help to determine the extent of tumor involvement in such cases.

Squamous cell carcinoma, a far more rapidly growing tumor, usually presents as an ulcerating raised nodule surrounded by inflammation. It does not usually have the pearly appearance that characterizes basal cell lesions. While metastases from these lesions are unlikely to occur, when present they require lymph node dissection. The parotid area should always be carefully examined. Lesions in the upper eyelid spread to this area and the cervical lymph node chain. Lower eyelid lesions drain to the submandibular and cervical nodes.

Meibomian gland adenocarcinomas are also quite rare and in their early manifestations can resemble a chalazion. A high index of suspicion should prevail, and a wide resection performed. Tumors of this type may spread to regional nodes in the pattern described above.

Malignant melanomas rarely occur in the eyelid or conjunctival region. On the other hand, pigmented nevi are more commonly seen and frequently require excisional biopsy. If these lesions prove to be malignant, surgical therapy is determined by the depth of invasion and presence of regional nodes. These patients should be carefully worked up for distant organ metastases.

GENERAL CONSIDERATIONS

Trauma

When examining any injury to the orbital area, it is essential to thoroughly appraise the patient and to determine whether any other injuries have occurred (abdominal, extremity, etc.). The patients past history, with particular reference to previous eye injury, the need for refractive correction, the use of contact lens, and the possibility of glaucoma, diabetes and other conditions that may affect the eye, should be evaluated. Vision should be examined utilizing funduscopy and visual acuity tests. Ophthalmalogical consultation should be obtained for all patients who have sustained a serious injury. It is important that these evaluations be made prior to administering any medications.

Anesthesia

The repair of acute traumatic defects as well as the majority of elective operative procedures can usually be performed under local anesthesia. Because of the natural anxiety associated with surgery in the region of the eye, parenteral sedation is advised. Lidocaine with epinephrine is preferred as the local anesthetic. The epinephrine provides a relatively bloodless field which allows more precise anatomical identification and repair. Regional block anesthesia can also be used effectively. The lower eyelid is innervated by the infraorbital and zygomaticofacial nerves which can be blocked by injecting directly into the region of respective foramina. The infraorbital foramen can usually be palpated and is located approximately 1.5 cm below the lower lid margin just medial to the pupil. The zygomaticofacial nerve can be anesthetized at a point approximately 1 cm directly below the lateral canthus. The entire upper lid can be blocked by injecting the roof of the orbit to anesthetize the frontal nerve. In most situations, however, local infiltration of the anesthetic directly into the operative site is preferred.

For major eyelid reconstruction, general endotracheal anesthesia is indicated. The injection of local anesthesia containing epinephrine facilitates the procedure.

Dressings and Medications

For most reconstructive procedures, occlusive eye dressings are not indicated. Such dressings are uncomfortable and keep the patient from seeing which can be a source of considerable anxiety. However, in specific circumstances, when eye rest or complete lid immobilization is required, occlusion with mild compression is beneficial. In these situations a double ophthalmic pad secured with adhesive tape extending from the forehead to the lateral cheek is satisfactory. Symptoms of eye irritation require the removal of the dressings and careful eye examination. Postoperative corneal abrasions are not uncommon.

Eye medications should be used sparingly and carefully. Prophylactic antibiotic ointments are rarely if ever indicated. Many of these ointments contain antibiotic mixtures as well as a steroid. Topical antibiotics, particularly neomycin, can be quite irritative, and whether or not they actually prevent infection is debatable. Steroid preparations raise intraocular pressure and should be avoided in patients with glaucoma. Moreover, in the presence of any viral infection they are definitely contraindicated.

The use of bland nonmedicated ophthalmic ointments is usually the best means of providing lubrication and preventing corneal disiccation. When an occlusive dressing is applied, bland petroleum-based ointments are preferred over those containing antibiotics.

When dressings are not used and the cornea needs to be lubricated, methyl cellulose drops are effective; they can be applied every hour and, unlike ointments, do not impair vision.

Radiation Therapy

Probably due to the general conservatism in dealing with lesions in the eyelid region and fear of surgery, radiation therapy is frequently recommended for the management of sensitive malignant tumors. It is mistakenly believed that surgery results in inordinate mutilation and scarring. On the other hand, radiation therapy is often believed to be free of the serious complications and risks. Both assumptions are false. It is unreasonable to assume that enough radiation can be given to destroy a tumor without significant damage to adjacent skin and other structures.

Regardless of which modality of therapy is chosen, similar rates of cure (exceeding 90%) are achieved in the management of basal cell carcinoma. In order to accurately compare the two methods, not only the advantages and disadvantages of each method during the period of therapy must be considered, but also the appearance and quality of the tissue after therapy has been completed. Before radiation therapy can be instituted, a biopsy must first be performed to identify the pathology. Radiation therapy is necessarily protracted over several weeks. In contrast, surgical excision and reconstruction can usually be performed as a one-stage procedure. In addition, surgery provides the substantial advantage of microscopic examination of the tumor margins so that clearance can be assured.

In the management of large tumors by irradiation, substantial residual scar deformity develops. In some instances, radiation can also damage other orbital structures resulting in complications such as irritative conjunctivitis, late appearance of cataracts, dry eyes, stenosis of the canalicular apparatus and epithelialization of the conjunctiva. However, perhaps the most significant disadvantage is that irradiated tissue is usually indurated and it is difficult to follow the patient for recurrent tumor. Should this occur surgical therapy is difficult at best. Tumor margins are ill defined and surgical reconstruction is compromised by the radiation fibrosis and small vessel occlusion in the area.

In the author's opinion, surgery is a more rapid and efficient method of dealing with malignant tumors of the eyelid. It not only assures similar cure rates when compared to radiation therapy, but also has the distinct advantages of microscopic confirmation of tumor margins as well as immediate reconstruction.

METHODS OF RECONSTRUCTION

The eyelid is composed of varying types of tissue. Reconstruction must consider these separate elements: skin (cover), tarsal plate (support) and conjunctiva (mucosal lining). If these anatomical elements cannot be approximated primarily after trauma or surgical resection of a tumor, they must be brought into the eyelid defect as a free graft, adjacent pedicle or interpolated flap (e.g., the Abbé principle).

In reconstructing any surgically created or traumatic defect, a limited number of options exist: (1) directly approximating the wound edges; (2) allowing the process of wound healing to close the defect, principally by wound contraction, without surgical intervention; (3) applying a split thickness graft; (4) applying a full thickness graft; (5) rotating a local adjacent pedicle flap into the defect; (6) introducing a more distant pedicle flap by interposition. Each of these methods has certain advantages and disadvantages and are frequently used in combination in reconstructing large eyelid tissue defects.

Primary Closure by Approximation

The vast majority of lacerations can be closed by approximating the wound in separate layers. Running fine absorbable sutures are effective when used to align the conjunctiva. The sutures are placed so that the knot is tied within the eyelid itself, thus preventing corneal irritation. A few delicately placed interrupted fine sutures can then approximate the tarsal plate. In some instances, approximation of the tarsal plate alone accurately opposed the conjunctival edges and precludes separate suturing of this layer. Interrupted fine silk is usually preferred as a means of skin closure. Silk suture ties easily and allows very precise adjustments in tension, compared to nylon which is considerably stiffer and more difficult to knot. Despite the theoretical criticism of greater inflammatory reaction to silk, removal of these sutures on the 3rd to 5th postoperative day precludes this response.

When tumors involve the margin of the eyelid, a full-thickness wedge of all layers of the eyelid must be removed. This defect usually is "V" shaped. If the defect is large, its closure tends to shorten the vertical height of the eyelid. Whenever possible, the excision should be shaped in the form of a shield so that closure can preserve as much of the vertical dimension of the eyelid as possible (Fig. 4.1). Once the excision has been performed the defect is closed in layers as described.

It is generally agreed that a defect of approximately one-quarter of the eyelid width can be excised and primarily closed without creating inappropriate tension. This obviously varies among individuals, particularly with age. The average width of the lower eyelid is approximately 3.0 cm. Therefore, malignant lesions measuring 3–4 mm can be excised with a 2-mm border on each side and usually primarily closed without difficulty. When necessary, additional mobility can be achieved by surgically dividing the lateral canthal ligament (Fig. 4.2). Depending on the inherent laxity of the tissue some defects greater than one-fourth of the eyelid width can be closed in this manner. Larger defects require the *addition* of tissue either by means of a graft or, more frequently, the introduction of a pedicle flap.

Full-Thickness Grafts

In general, lesions of the eyelid that do *not* involve the free margin should be excised to the depth of the orbicularis oculi muscle. If primary closure cannot be achieved by mobilizing the comparatively lax eyelid skin, a full thickness graft from the redundant skin of the upper eyelid or the retroauricular area is usually the reconstructive method of choice. Split thickness

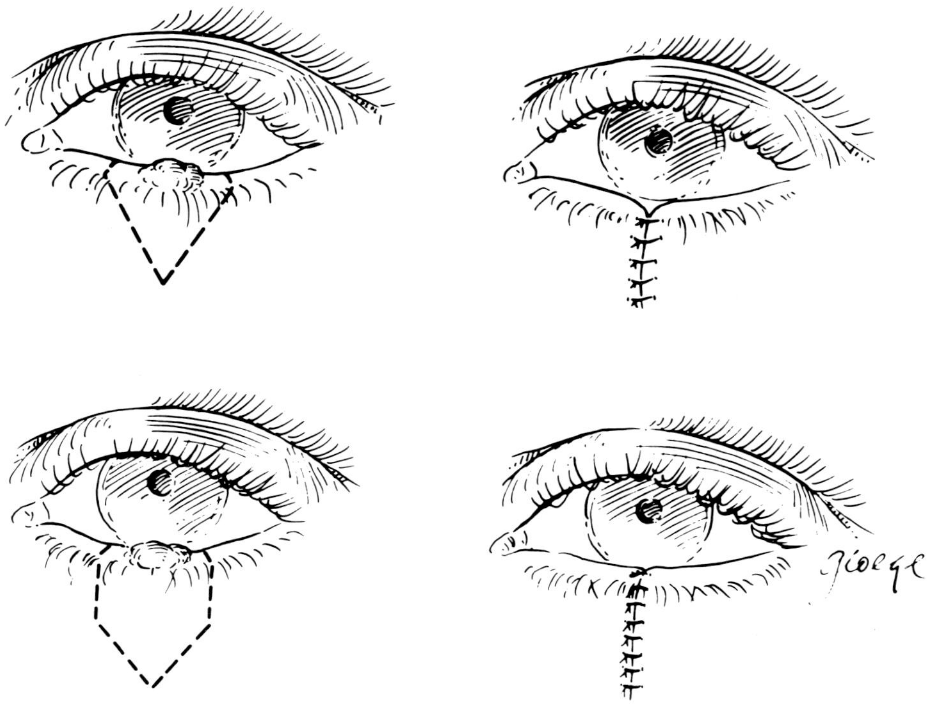

Figure 4.1 In most individuals, one-quarter of the total width of the eyelid can be excised and primarily closed. Closure of shield-shaped defects tends to preserve verticle height as opposed to "V" type excisions.

grafts, although easily obtained, allow marked contraction of the wound and because of the eventual anatomic distortion and poor color match are generally unsuited to use around the eyelid. Full thickness grafts, on the other hand, suppress wound contraction and blend quite well with the texture and color of eyelid skin. Whenever possible, therefore, this comparatively simple method of reconstructing skin defects around the eyelids should be employed.

Successful vascularization of the graft is assured by careful attention to intraoperative hemostasis, thinning of the graft and application of a bolster, tie-over dressing. This type of dressing is sometimes misunderstood; the assumption is often made that its purpose is to apply pressure on the wound surface and prevent bleeding. Hemostasis is the responsibility of the surgeon, not the dressing. The principal function of the tie-over dressing is to contour the graft to the wound surface and provide a means of immobilization. It should be left in place for 5 days, at which time all sutures can be removed. Full thickness grafts obtained from areas above the clavicle match the texture and color of eyelid skin extremely well.

Pedicle Flap Reconstruction

Almost all tumors of the eyelid and surrounding orbital skin can be excised and either primarily closed or grafted without performing more major reconstructive procedures. When over one-quarter of the width of the eyelid requires resection, however, a pedicle flap should

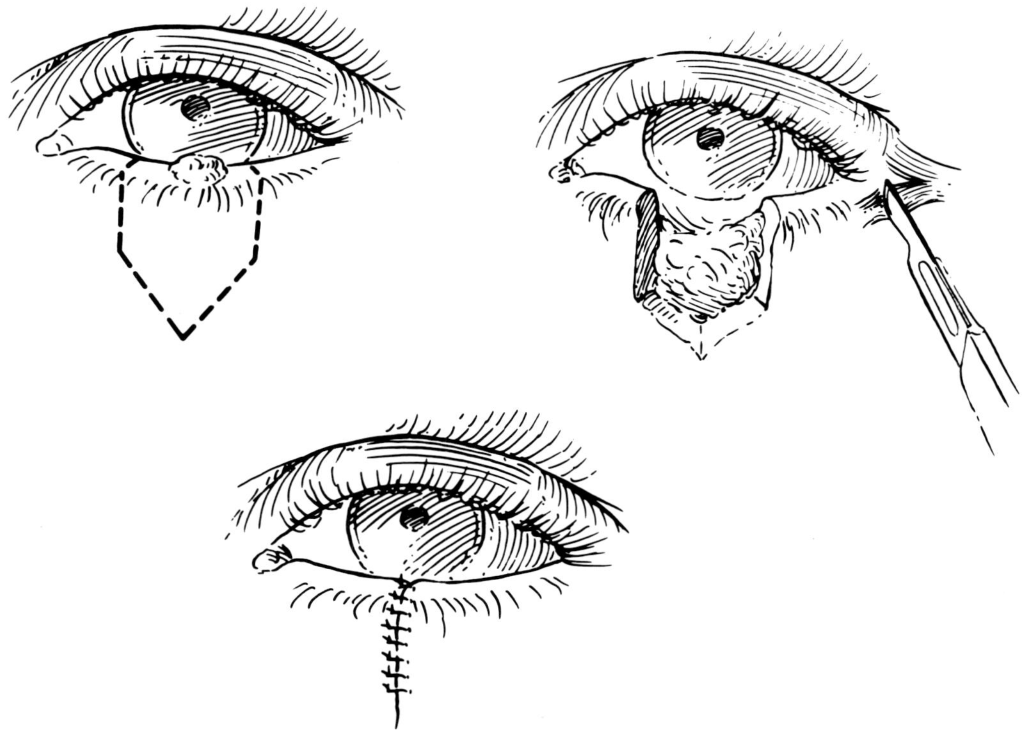

Figure 4.2 When the excision of a lesion exceeds one-quarter of the width of the eyelid, or when there is considerable tension on wound approximation, the division of the inferior portion of the lateral canthal ligament can facilitate closure.

be used. Techniques for the reconstruction of large eyelid defects are sufficiently challenging and difficult that different concepts and divergent philosophies have developed concerning the best way to reconstruct a given eyelid defect. In the author's opinion, the clearest scheme and most reasonable approach to these complex reconstructive problems has been developed by Mustarde. In this regard, several basic principles apply:

1. The upper eyelid (not the lower) is responsible for corneal protection, lubrication and closure. It has definite anatomical and functional differences which distinguish it from the relatively immobile lower lid. Because of this greater functional importance, its structure should never be sacrificed or jeopardized when reconstructing the lower eyelid defects. Conversely, however, the lower eyelid can and should be used as donor tissue to reconstruct larger composite defects in the upper lid.
2. Because of the obvious anatomical differences of the two eyelids, the lower is much more easily reconstructed. There are several reasons for this difference. The presence of the canalicular apparatus medially requires that additional tissue be brought in by rotation of more lateral tissue. However, owing to the presence of the hair-bearing brow and lacrimal gland, lateral rotation is impossible in the upper eyelid. When reconstructing the lower eyelid, however, a flap can be developed from the cheek and moved medially (Fig. 4.7). This allows the lower lid to be used as a donor for upper eyelid reconstruction by the Abbé (180° interpolation) principle (Fig. 4.8).
3. Because of the inherent elasticity of the upper eyelid, only three-quarters of the total width of the lid needs to be reconstructed.

RECONSTRUCTION OF THE LOWER EYELID

Upper Eyelid Pedicle

Occasionally malignant tumors, particularly basal cell carcinoma, extend horizontally along the lower eyelid margin. Resection may require removal of over half of the lid width but little of the vertical height (Fig. 4.3). In this situation, the conjunctiva of the remaining lower lid can be mobilized inferiorly to the fornix and advanced superiorly. Reconstruction is accomplished by the creation of a laterally based flap of upper lid skin. This procedure is possible when there is some natural redundancy of skin overlying the upper eyelid (as is common in older patients who tend to develop such tumors). This does not constitute a violation of the previously outlined principle of preserving the upper eyelid, in that the basic structural integrity of the upper eyelid has not been altered.

In larger horizontal defects, particularly when they are medial, a bipedicle flap of upper eyelid skin can be employed (Fig. 4.4). To avoid the natural tendency of the flap to curl, considerable surgical thinning of the flap can be performed during the procedure. In addition, a small tie-over dressing can be applied to approximate the pedicle to the lining of the advanced conjunctiva.

Cheek Flap Reconstruction

Medial rotation cheek skin can be effectively employed as a means of lower eyelid reconstruction. Lining and structural support can be provided by a free composite graft of nasal mucosa and cartilage, thus leaving the more structurally important upper eyelid undisturbed.

In this method the cheek is mobilized from an incision beginning in the lateral canthal region and extending laterally and superiorly. The superior extension of the flap should progressively ascend due to the fact that as the cheek flap is rotated medially, height is lost. Therefore, the flap will be developed *above* the level of the lower lid margin. The extent of the cheek flap undermining can be variable. Only enough cheek tissue needs to be undermined to facilitate rotation and closure of the undivided defect. Particularly in older patients with lax tissues, defects can be closed without completely mobilizing the entire cheek flap. Frequently a Z-plasty can be used to close the horizontal incision in the temple region. To facilitate medial rotation, a triangle of normal lower eyelid and mid-cheek skin must be excised (Fig. 4.5).

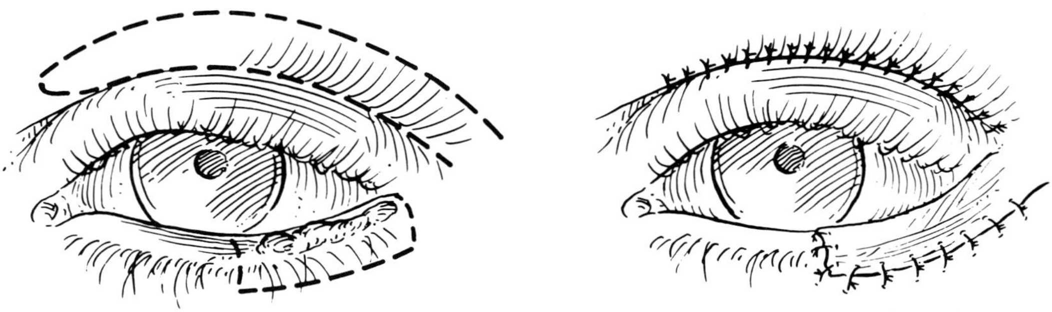

Figure 4.3 A lesion which does not occupy a significant verticle height of the eyelid can be resected (full thickness of the lid) and reconstructed by the interpolation of a flap of redundant upper eyelid tissue. Lining is provided by undermined conjunctiva which is advanced superiorly. The procedure can be performed in one stage.

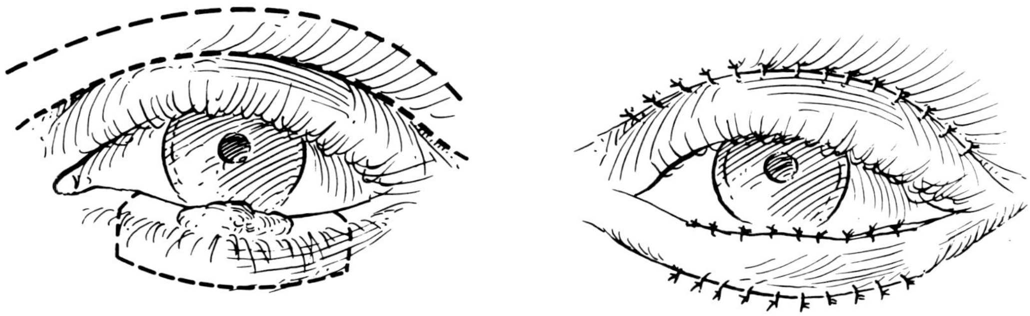

Figure 4.4 Medial and central defects of the eyelid margin can be reconstructed by a bipedicle flap from the upper eyelid. Lining is provided by mobilization of the conjunctiva advanced superiorly. After 3 weeks, the medial and lateral base of the flap can be excised and primarily closed quite similar to an upper lid blepharoplasty.

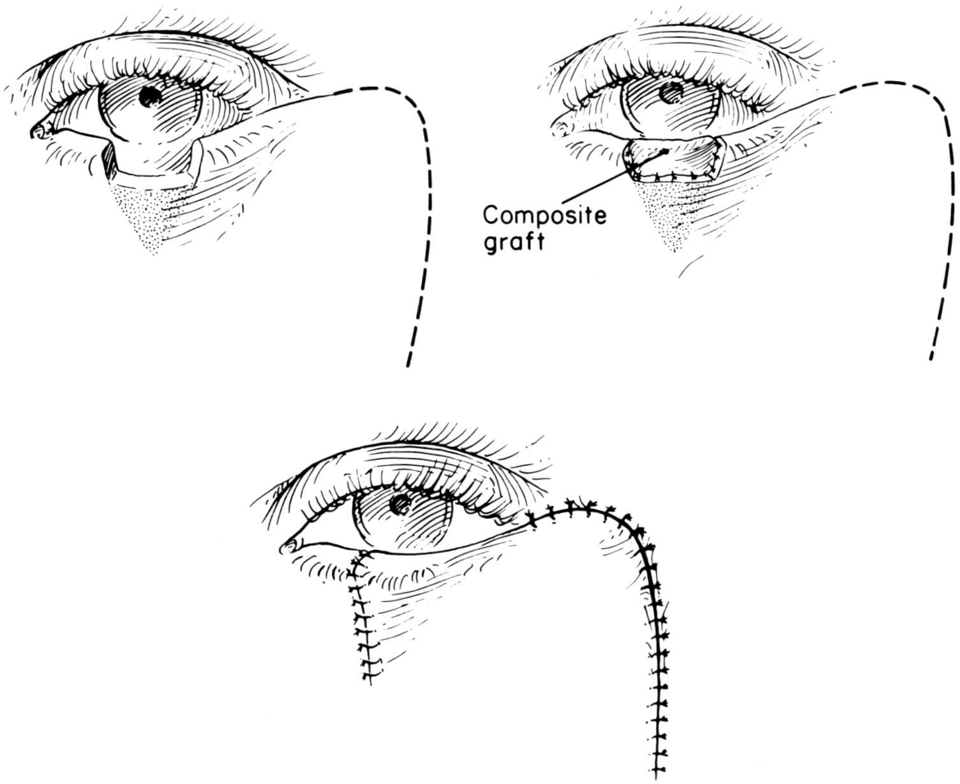

Figure 4.5 The Mustarde cheek flap for reconstruction of the lower eyelid. It is important to design the cheek flap so that the incision is at a higher level than the lateral canthus and margins of the lower eyelid. As the cheek is rotated medially, height is lost. If lining is required a composite graft (usually nasal septum mucosa-cartilage) is employed. To facilitate closure when rotation is completed, a triangle of skin (*stippled area*) should be excised.

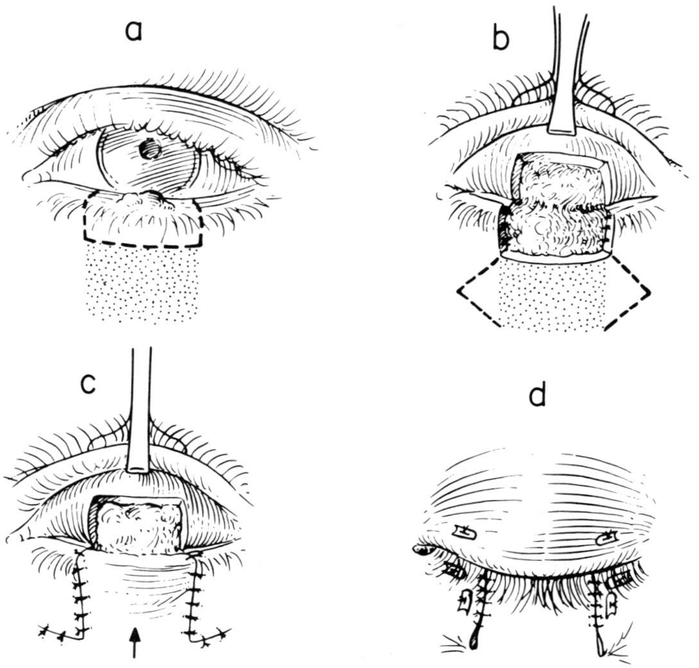

Figure 4.6 The lid sharing procedure: (*a*) Following the full thickness excision of a lower eyelid tumor a composite flap of conjunctiva and tarsal plate is created sutured into the lower eyelid defect. (*b*) Care is taken to preserve the integrity of the distal 2–3 mm of tarsal plate at the upper eyelid margin. Skin coverage for the exposed, partially reconstructed lower eyelid can be provided as shown by superior advancement of lower eyelid skin. (*c, d*) In order to advance this skin, triangles must be excised on either side. Skin coverage can also be provided by a full thickness graft or by methods shown in Figures 4.3 or 4.4.

Lid Sharing Procedures

There is an alternative to the concept that the structural integrity of the upper eyelid must not be jeopardized to reconstruct a lower lid defect. In this procedure, the conjunctival lining and portions of the upper tarsal plate are "borrowed" to restore the lining and structural support of the lower eyelid (Fig. 4.6). If this procedure is employed, it is imperative to preserve the structural integrity of the distal 3 mm of the upper tarsal plate.

The skin covering is reconstructed by applying a graft, an upper eyelid skin pedicle (as previously described), or by advancing a flap of lower eyelid skin superiorly. However, this method of reconstructing large lower eyelid defects has certain disadvantages. The period of immobilization and occlusion of the eye during the sharing place is often approximately 2–3 months. It is obvious, moreover, that a considerable degree of the structural integrity of the upper eyelid must be sacrificed. In addition, in large defects the advancement of lower eyelid and orbital skin often tends to pull the reconstructed eyelid interiorly when the two lids are surgically separated.

Medial Based Pedicle

One of the shortcomings of the lateral cheek flap rotation is that frequently the reconstructed eyelid is lower than normal. An alternate method which can preserve the height of the lower lid utilizes a medial based superiorly rotated cheek flap (Fig. 4.7).

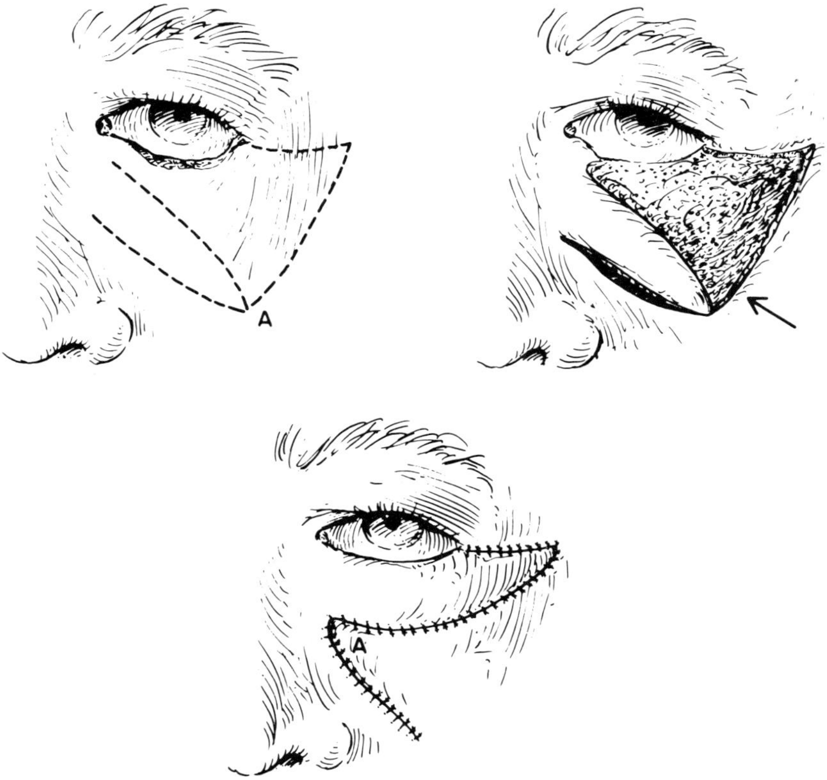

Figure 4.7 In large lower eyelid defects a superiorly and medially based cheek flap can be moved superiorly. When sutured into the lateral canthal region, it has the advantage of preserving the height of the reconstructed lower eyelid (a problem which is not uncommonly seen followed the medial rotation of cheek skin). Cheek skin (*A*) is undermined and mobilized superiorly to close the donor defect.

UPPER EYELID RECONSTRUCTION

The ability to reconstruct the lower eyelid by cheek flap rotation has made the lower eyelid itself an available source of upper eyelid reconstruction when the defect exceeds one-quarter of the width. Because of the inherent elasticity of the tissues, only three-quarters of the total width of the eyelid need be reconstructed. Defects up to one-quarter of the width (7–8 mm+) can be primarily closed. Theoretically, therefore, the extent of reconstruction of any given defect can be reduced by approximately one-quarter of the eyelid width. In reconstructing a defect measuring 15 mm, a flap of only 8 mm need be introduced from the lower eyelid. Because the donor defect involves only one-quarter of the lower eyelid width, it can be closed by primary approximation (Fig. 4.8). The pedicle of composite lower eyelid tissue is nourished by the marginal artery of the eyelid which lies approximately 2–3 mm below and parallel to the rim. A pedicle of approximately 3–4 mm is therefore preserved and the composite flap is rotated 180° into the upper lid defect. Usually the vascular base is designed to originate on the lateral aspect of the lower eyelid pedicle. For medial upper eyelid defects, the pedicle can

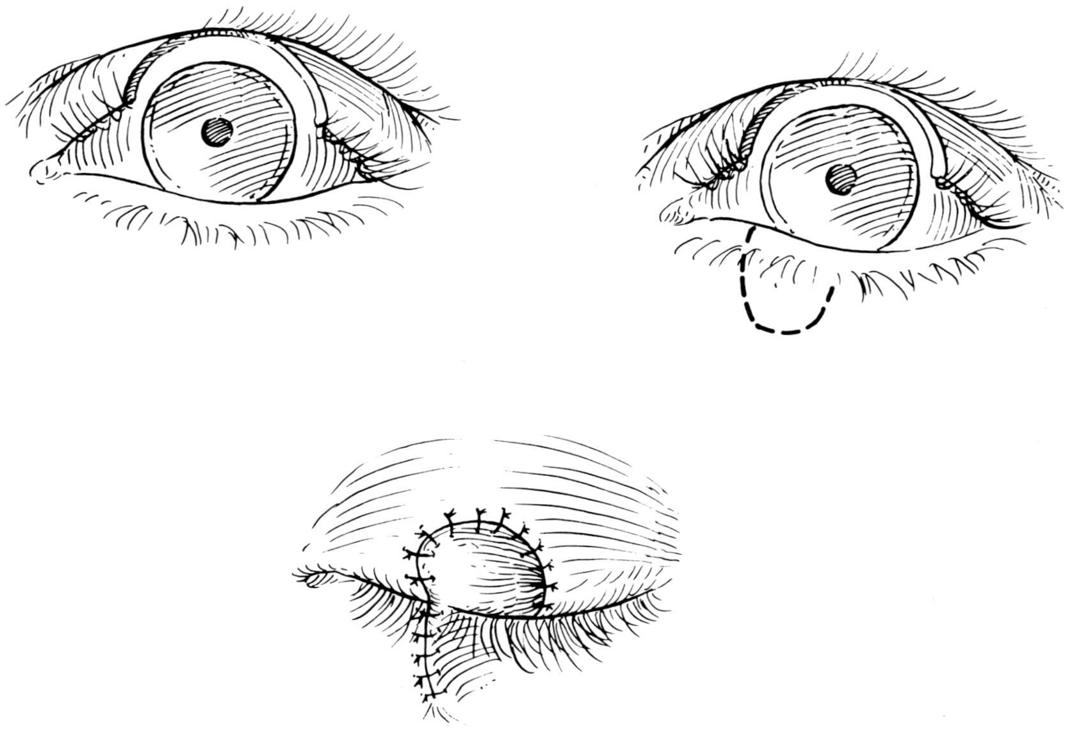

Figure 4.8 In the reconstruction of a defect of the upper eyelid which exceeds one-quarter of the total width, a composite pedicle of lower eyelid can be rotated 180°. Usually a loss of one-quarter of the width of either eyelid can be closed primarily. Therefore, if the upper eyelid defect measures one-half of the total width, only one-quarter of the width of lower eyelid need be used for reconstruction. The lower eyelid can be closed primarily.

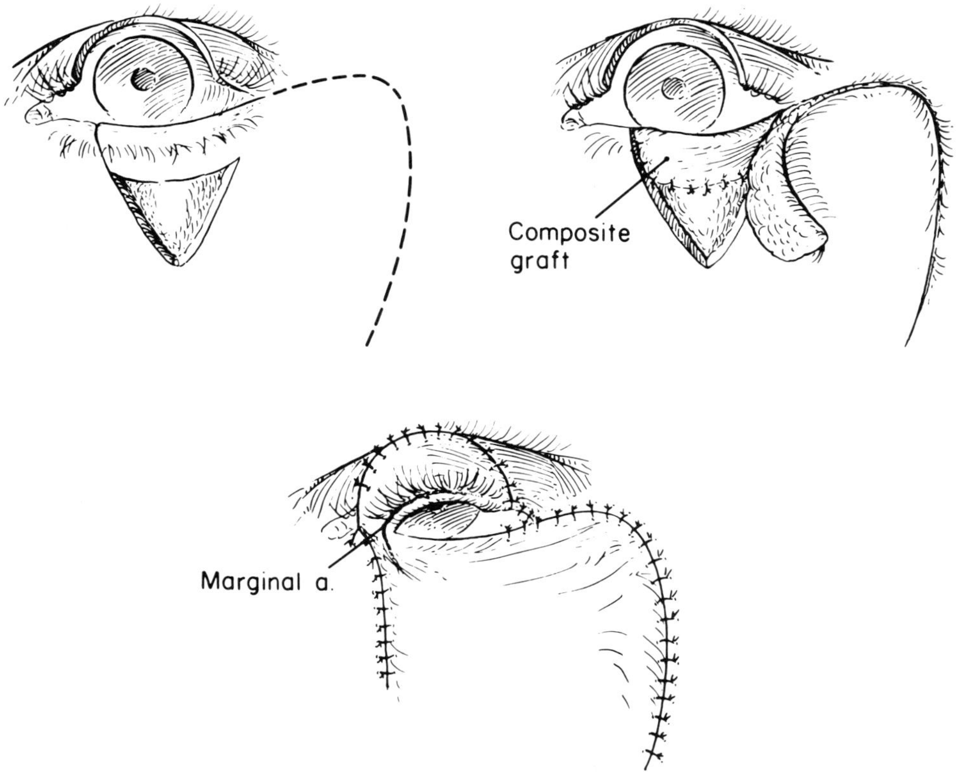

Figure 4.9 In large upper eyelid defects (requiring more than one-quarter of the lower lid for reconstruction) a cheek flap is elevated and rotated medially to reconstruct the lone eyelid defect. Lining and structural support can be effectively provided by a composite graft of nasal mucosa and septal cartilage.

arise from the medial aspect of the lower lid. In either case, the vascular base can be divided and the pedicle inset under local anesthesia, usually without hospitalization, 3 weeks after the initial procedure.

When the surgical defect in the upper eyelid exceeds 15 mm (about one-half eyelid width), the reconstruction becomes more challenging. The upper lid defect is reconstructed by the introduction of a composite pedicle of the lower eyelid tissue and simultaneous creation of a lateral cheek flap used to reconstruct the lower eyelid defect (Fig. 4.9). The lower eyelid pedicle is rotated 180° and its base moved medially with the cheek flap. It is usually necessary to create the lower lid pedicle on the advancing edge of the cheek flap rather than on the stationary medial aspect of the lid. The medially rotated cheek skin reconstructs the skin cover of the lower eyelid. A composite graft of nasal mucosa and cartilage is used to provide structural support and lining.

The obvious advantage of this method is that lining, structural support and skin coverage are all introduced into the upper eyelid simultaneously. During the excision of the tumor, care should be taken to identify the levator muscle and carefully reconstruct its attachments to the portion of tarsal plate within lower pedicle whenever possible. As mentioned previously, equal amounts of lower eyelid do not have to be used in upper eyelid reconstruction. Approximately one-quarter of the upper lid width (±7 mm) can be substrated when calculating reconstruction needs.

Because of the reliability of these reconstructive concepts eyelid lesions can be aggressively excised with the anticipation of very satisfactory esthetic and functional results following immediate reconstruction.

References

1. Converse, J. M., and Smith, B.: The eyelids and their adnexa, in *Reconstructive Plastic Surgery*, edited by J. M. Converse, pp. 858–1039, W. B. Saunders, Philadelphia, 1977.
2. Hughes, W. L.: New method for rebuilding lower lid. *Arch. Ophthalmol.*, *17*:1008, 1937.
3. Kazanjian, V. H.: Deformities of the eyelids, orbital and zygomatic regions, in *The Surgical Treatment of Facial Injuries*, edited by V. H. Kazanjian and J. M. Converse, p. 548, Williams & Wilkins, Baltimore, 1949.
4. Mustarde, J. C.: *Repair and Reconstruction in the Orbital Region. A Practical Guide.* Williams & Wilkins, Baltimore, 1966.
5. Reese, A. B.: *Tumors of the Eye*, Hoeber-Harper, New York, 1953.
6. Whitnall, E.: *Anatomy of the Human Orbit*, Milford, London, 1932.

CHAPTER 5

Nasal Reconstruction

Malcolm A. Lesavoy, M.D., F.A.C.S., Timothy A. Miller, M.D., F.A.C.S., and S. Anthony Wolfe, M.D., F.A.C.S.

Reconstruction of the nose is one of the most challenging aspects in plastic surgery. The nose, sitting high on a pedestal of the human face is the first part of our anatomy to come around the corner and the most obvious projection of our face. It is still unclear in history when nasal reconstruction began, but the importance of the nose was realized in India centuries ago. Loss of the nose from either amputation from punishment for adultery or trauma inflicted in battle must have been a relatively frequent sight. The Suśrutae Áyrvédam was a medical system taught by Dhanwantari centuries ago. It is said that within these Sanskrit writings, orginating only several hundred years after the birth of Christ, the first documentation of nasal reconstruction could be found. With this evidence, it is interesting to conceive that the preeminence of the nose on the human face and nasal reconstruction has been with us for almost two thousand years.

Because of the prominence and preeminence of the human nose, much importance in untold realms of literature has been accumulated on nasal surgery. It is not within the confines of this textbook and this chapter to discuss aesthetic rhinoplasty, and for that reason this chapter will be limited to basic reconstruction. The reconstructive surgeon, however, must have an appreciation for "the normal" and understand that the anatomy of the nose is extremely complex and consists of more than just two nostrils, a midline septum, and paired nasal bones. When planning nasal reconstruction, one must constantly keep in mind the basic mechanical configuration of nasal tissue: lining (nasal mucosa), support (bony skeleton), and cover (nasal skin). If any one of thse anatomic parts is missing, reconstruction of the nose will be unsuccessful. Adequate plans must be made for all three components before nasal reconstruction should be commenced. Nasal deformities can be either congenital or acquired. Congenital deformities can range all the way from small hemangiomas of the nose, gliomas, dermoid cysts and lymphangiomas, to large frontal encephaloceles. These deformities of the nose must be evaluated in their entirety with facial x-rays to rule out underlying bony abnormalities with special concentration toward the ruling out of intracranial communication with the nose. Congenital deformities can range from complete absence of the nose to development of only one half of the nose (Fig. 5.1) and subsequently to variable formations of the cleft lip nose (Fig. 5.2). Infections of the nose such as blastomycosis (Fig. 5.3) are rare but can give rise to a puzzling diagnostic dilemma. Malignant tumors of the nose such as basal cell carcinoma

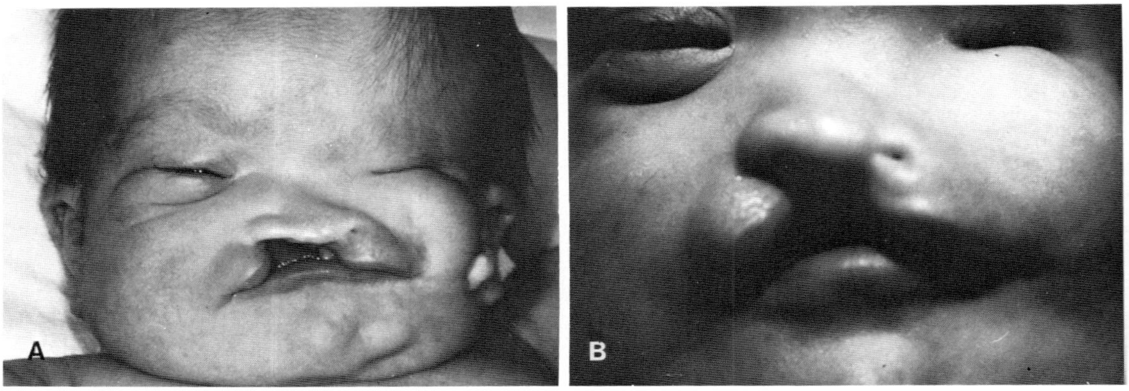

Figure 5.1 (*A* and *B*) Congenital absence of at least one half of the nose.

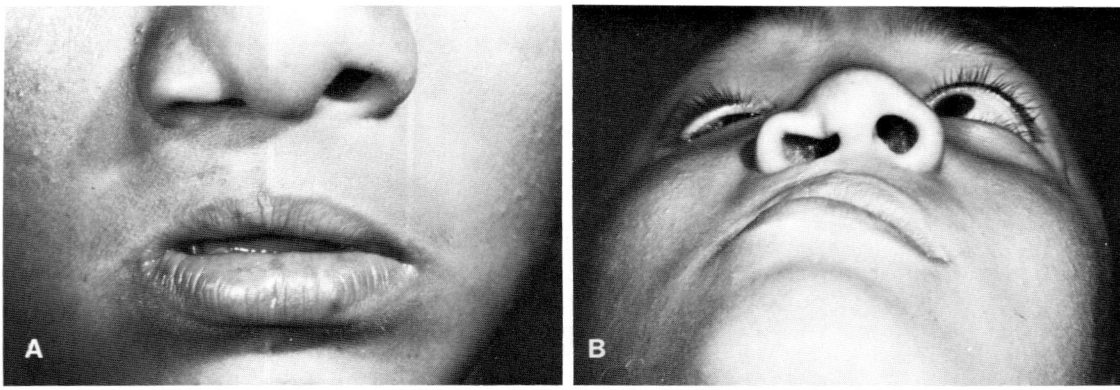

Figure 5.2 (*A* and *B*) Cleft lip nose.

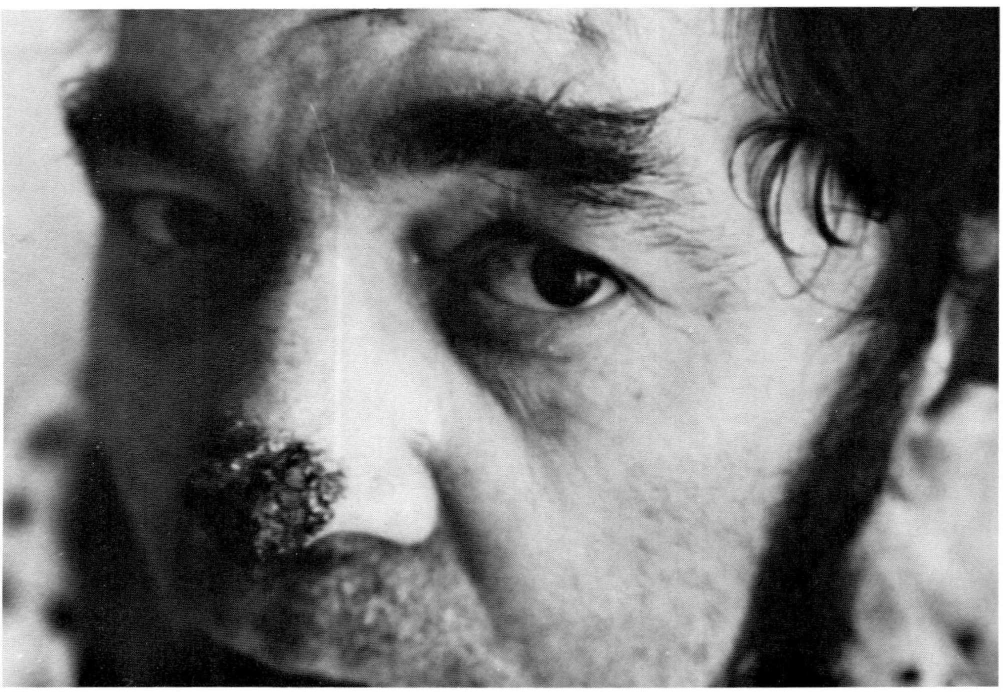

Figure 5.3 Blastomycosis of the nose.

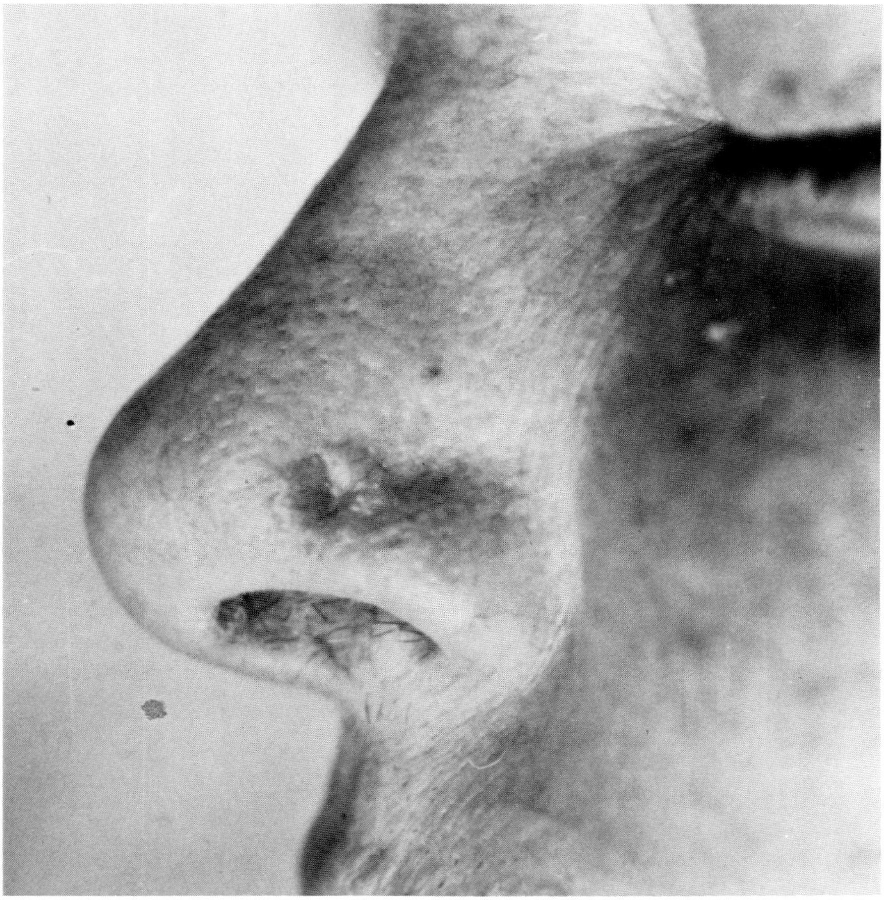

Figure 5.4 Basal cell carcinoma of the nose.

(Fig. 5.4), squamous cell carcinoma (Fig. 5.5), and melanoma (Fig. 5.6) present different reconstructive challenges depending on the size and nature of the tumor. Extirpation of these various tumors will vary from simple elipse excisions to total rhinectomy (Fig. 5.7). Reconstruction is tailored to the particular ensuing defect. In general, defects that are confined to the skin and are not amenable to direct closure, can be nicely reconstructed with the use of full thickness skin grafts (Fig. 5.8). These grafts are generally taken from a postauricular area because of the excellent color match and minimal donor defect. The use of local flaps for coverage is sometimes misused, however, bilobed flaps, nasolabial flaps, island-pedicle flaps, and small banner flaps can be most useful for local coverage.

In some instances, lining and cover are present, but traumatic loss of the bony structure is deficient (Fig. 5.9 *A*). In these cases, replacement of the tissue with either iliac or rib bone grafts can be most helpful (Figs. 5.9, *B* and *C*, and 5.10). It should be pointed out, however, that lining and cover must be adequate to house this bone graft, because frequently with the absence of good solid support, the cover, and specially nasal lining, will contract and shrink and subsequently be deficient (Fig. 5.11).

At times, total resurfacing of the nose is indicated and full thickness skin grafts may fail. Although full thickness skin grafts have the advantages of ease of technique, one-stage procedure, minimal donor defect, and moderate cosmetic appearance, sufficient results may

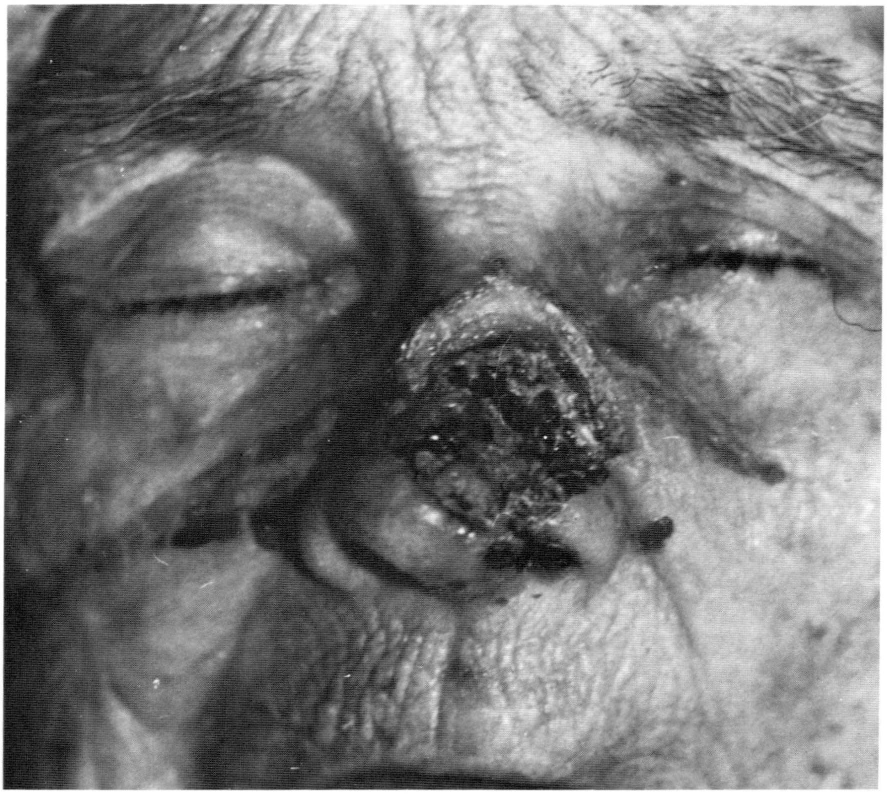

Figure 5.5 Squamous cell carcinoma of the nose.

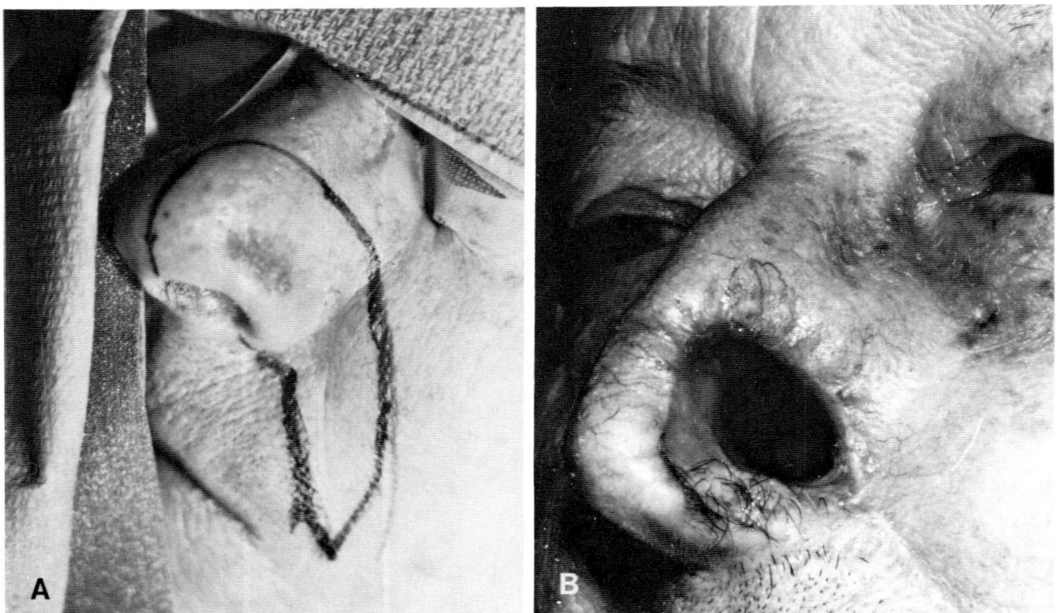

Figure 5.6 (*A*) Melanoma of left ala. (*B*) Wide excision of ala and nasolabial fold and discontinuous radical neck dissection. Prior to heminasal reconstruction with midline forehead flap.

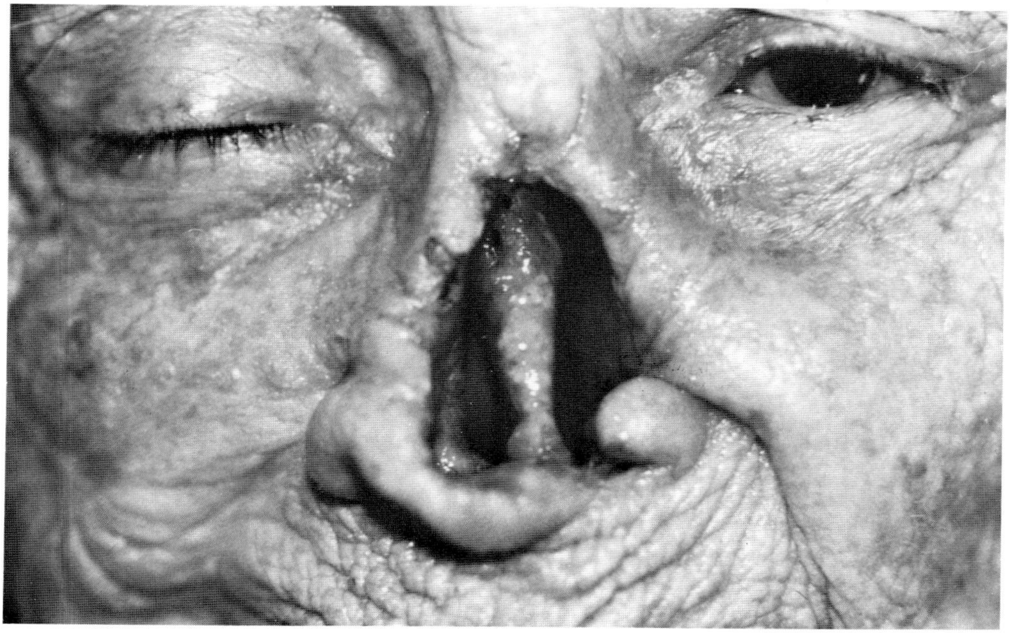

Figure 5.7 Total rhinectomy.

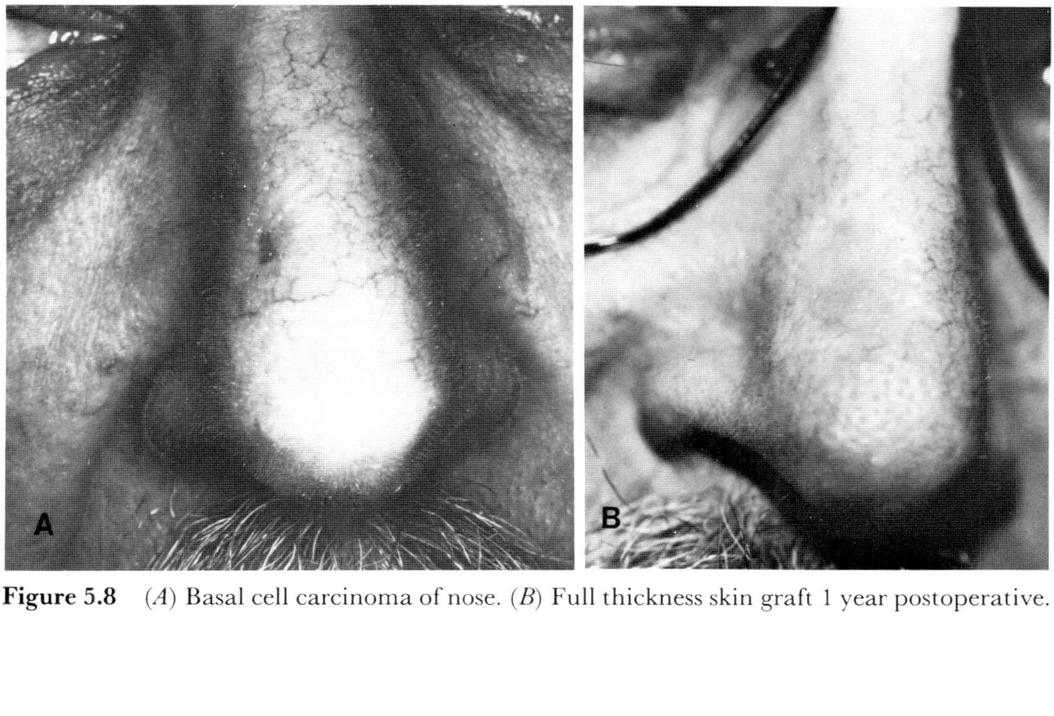

Figure 5.8 (*A*) Basal cell carcinoma of nose. (*B*) Full thickness skin graft 1 year postoperative.

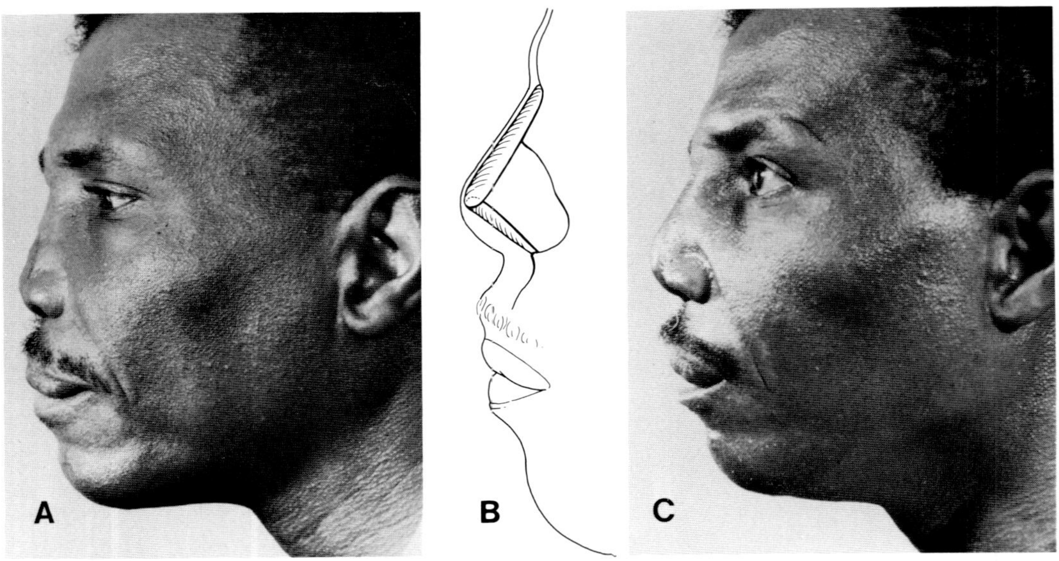

Figure 5.9 (*A*) Deficient bony structure. (*B*) Rib grafts to nose. (*C*) Postoperative.

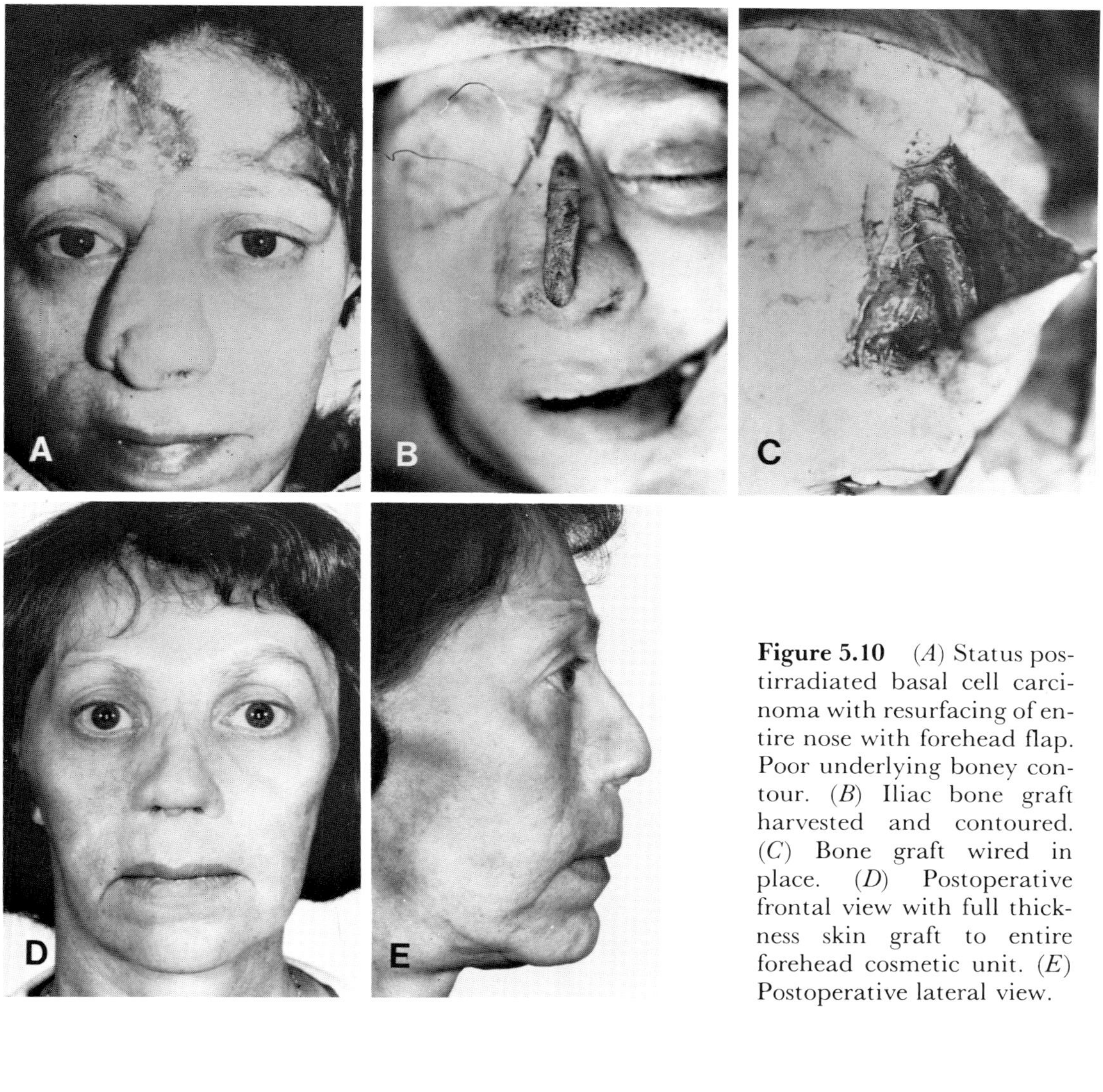

Figure 5.10 (*A*) Status postirradiated basal cell carcinoma with resurfacing of entire nose with forehead flap. Poor underlying boney contour. (*B*) Iliac bone graft harvested and contoured. (*C*) Bone graft wired in place. (*D*) Postoperative frontal view with full thickness skin graft to entire forehead cosmetic unit. (*E*) Postoperative lateral view.

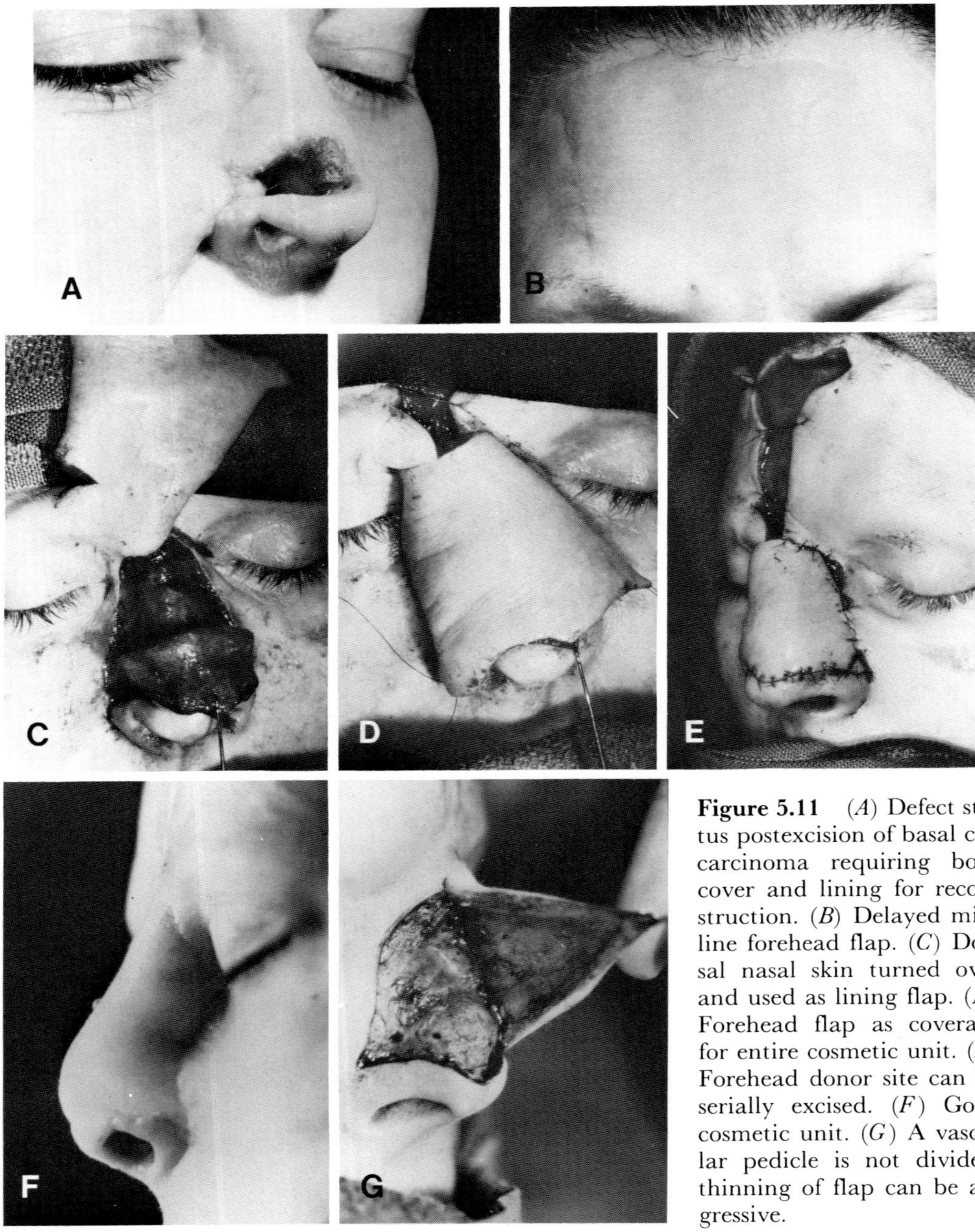

Figure 5.11 (*A*) Defect status postexcision of basal cell carcinoma requiring both cover and lining for reconstruction. (*B*) Delayed midline forehead flap. (*C*) Dorsal nasal skin turned over and used as lining flap. (*D*) Forehead flap as coverage for entire cosmetic unit. (*E*) Forehead donor site can be serially excised. (*F*) Good cosmetic unit. (*G*) A vascular pedicle is not divided, thinning of flap can be aggressive.

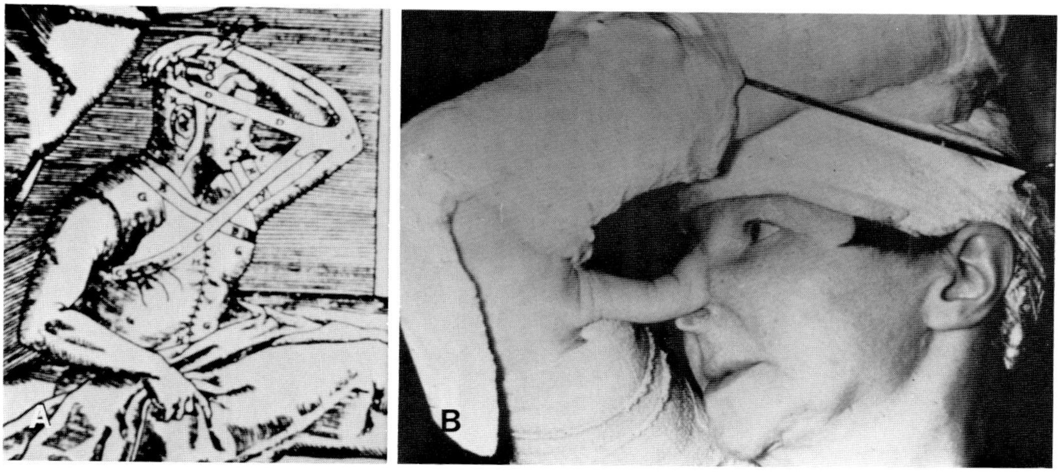

Figure 5.12 (*A*) Drawing by Tagliacozzi. (*B*) How far have we come?

not be forthcoming. Total resurfacing of the nose can then be carried out with median forehead flap coverage.

ARM FLAP NASAL RECONSTRUCTION

When pedicle flap reconstruction of the nose is required it is generally agreed that the forehead provides the best source of tissue. In certain circumstances, however, the forehead may not be suitable or available: (1) if there are malignant or potentially malignant skin lesions on the forehead, (2) if the forehead is extremely narrow or severely scarred and (3) if a patient refuses to accept additional facial scarring. In such situations the surgeon must consider distant pedicle flaps for reconstructing the nose.

The tissue of the upper medial arm is relatively thin and elastic and can be effectively used to completely resurface the nose and reconstruct the alar rims. This method dates back to its original description in 1957 by Gaspar Tagliacozzi (Fig. 5.12). Principally because of the problems of immobilizing the arm flap to the nose and disparity of color match between arm and facial tissue, this technique has not gained wide acceptance. In patients who require total nasal resurfacing and alar rim reconstruction, this flap can be employed as a valuable alternate method when the forehead cannot be used.

Operative Technique

The average adult nose measures approximately 7 ± 1 cm from one lateral alar groove to the other, and approximately 7 ± 1 cm from glabella to base of columnella. This roughly quadrangular shaped area is outlined on the proximal portion of a distally based upper arm flap. The flap measures approximately 8×16 cm and is oriented in a slightly oblique angle toward the medial upper arm; this obliquity prevents the flap from kinking when it is inset into the nose and minimizes tension. To interrupt the muscular perforating branches from the

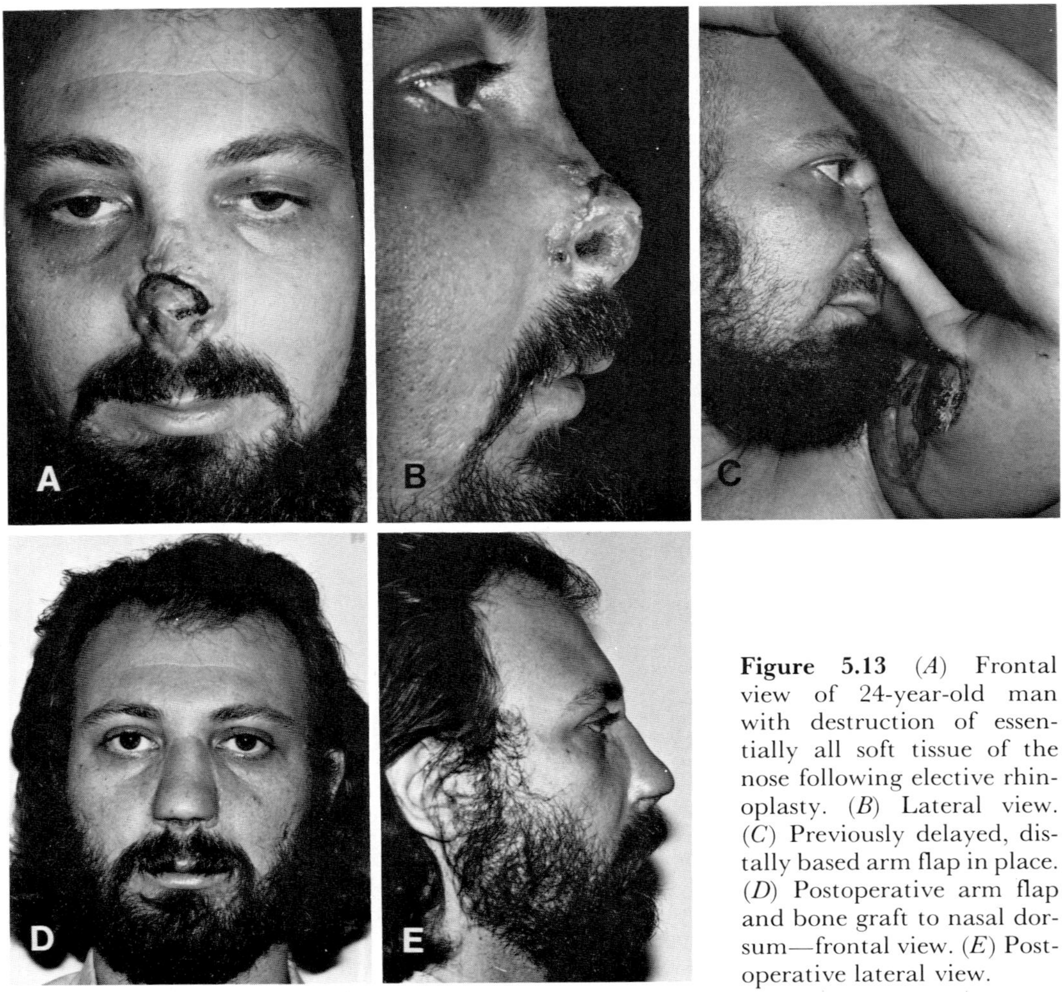

Figure 5.13 (*A*) Frontal view of 24-year-old man with destruction of essentially all soft tissue of the nose following elective rhinoplasty. (*B*) Lateral view. (*C*) Previously delayed, distally based arm flap in place. (*D*) Postoperative arm flap and bone graft to nasal dorsum—frontal view. (*E*) Postoperative lateral view.

underlying biceps muscle, two delay procedures are performed. This first is the creation of a bipedicle flap. Two weeks later, the proximal portion of the flap is incised. Both of these procedures can be done on an out-patient basis using a local anesthetic.

After 2 additional weeks, the flap can be inset into the nasal area. Although the entire procedure can be performed under local anesthesia, the flap is usually elevated and the donor site grafted under general anesthesia. The flap is sutured into the nasal area under local anesthesia *after* the patient has recovered from anesthesia and can assist in the positioning of his arm. Care must be taken to avoid any tension on the flap.

Available paranasal skin is elevated and turned down to provide internal lining for the arm flap. During the inset procedure, all exposed tissue on the undersurface of the arm pedicle and the donor site are covered by split thickness skin grafts taken from the upper thigh or lateral hip area. When the procedure has been completed, no subcutaneous tissue is exposed.

The patient's arm and head can be immobilized by applying circumferential adhesive tape around the occipital area and extensor aspect of the upper arm. While tape is also used over the forearm, it can be loosened each day to allow elbow extension and flexion. During the immobilization period, small doses of muscle relaxants are very helpful. In receptive patients, hypnosis and training in self-hypnosis has been very helpful.

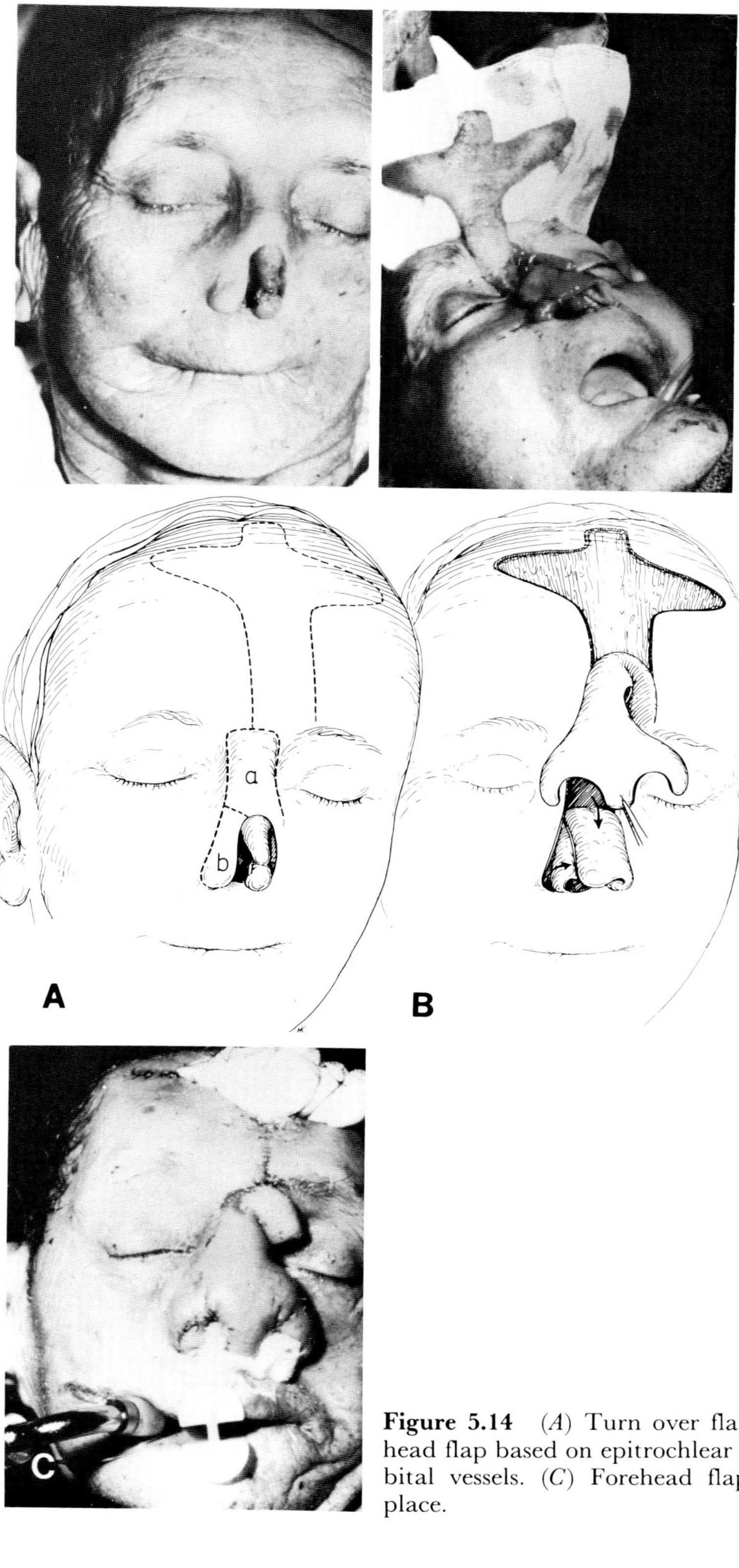

Figure 5.14 (*A*) Turn over flaps. (*B*) Forehead flap based on epitrochlear and supraorbital vessels. (*C*) Forehead flap sutured in place.

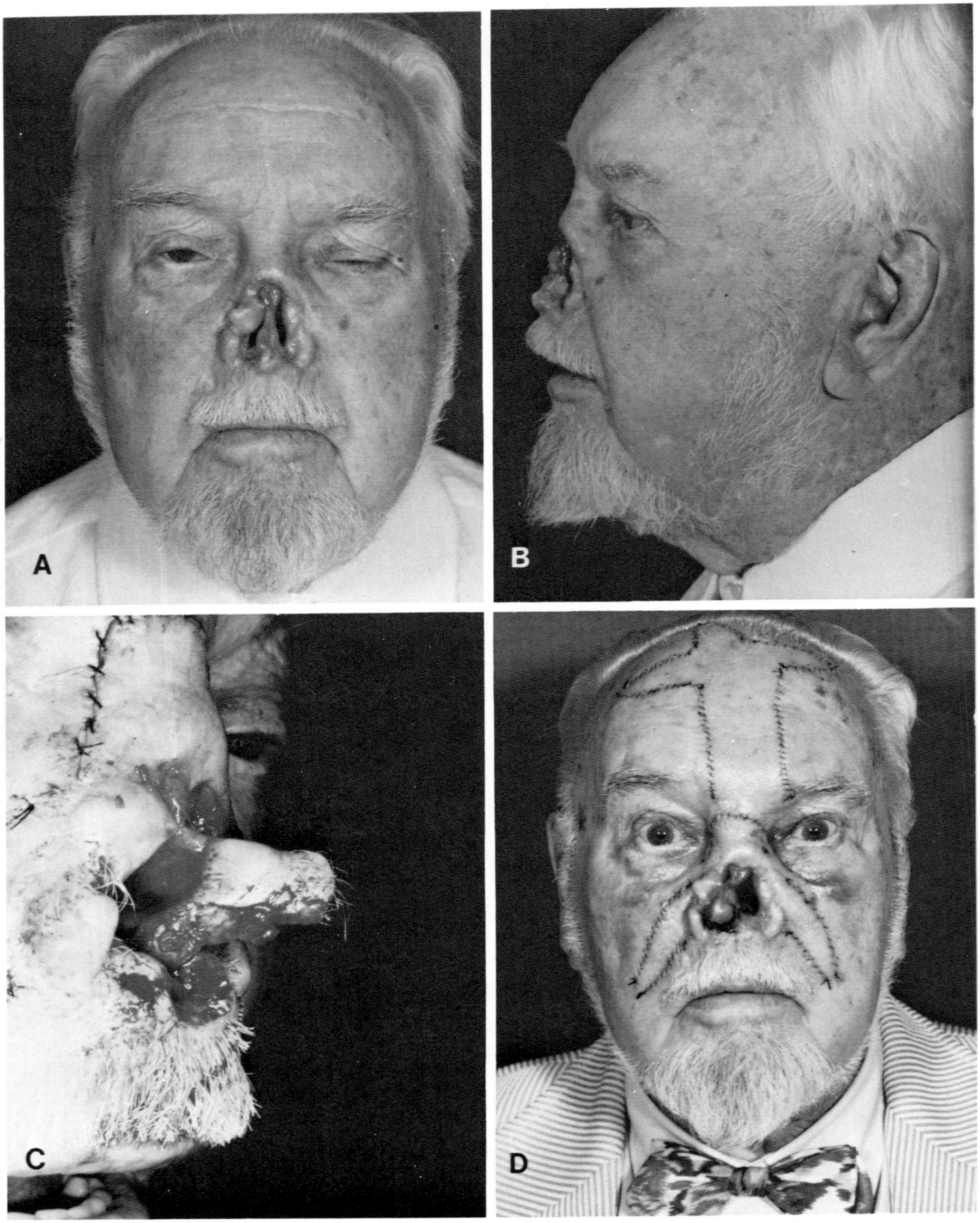

Figure 5.15 (*A*) Frontal view of patient after removal of basal cell carcinoma with Mohs' chemosurgery. (*B*) Lateral view. (*C*) L-shaped septal advancement flap is based superiorly, and mucosa is carefully sewn to mucosa along the posterior edge of the cartilage. Inferiorly, a small split thickness skin graft covers the raw area. (*D*) After septal advancement, and delay of seagull-shaped forehead flap for cover, and turnover flaps from the remaining nose and nasolabial areas for lining.

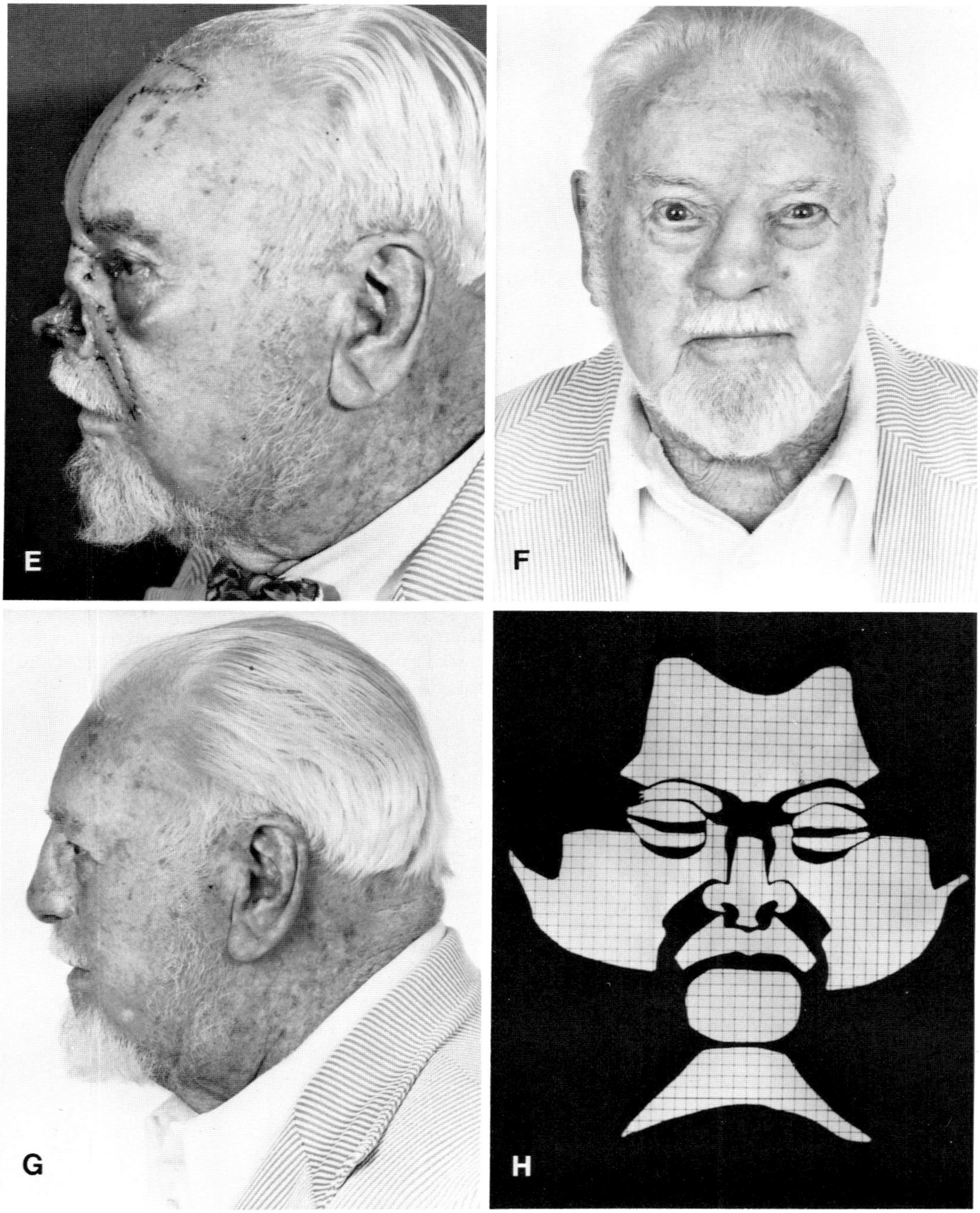

Figure 5.15 (*E*) Lateral view of patient as shown in (*D*). (*F*) Final result 1 year after completion of the reconstruction a scalp rotation flap aided in the closure of the forehead defect. (*G*) Lateral view of patient as shown in (*F*). (*H*) The "aesthetic units" of the face (from a cadaver dissection). The alae and midportion of the nose may constitute "subunits." Better results in nasal reconstruction will be obtained if one replaces the entire unit or subunit rather than simply replacing just the missing tissue.

In 9 days, the pedicle flap is completely transected at the level of the upper lip vermillion and the remainder of the flap is reinset in the upper arm. After a 3- to 4-week interval, the nasal pedicle flap softens considerably. The resolution of edema during this time facilities the thinning and infolding of the flap to reform the alar rims (Fig. 5.13).

Discussion

Undoubtedly the greatest advantage of the arm flap method of nasal reconstruction is the avoidance of additional facial scarring such as that encountered when the forehead flap is employed. The upper arm tissue is particularly adaptable to complete nasal resurfacing and alar rim reconstruction in patients who have intact nasal bone and septum.

Ever since this technique was introduced in 1597, it has been subject to criticism because of the discomfort associated with the prolonged immobilization. In our small series of five patients, the arm pedicle was transected on the 9th postoperative day, rather than the 21st, and, although two patients were in the 60s, they experienced minimal difficulty. The shorter period of immobilization, the good health of the patients, the opportunities for regular elbow motion, and the use of muscle relaxants were all highly beneficial factors.

There is a significant disadvantage of the Tagliacozzi flap: the match of color and texture of the reconstructed nose. With regard to texture, forehead skin is comparatively thicker and inelastic and holds a given form well. By contrast, arm tissue is relatively elastic, thin, very pliable and requires bony or cartilaginous support to maintain a given shape. In addition, the color match of arm pedicle tissue is unpredictable. Arm tissue does not have the characteristic red tones of facial skin and therefore frequently appears hypopigmented.

In our series of four cases, the one black patient had an excellent color match. In the Caucasian patients there was a general lack of red tones with relative hypopigmentation. These differences in color match were quite acceptable to the patients however.

Despite these disadvantages, however, the Tagliacozzi arm flap provides a very acceptable *alternative* when the forehead is not available as a source of nasal reconstruction.

NASAL RECONSTRUCTION WITH MIDLINE FOREHEAD FLAPS

The nose has three components: lining (mucous membrane), support (bone and cartilage), and cover (skin), and any or all of these components may require replacement in nasal reconstruction.

Lining can generally be provided by turn-over flaps of remaining nasal skin (Fig. 5.14 *A*), or flaps from the nasolabial region. Support can be provided by L-shaped advancement of the remaining septum, or cantilevered bone grafts. In most cases, the best material for cover is a midline forehead flap. The flap is based on the epitrochlear vessels (Fig. 5.14 *B*), and because of its high vascularity, is a safe flap. Coming from an adjacent area, it does not require a long period of immobilization in an uncomfortable position. The donor scar, in properly selected patients, is innocuous, and a small price to pay for the superb color and texture match of forehead skin. Most of the time the donor area can be closed primarily, and occasionally scalp and forehead rotation flaps will be necessary to ensure that no "patches" of skin graft be left on the forehead. If large amounts of forehead skin must be used, it is better to graft the entire forehead as a homogeneous "aesthetic unit."

In patients with moderately short foreheads, the flap may be taken obliquely and still based on the epitrochlear vessels. However, in children and black patients, both of whom may have very short foreheads and a tendency to form heavier scars, greater consideration should be

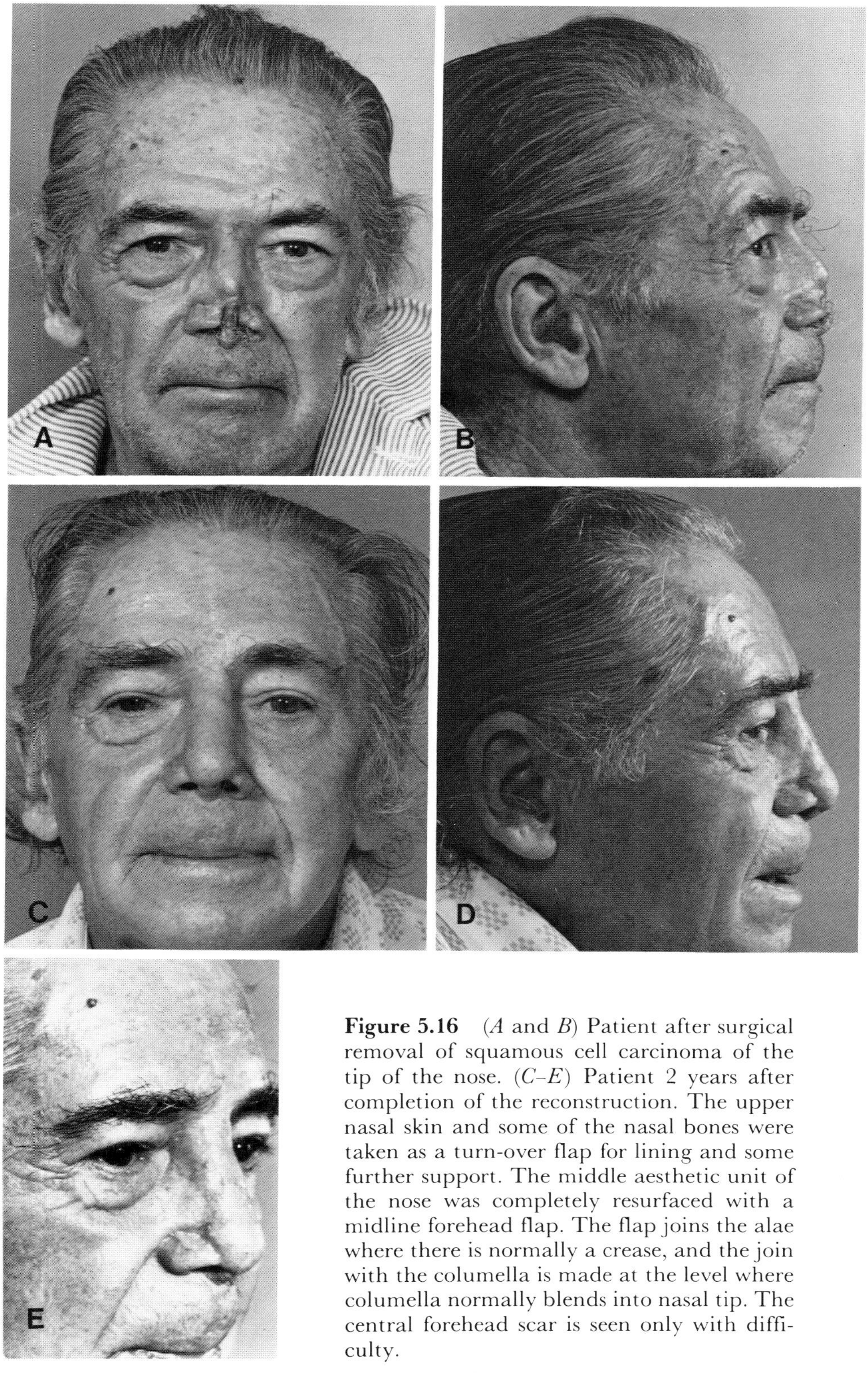

Figure 5.16 (*A* and *B*) Patient after surgical removal of squamous cell carcinoma of the tip of the nose. (*C–E*) Patient 2 years after completion of the reconstruction. The upper nasal skin and some of the nasal bones were taken as a turn-over flap for lining and some further support. The middle aesthetic unit of the nose was completely resurfaced with a midline forehead flap. The flap joins the alae where there is normally a crease, and the join with the columella is made at the level where columella normally blends into nasal tip. The central forehead scar is seen only with difficulty.

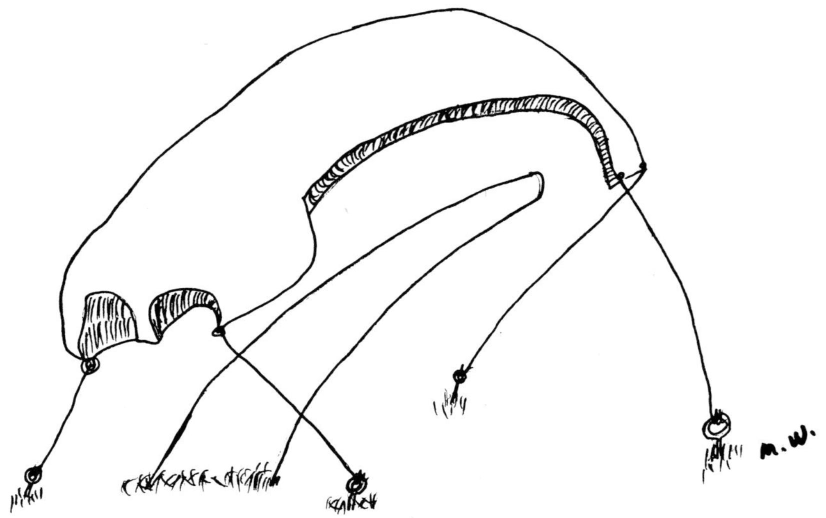

Figure 5.17 A patient's preoperative schematic interpretation of the surgeon's explanation of total nasal reconstruction using a midline forehead flap.

given to methods which bring in distant tissue, such as the Tagliacozzi flap from the inner brachial area.

Total nasal reconstruction must consider and plan for addition of lining, bony skeleton, and adequate cover. A number of methods have been described that surgeons have to choose from, but principles of reconstructive surgery should always prevail and imagination and tailoring of each case is imperative (Figs. 5.15–5.17).

References

1. Almast, S. C.: History and evolution of the Indian method of rhinoplasty, in *Transactions of the 4th International Congress of Plastic and Reconstructive Surgeons; Rome, October 1967*, p. 19, Excerpta Medica Foundation, Amsterdam, 1967.
2. Antia, N. H.: The scope of plastic surgery in leprosy: A ten-year progress report. *Clin. Plast. Surg.*, *1:*69, 1974.
3. Aufricht, G.: Combined nasal plastic and chin plastic; correction of microgenic by osteocartilaginous transplants from large hump nose. *Am. J. Surg.*, *25:* 292, 1934.
4. Blair, V. P.: Total and subtotal restoration of the nose. *J.A.M.A.*, *85:*1931, 1925.
5. Blair, V. P., and Brown, J. B.: Nasal abnormalities, fancied and real. *Surg. Gynecol. Obstet.*, *53:*797, 1931.
6. Blocksma, R., and Innis, C. O.: Reconstruction of the amputed nose. *Plast. Reconstr. Surg.*, *15:*390, 1955.
7. Brown, J. B., and Cannon, B.: Composite free grafts of skin and cartilages from the ear. *Surg. Gynecol. Obstet.*, *82:*253, 1946.
8. Carpue, J. C.: *An Account of Two Successful Operations for Restoring a Lost Nose from the Ineguments of the Forehead in the Cases of Two Officers of His Majesty's Army*, Longman, London, 1816.
9. Converse, J. M.: New forehead flap for nasal reconstruction. *Proc. R. Soc. Med.*, *35:*811, 1942.
10. Converse, J. M.: Reconstruction of the nose by the scalping flap technique. *Surg. Clin. North Am.*, *39:*335, 1959.
11. Converse, J. M. (Ed.): *Reconstructive Plastic Surgery*, W. B. Saunders, Philadelphia, 1977.
12. Converse, J. M.: Clinical applications of the scalping flap in reconstruction of the nose. *Plast. Reconstr. Surg.*, *43:*247, 1969.
13. Converse, J. M., and Wood-Smith, D.: Experiences with the forehead island flap with a subcutaneous pedicle. *Plast. Reconstr. Surg.*, *31:*521, 1963.
14. Gillies, H. D., and Millard, D. R., Jr.: *Principles and Art of Plastic Surgery*, Little Brown, Boston, 1957.
15. Heanley, C.: The subcutaneous tissue pedicle flap in columellar and other nasal reconstruction. *Br. J. Plast. Surg.*, *8:*60, 1955.
16. McDowell, F. (Ed.): *The Zeiz Index and History of*

Plastic Surgery 900 B.C.—1863 A.D., Williams & Wilkins, Baltimore, 1977.
17. Millard, D. R., Jr.: Total reconstructive rhinoplasty and a missing link. *Plast. Reconstr. Surg.*, *37:*167, 1966.
18. Millard, D. R., Jr.: Hemirhinoplasty. *Plast. Reconstr. Surg.*, *40:*440, 1967.
19. Millard, D. R., Jr.: Reconstructive rhinoplasty for the lower half of a nose. *Plast. Reconstr. Surg.*, *53:*133, 1974.
20. Natvig, P., Sether, L. A., Gingrass, R. P., and Gardner, W. D.: Anatomical details of the osseous-cartilaginous framework of the nose. *Plast. Reconstr. Surg.*, *48:*528, 1971.
21. Penn, J.: The reconstruction of the nose. *Br. J. Plast. Surg.*, *20:*369, 1967.
22. Skoog, T.: *Plastic Surgery—New Methods and Refinements.* W. B. Saunders, Philadelphia, 1974.
23. Tagliacozzi, G.: *De Curtorom Chirurgia*, G. Bindonus, Venice, 1597.

CHAPTER 6

Ear Reconstruction

Jon A. Perlman, M.D., and Harvey A. Zarem, M.D., F.A.C.S.

Few structural abnormalities provide the plastic surgeon as difficult a challenge, as does external ear reconstruction. The auricle has a delicate and complex form which is not only difficult to reproduce, but requires precise positioning to provide symmetry with the opposite side. The continuing evolution of different techniques of ear reconstruction testifies to the fact that no single method has yet been found to produce reliably a satisfactory result. When one considers the psychologic burden of a severe ear deformity, and the extreme difficulty of secondary ear reconstruction, one sees that the procedure warrants being performed only by skilled surgeons experienced in such techniques.

ANATOMY AND EMBRYOLOGY

The external ear is a delicate structure that is composed of a fine fibroelastic cartilaginous skeleton covered by a thin well fitting integument (Fig. 6.1). Structurally, the auricle is best thought of as existing in four planes, each at right angles to that adjacent to it: conchal floor, conchal wall, scapha-antihelix, and helix[18] (Fig. 6.2). With the exception of the lobule, every structure of the external ear derives its shape from the underlying cartilage. Through experience, it has been learned that a normal ear maintains its shape, height and position with intact helical arch and crus, the Y of the antihelix, the cartilage of the tragus and antitragus, as well as the cartilage surrounding the ear canal.[11] As a result, the normal ear has been well mapped for use as a cartilage or composite graft donor (Fig. 6.3).

Even more critical to successful ear reconstruction than ear structure is three dimensional positioning. The best ear reconstruction improperly positioned falls short of a less elaborately formed ear symmetric in size and position with the opposite side. Normally the ear protrudes 30° from the side of the head with the top of the auricle located at a point parallel to the top of the brow, and the midpoint of the tragus corresponding to the alar groove. The anterior border of the auricle is ordinarily one ear length from the lateral orbital rim with its long axis offset from the vertical by 20–30°, roughly paralleling in the adult the nasal dorsum. The latter cannot be used as an

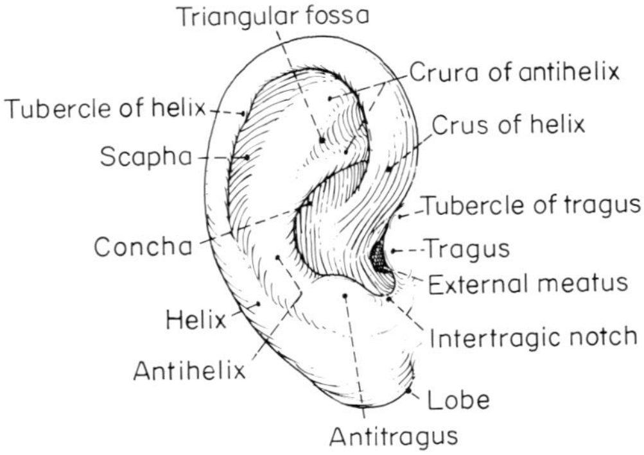

Figure 6.1 Normal external ear anatomy.

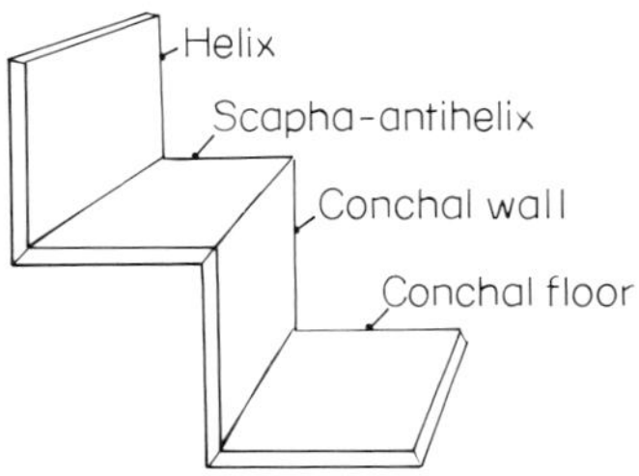

Figure 6.2 The four perpendicular planes of the external auricular structure.

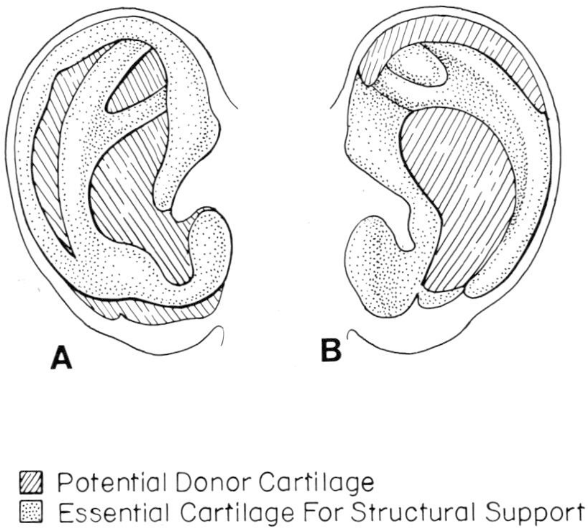

Figure 6.3 Outline of potential cartilage donor sites on (*A*) anterior or lateral, and (*B*) medial or posterior auricular surfaces. (Reproduced with permission from M. Gorney: *Symposium on Reconstruction of the Auricle*. C. V. Mosby, St. Louis, 1974.[11]).

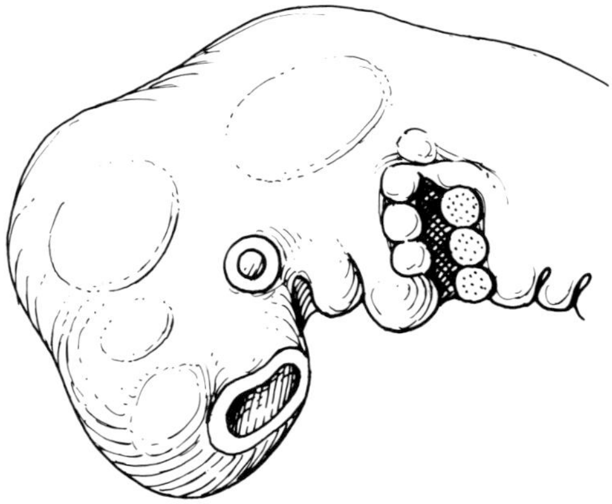

Figure 6.4 Thirty-eight day human embryo showing the prominent first branchial cleft surrounded by the mandibular and hyoid arches and their six hillocks. The hyoid arch is stippled and is destined to account for the majority of the auricular substance. The otic vesicle can be appreciated dorsal to the first and second arches. (Reproduced with permission from J. M. Converse (Ed.): *Reconstructive Plastic Surgery*, W. B. Saunders, Philadelphia, 1977.)

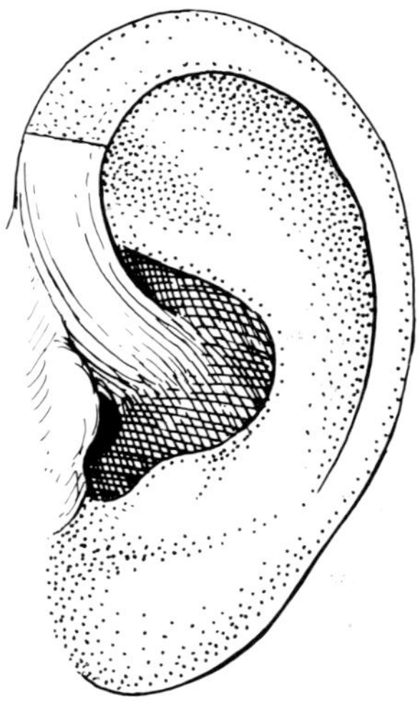

Figure 6.5 The proportional contribution of the mandibular (*non-stippled*) and hyoid arches to the fully developed auricle. The mandibular arch accounts for only the helical crus and the tragus of the auricle. (Reproduced with permission from J. M. Converse (Ed.): *Reconstructive Plastic Surgery*, W. B. Saunders, Philadelphia, 1977.)

accurate reference point in the child whose nasal bridge is flat and not fully developed until puberty.

Vertical ear growth parallels body growth until the age of 10, after which growth is nominal. The horizontal ear dimension probably does not increase after the age of 4. The normal male ear is 55–60 mm in height, whereas the female is in the range of 50–55 mm.

Embryologically the external and middle ear have shared origins explaining the frequent associations of external and middle ear abnormalities (Fig. 6.4). The inner ear, however, derives from an ectodermal thickening, the otic placode. This structure appears in the 3-week embryo dorsal to the future site of the ear and becomes the otic vesicle or otocyst after sinking into the underlying mesenchyme. The middle and external ears derive from the first brachial cleft or groove, and the surrounding first and second brachial arches. The malleus and incus derive from the first, and the stapes from the second brachial arch. The first endodermal pharyngeal pouch enlarges to form the auditory tube and the tympanic cavity of the middle ear.

In early phases of auricle development the first (mandibular) and second (hyoid) arches contribute equally. At approximately embryonic day 38, 6 prominences or hillocks appear on the arches surrounding the first branchial cleft. These were originally felt to be responsible for pre- and postauricular tags or sinuses, but are now felt to contribute to individual components of the external ear. During the 7th embryonic week, growth of the face and lower jaw causes a dorsolateral migration of the primitive auricle from the developing mandible toward its normal position. The hillocks are once again smooth by the 45th day and precartilage cells appear in the auricle aligned as in a normal adult ear cartilage. The ventral third of the brachial groove deepens and eventually forms the external auditory meatus. The concha is the last structure of the auricle to appear. Up to this point, the mandibular and hyoid arches contributed equally to development; however, by the 8th week the proportion of mandibular arch tissue present gradually diminishes until 85% of the auricle is composed of hyoid arch mesenchyme with the mandibular arch contributing only to the formation of the anterior helical crus and the tragus[14] (Fig. 6.5). Further shaping and positioning of the ear occurs subsequently, with gradual protrusion from the side of the head occurring in the 3rd embryonic month, with folding of the helical margin and the antihelix and its crura by the 6th month.[14]

CONGENITAL EAR DEFORMITY

External ear deformities are a common head and neck anomaly, occurring in approximately 1 in 3500 live births.[12] One half of these defects are nothing more than preauricular tags or sinuses; however, it is important to emphasize that any congenital auricular deformity requires careful investigation because of the frequent association with hearing deficits. This becomes particularly important when one considers the key role auditory perception plays in stimulation of speech as early as the first year of life.[8] In addition, the pediatrics literature has well documented the association between congenital ear and urologic abnormalities. There is no association between the severity of the external ear deformity and the presence of middle ear malformation; however, such a correlation has been made with the presence of mandibular dysmorphia or 7th nerve dysfunction.[8, 12]

Terminology used to define congenital ear anomalies has been inconsistent and confusing. There is a moderate degree of overlap among the deformities and in 1968

Rogers supported the concept that microtic ears as well as ears with cupping, protrusion or lop deformities, represented variable penetrance of an abnormal group of genes, and each represented an arrest of development at a different embryologic stage.[14]

The most severe deformity, next to the very rare anotia, microtia. The microtic ear is distinctly malformed and always smaller than normal, as its name implies. Usually, only a malpositioned rudiment of the ear, such as the lobule, remains. According to Converse, close examination will always reveal an associated mandibular malformation, not surprising when one considers their close embryonic association.[21]

Marx divided microtia into 3 subgroups dependent on the severity and degree of malformation[15]:

Grade 1. Small auricle with recognizable individual structures.

Grade 2. Small auricle with some remnants resembling a helix in configuration.

Grade 3. No auricular configuration with only a ridge of tissue or lobule present.

Multiple syndromes have been associated with microtia and should be kept in mind when assessing a patient so affected (Fig. 6.6).

The reconstruction of the microtic auricle is particularly challenging, as one faces the difficult decision as to what use to make of the deformed and malpositioned tissue remnants. Before setting out on the project of reconstruction, one must carefully assess bilateral hearing function. With normal contralateral hearing function, there is no practical gain in middle ear surgery on the affected side, as normal binaural hearing could not technically be achieved. With bilateral middle ear deafness, early otic surgery may be necessary on one side, followed by middle ear surgery on the second ear after completion of temporal bone growth. In such a case, auricle reconstruction would need to be delayed, or at least planned inconjunction with the otologist due to difficulties with middle ear operative exposure following auricular reconstruction, external canal positioning, and the chronic drainage so frequent following middle ear surgery.[20]

The lop ear deformity or "limp ear" is characterized by a downward folding of the helix and scapha occurring at the level of Darwin's tubercle, producing a flattening of the superior helix. This is often associated with a malformation of the superior antihelical crus and may result in such severe hooding as to cover the conchal cavity. The ear lacks normal vertical height secondary to the folding and compression of the fossa triangularis and scapha. A probable variant of the lop ear deformity, most commonly seen in the Oriental and rare in Caucasians, is cryptotia or "pocket ear." Here the deficient upper portion of the auricle is unnaturally adherent to the head covered by temporal skin. There is an absence of the retroauricular sulcus with scaphal underdevelopment and an abnormally sharp antihelix and/or inferior antihelical crus.

The cup ear is a malformed protruding ear secondary to an exaggerated cup-shaped concave concha. The ear height and circumference are reduced and commonly there are features of both lop ears and protruding ears.

The protruding ear is normal in size and shape and is often a bilateral deformity. Its protrusion is secondary to any combination of the following mechanisms: (1) unfurling

---

Atretic Auditory Canal
Otomandibular Dysplasia (First and Second Branchial Arch Syndrome)
Mandibulofacial Dysostosis (Treacher-Collins Syndrome)
Pierre Robin Syndrome
Goldenhar's Syndrome

Figure 6.6 The most common of the large number of syndromes associated with microtia.

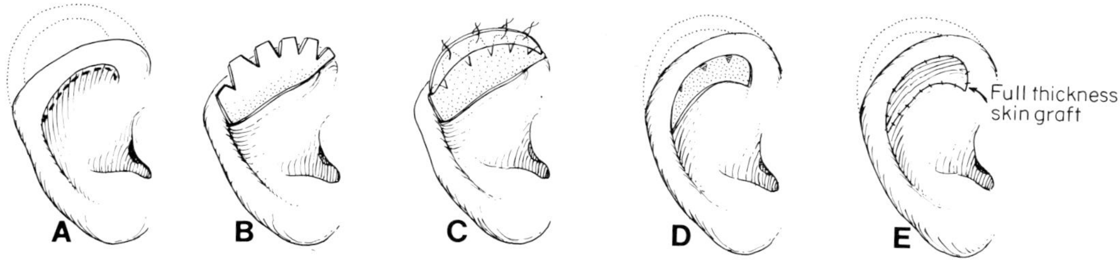

Figure 6.7 Musgrave correction of cup ear deformity. Using this technique, through a posterior auricular incision a strip of cartilage including helical tail and conchal cartilage is excised in a line corresponding to the desired antihelix and superior crus. This excision crosses the helical rim, which is further uncurled and expanded through a lateral auricular incision (*A*), by radial incisions in the rim (*B*). The resultant expansion is maintained by the previously obtained cartilage strip (*C*). A full thickness skin graft is usually required to cover the lateral auricular deficit (*D*, *E*). Normal vertical ear height can be approached but rarely obtained. (Modified from B. Cosman: *Symposium on Reconstruction of the Auricle*, edited by R. C. Tanzer and M. T. Edgerton, C. V. Mosby, St. Louis, 1974.).

of the antihelix and its superior crus, (2) excessive conchal cartilage, (3) increased angle of lobule protrusion or excess lobule size, (4) inadequate folding of helical margin ("shell ear").[14]

The primary repair of congenital auricular deformities can be extremely rewarding and gratifying to both patient and surgeon. Techniques available allow one to anticipate very acceptable results if good judgment and skill and caution are combined. A careful analysis of the anatomic deformities is necessary in each individual case, along with a determination of the presence of a true skin or cartilage deficit, and, in the most severe cases, a determination of the usefulness of the remnants of the auricular skin and cartilage present.

Beginning with the mildest form of lop ear where the superior helical rim forms only a small lid covering the scapha, minor skin and cartilage excision can provide a satisfactory rim contour. More severe lidding is usually associated with significant loss of height in the superior helical area, and requires freeing of the helical rim as either anteriorly or posteriorly based banner flaps, or as a free cartilage graft, reoriented and sutured in proper position at the top of the scapha. Musgrave described a series of radial cartilaginous incisions across the superior helical rim which uncurl the lidding and expand the helix (Fig. 6.7). This is supported by a free graft of conchal cartilage strip sutured to the ends of the helical rim to stabilize them and give a smooth contour. A full thickness skin graft is often needed for soft tissue coverage. The resultant ear usually lacks full vertical height, but the frequent bilateral nature of the deformity makes this acceptable.

Severe lop and cupping deformities with adequate skin coverage require radical cartilage reorientation to expand the helix. Barsky described a Y-V advancement of the superior helical insertion coupled with posterior antihelical cartilage scoring using mattress sutures as described by Luckett (Fig. 6.8). He later modified his technique by incising superior auricular skin and cartilage for expansion, coupled with a posterior skin flap (Fig. 6.9). Erich combined a Z-plasty to elevate the facial attachment of the anterior helix with a modification of the Luckett antihelical fold formation to uncurl the ear and improve the superior helical contour.

In the cryptotic ear, a retroauricular sulcus must be created with either release and full thickness skin graft, or with local pedicle flap tissue. A triangular temporal flap has been described by Washio which can be rotated onto the posterior auricle with donor

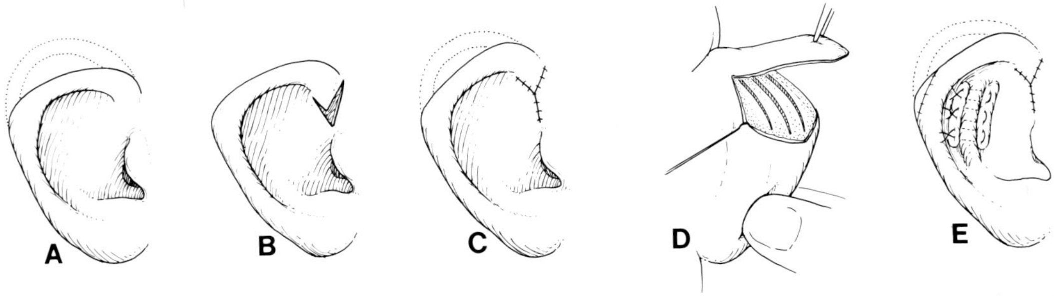

Figure 6.8 Technique of Barsky (1950) to treat severe cup deformity (*A*). The height of the helical crus is increased using a V-Y advancement (*B*, *C*). The antihelical fold is created by posterior cartilage incision (*D*), and Luckett type mattress sutures tied over bolsters (*E*). The severe cupping and excessive ear concavity are improved; however, the flatness of the helix and lack of vertical height are unaffected. (Modified with permission from B. Cosman: *Symposium on Reconstruction of the Auricle*, edited by R. C. Tanzer and M. T. Edgerton, C. V. Mosby, St. Louis, 1974.).

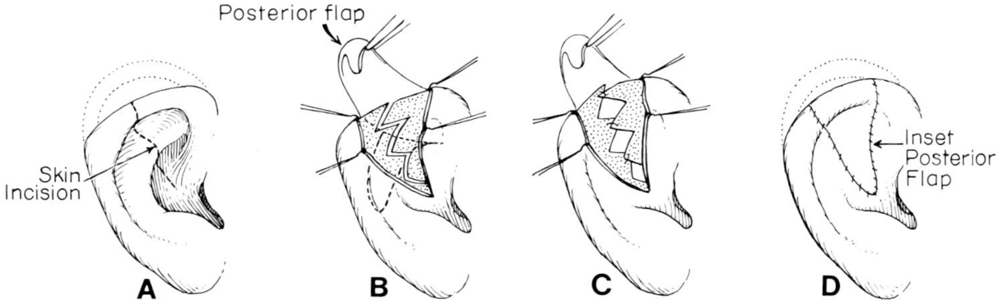

Figure 6.9 Technique of Barsky (1964) for cup ear deformity (*A*), permitting expansion of the auricle via cartilaginous incisions (*B*, *C*) requiring coverage with a posterior auricular skin flap (*D*). (Modified with permission from B. Cosman: *Symposium on Reconstruction of the Auricle*, edited by R. C. Tanzer and M. T. Edgerton, C. V. Mosby, St. Louis, 1974.).

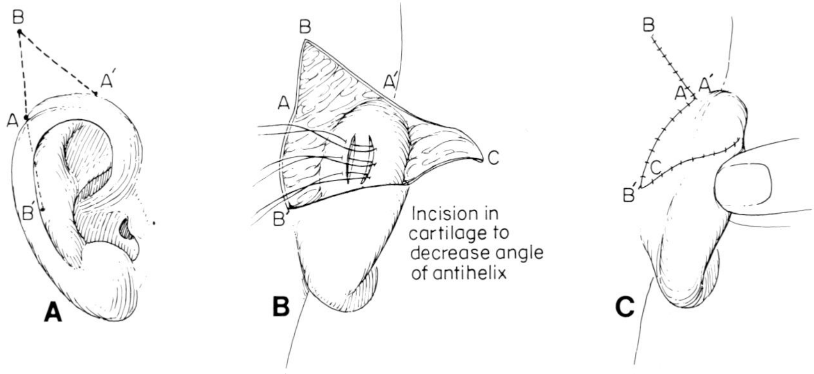

Figure 6.10 In the cryptotic ear (*A*) an absence of retroauricular sulcus is combined with sharp angulation of the antihelix. A triangular skin flap is designed (*B*) based on the helical rim and elevated from the scalp above the ear (*A-B-A′*). Medial cartilaginous incisions are made and sutured to decrease antihelical angulation and project the ear away from the scalp. The triangular flap is sutured in place (*C*) creating a retroauricular sulcus with the donor site closed primarily via advancement, or grafted. (Reproduced with permission from H. Washio: *Plastic & Reconstructive Surgery*, *52*:648, 1973.[24])

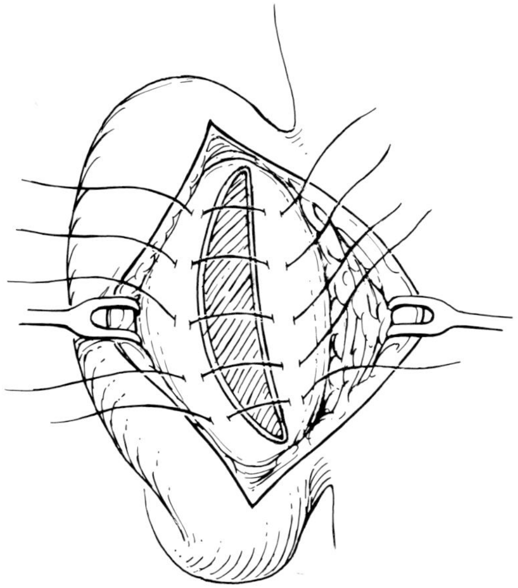

Figure 6.11 Luckett method of creating an antihelical fold in the protruding ear through excision of an ellipse of conchal cartilage and medial skin and placement of mattress sutures. The shortcoming of this procedure was the resultant sharp angulation. (Reproduced with permission from J. M. Converse (Ed.): *Reconstructive Plastic Surgery*, W. B. Saunders, Philadelphia, 1977.)

wound coverage using local flap advancement (Fig. 6.10). This method of creating the retroauricular sulcus is combined with parallel cartilage incisions adjacent to the antihelical fold permitting resuturing of the cartilaginous edges at an angle which lessens the acuity, and which projects the ear away from the head.[24]

The usual protruding ear lacks adequate concho-scaphal angle due to flatness of the antihelix. To restore bilateral protruding ears to a normal position, one must aim to have the most lateral portion of the auricle 17–20 mm from the side of the head.[9] This is best accomplished by a procedure which combines resection of excess posterior skin with creation of an antihelical fold or tube. Luckett was the first to describe excision of an ellipse of cartilage in the area of the proposed antihelix, with formation of the proper angulation using permanent mattress sutures (Fig. 6.11). The resultant conspicuous sharp angulation was improved by Erich's use of parallel incisions providing a cartilage strip which was displaced forward covering the angulation at the junction of the cartilages. Tanzar makes vertical incisions adjacent to the anticipated antihelix and superior crus, creating a broad cartilage band which tubes when the adjacent cartilage margins are sutured together behind it[21] (Fig. 6.12). Stenstrom[17] described a technique of scoring the anterior cartilage at the proposed antihelical fold which is simple and effective in creating a natural appearance. When the patient has an adequate antihelical fold and the concha itself is deep and responsible for the protrusion, tacking of the concha to the mastoid fascia is a procedure that is thought adequate by some surgeons; alternatively, excision of a long conchal ellipse of skin and cartilage can be corrective.

TOTAL EAR RECONSTRUCTION

The severity of the deformity requiring total ear reconstruction coupled with the difficulty of proper positioning of the auricle makes total reconstruction of the ear a technical challenge. The potential gains in reconstruction for microtia, traumatic, or surgical ear loss are so great as to warrant meticulous attention to detail and planning.

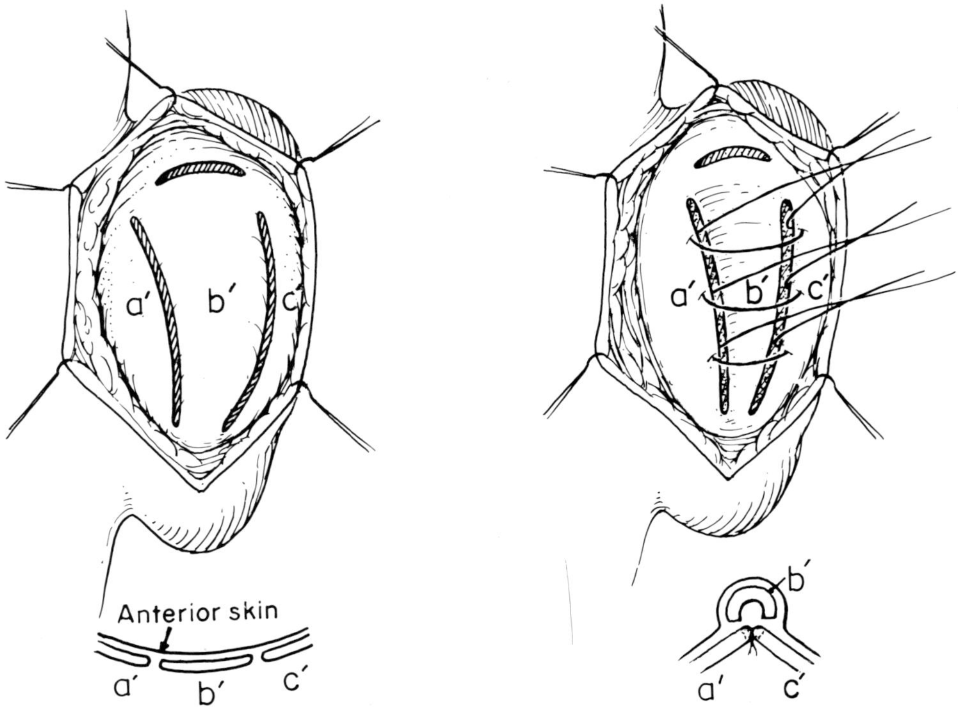

Figure 6.12 Tanzer's method of creating a more natural cartilage fold of antihelix without sharp angulation. The central cartilage strip (*b*′) is displaced forward beneath the anterior (or lateral) skin. A gentle roll is created camouflaging the cartilaginous angulation as shown. (Modified from J. M. Converse (Ed.): *Reconstructive Plastic Surgery*, W. B. Saunders, Philadelphia, 1977.)

The first step in beginning a total ear reconstruction involves the assessment of the usefulness of not only the ear remnants, but the surrounding tissues. One must assess whether the local soft tissue is of adequate quality to accept an ear framework and provide for the construction of a retroauricular sulcus, and whether the helical or lobular remnant is positioned such that it can be of use. One also needs to consider whether there is adequate glabrous skin for ear coverage. If not, a scalp roll with full thickness skin graft may be needed to precede insertion of the ear framework. In a hemifacial microsomia patient, mandibular bone grafts or dermal fat grafts may be necessary to build up facial contour and add symmetry prior to ear reconstruction.

Next comes the crucial step of selecting proper position and orientation of the auricle. Here the use of two-dimensional designs copied on clear x-ray film from the opposite ear have proven valuable for orientation and sizing of the new ear. In dealing with hemifacial microsomia, the surgeon must give priority to avoiding the construction of an ear in the anterior and inferiorly displaced position of the microtic ear remnant.

Ears constructed with autogenous cartilage have been shown to grow in size by Tanzer, nearly paralleling the opposite side (with the exception of the child operated upon at the age of 6–7 when the eventual growth of the reconstructed ear lags the normal ear by 2–3 mm).

One unsettled controversy that seems likely to persist is the choice of framework material. Early attempts at ear reconstruction included use of preserved cartilage, maternal cartilage, bone, and homogenized cartilage substance. These all proved unsat-

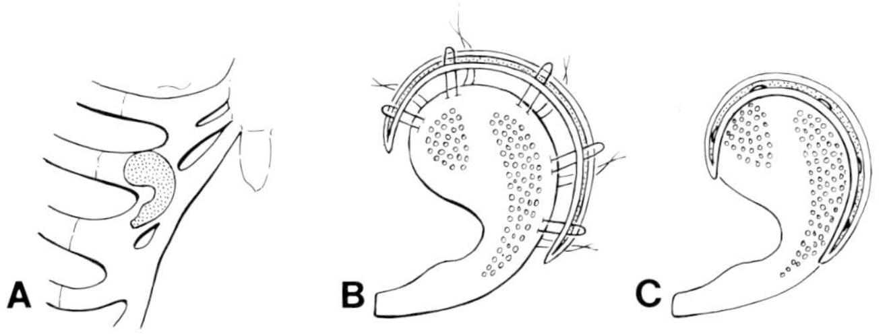

Figure 6.13 Tanzer's method of harvesting a cartilage ear framework from costal cartilages 6 and 7 (*A*). Multiple perforations (*B*) are placed to permit tissue ingrowth within the framework, and a strip of cartilage harvested from the 8th costal cartilage is positioned with sutures to provide a helical rim (*C*). (Reproduced with permission from R. C. Tanzer and M. T. Edgerton (eds.): *Symposium on Reconstruction of the Auricle.* C. V. Mosby, St. Louis, 1974.)

isfactory and suffered high rates of resorption. Tanzer was instrumental in first designing a technique using autogenous hyaline rib cartilage using 4–6 stages for total ear reconstruction.[18] This has now been reduced by Tanzer to only 3 or 4 stages,[19] and rapidly became and remains the standard of excellence of total ear reconstruction. Others have found shortcomings in use of rib cartilage and have derived other approaches. Steffensen preferred conchal cartilage, feeling that the fibroelastic conchal cartilage is probably metabolically and physically better suited to ear reconstruction than is rib cartilage.[16] This is logical when one considers the unprotected location of the delicate ear framework and all the trauma and temperature changes to which it is subjected. However, today rib cartilage remains the most common choice of experienced surgeons in ear reconstruction.

Total Ear Reconstruction Using Rib Cartilage

As mentioned above, Radford Tanzer has been the founder and strongest advocate of the use of costal cartilage for total ear reconstruction. His technique has been refined over two and a half decades and with such excellent long term results free of significant absorption or extrusions this has become the method by which all other total ear reconstructions are compared.[22] Tanzer enumerated he critical components of total ear reconstruction and began by emphasizing the need to provide adequate skin coverage matching the color and texture of normal auricular skin. This he felt could be accomplished through full thickness skin grafts. The requirements of a permanent inert framework with delicacy and contour, he felt, could best be provided by a carefully carved pattern of 6th and 7th costal cartilage to create antihelix and scapha with a portion of the 8th rib carved and wired in place for the helix (Fig. 6.13). Tanzer was also immersed in the production of the refined ear, and incorporated techniques in his reconstruction for creation of an adequate tragus and conchal floor (method of Kirkham) (Fig. 6.14), and conchal wall (valise handle technique).[18]

In a report of his 3- or 4-stage technique, Tanzer[19] commenced with the patient age of 6 by relocating the lobular remnant from its superior position transposing it into a useable position by modified Z-plasty flap transfer. This procedure may precede or be combined with the insertion of the costal cartilage ear framework with a cartilage

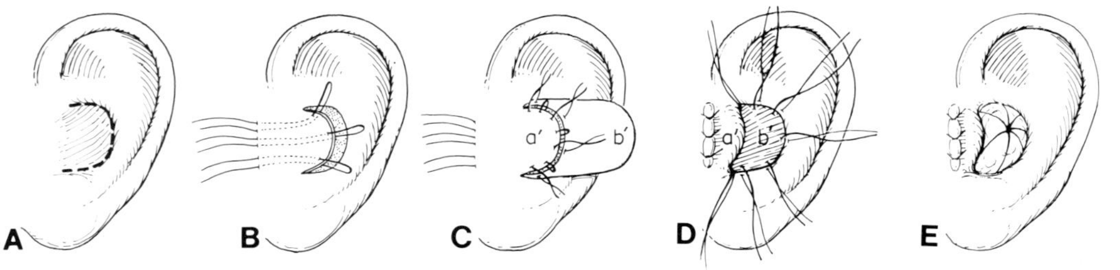

Figure 6.14 The method of Kirkham to create a tragus and deepen the conchal floor in the reconstructed ear (*A*). A full thickness flap is elevated (*B*) and sutures placed permitting inversion of the flap upon itself (*C*). A full thickness skin graft is sutured in place (*D*, *E*), and all sutures tied over bolsters. (Reproduced with permission from R. C. Tanzer and M. T. Edgerton (eds.): *Symposium on Reconstruction of the Auricle*. C. V. Mosby, St. Louis, 1974.)

extension into the lobule used to serve as a stabilizer. Tanzer prefers insertion of the framework through a central incision, believing that skin vascularity in the helical rim area is less affected (compared to a posthelical rim incision), permitting safer placement of horizontal mattress sutures in the area of helix and antihelix, consequently obtaining better skin confirmation to the framework. The 3rd stage involves elevation of the auricle from the side of the head, combined with temporary creation of a valise handle of helix, scapha and antihelix. This handle is closed at the 4th stage using a skin graft, and results in an enlarged conchal wall. At this stage a Kirkham flap with skin graft can be used to create the tragal skin fold while thinning the conchal floor. Using this technique Tanzer reported on 44 patients followed up to 19 years.[22] He found an extraordinary ability of the reconstructed auricle to grow fairly symmetrically with the opposite side, and had no extrusions of cartilage framework. Eleven percent of patients complained of loss of definition of the auricular form (particularly in secondary reconstruction); however, this could be prevented by deepening all sulci at the initial reconstruction, avoiding all undue skin tension on the cartilage, and by keeping the skin flap over the framework as thin as possible. Tanzer commenced his primary reconstructions at the age of 6, feeling that the majority of ear growth had occurred at this time, and wishing to spare the child as much psychologic trauma as possible. Operating at this early age adds somewhat to the difficulty of the procedure, inasmuch as the costal cartilage is frail until the age of 10. Consequently, variations of Tanzer's rib harvest technique have arisen hoping to refine the definition of the framework as well as to allow its development from the small 6th, 7th and 8th costal cartilages present in the young child. The cantilever design of Furnas[10] (Fig. 6.15) and the "expansile framework" of Brent[2] (Fig. 6.16) are examples of how definition of folds and surfaces is obtained by removing cartilage from the scapha, fossa triangularis, and concha. Brent's modified "expansile framework" enables cartilage harvest in 3 pieces utilizing portions of the 7th and 8th costal cartilages.

Brent[3] has also made two modifications for total ear reconstruction: 1) Leave the reconstruction of the lobule for last. Brent feels it is easier to construct an ear and bring the lobule to it, rather than the reverse. 2) The manual carving of the autogenous rib cartilage framework should include thickness and lateral height (away from the mastoid) so that a later stage requiring full thickness skin graft in the retroauricular sulcus to bring the ear out and away from the mastoid is not needed.

Total Ear Reconstruction with Silicone Framework

Despite the degree of success obtainable with costal cartilage framework ear reconstruction, several shortcomings lead to the use of preformed silicone frameworks by some reconstructive surgeons. The difficulty of harvesting adequate rib cartilage in a

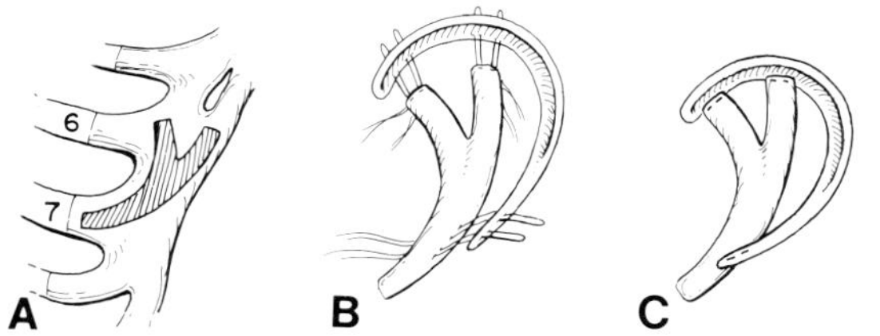

Figure 6.15 The cantilever framework design of Furnas using 6th and 7th costal cartilage to form the antihelix (*A*) and 8th rib for the helix (*B*). The helix and antihelix framework are assembled (*C*) and ready for positioning. (Reproduced with permission from D. W. Furnas: *Symposium on Recostruction of the Auricle*, C. V. Mosby, St. Louis, 1974.[10])

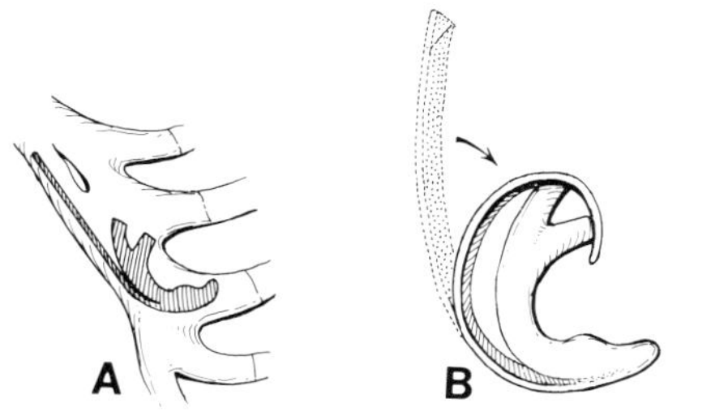

Figure 6.16 The "expansile framework" of Brent was designed for totol ear reconstruction in the adult obtaining the complete framework from the 7th costal cartilage (*A*). The cartilage strip is sutured to the antihelical crura to form the helix (*B*).

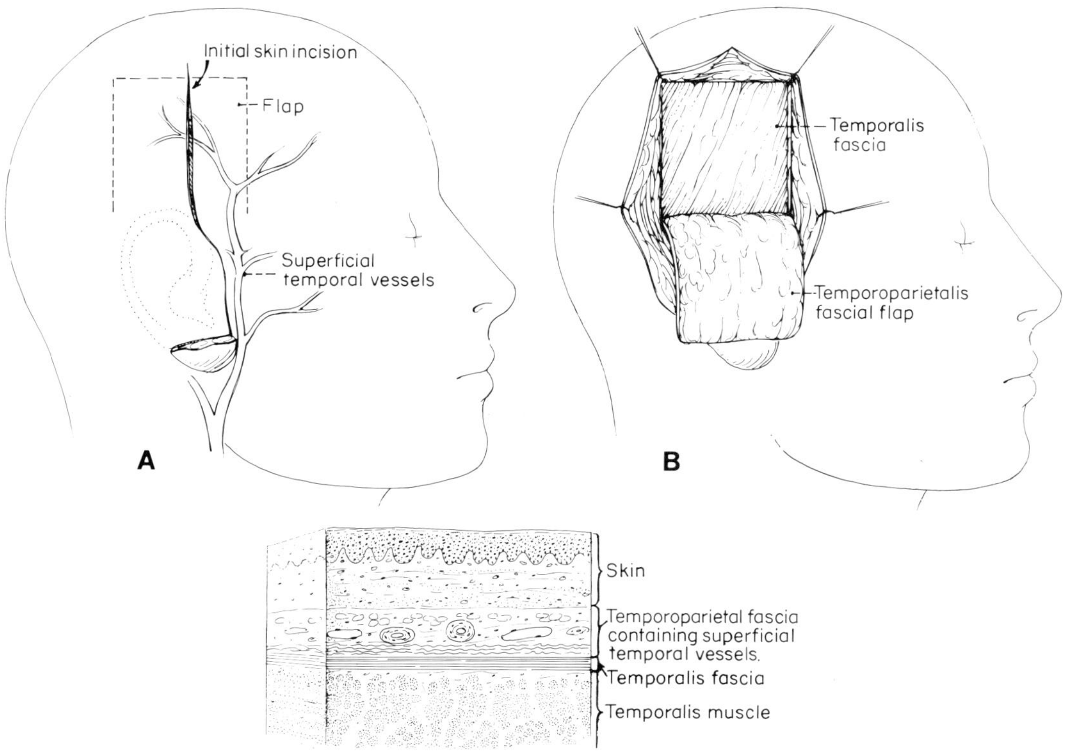

Figure 6.17 Tegtmeier's temporoparietalis flap is a thin, strong fascial layer containing superficial temporal vessels. Through a preauricular incision extended into the scalp (*A*), a rectangular flap of vascularized fascia can be turned to cover a synthetic ear framework (*B*). The flap can be seen to be superficial to the temporal muscle fascia.

child, the intraoperative time spent fabricating the ear framework, as well as the occasionally reported absorption of hyaline cartilage encouraged such trials. Silicone requires special handling but has been found to be reasonably reliable and dependable when careful attention to detail and surgical principles are followed.[6, 8] A prosthetic implant has the advantage of greater softness, flexibility, and more natural contour than costal grafts, and avoids donor site wounds and lengthy and sometimes difficult framework fabrication.[7] The procedure can also be accomplished in fewer stages. A major drawback to this synthetic ear framework is its decidedly higher rate of extrusion. Nonetheless, in large series, extrusion rates of approximately 15% have been reported with most implants being eventually successfully reinserted. Improved results with silicone have been obtainable by covering the prosthesis with dacron mesh or fascia lata enhancing fibrous ingrowth. In addition, the avoidance of thin anesthetic or excessively stretched skin coverage, careful avoidance of seroma, hematoma or sepsis, and the use of soft implants have reduced extrusion significantly. Also, multiple perforations in the silicone have improved implant fixation secondary to tissue ingrowth.

One recent advance facilitating coverage of the synthetic framework by a thin, yet strong and well vascularized tissue, has been a temperoparietalis fascial flap (dependent on superficial temporal artery circulation) reported by Tegtmeier[23] (Fig. 6.17). This fascial flap can be turned to cover an implant and in turn itself accept a skin graft. The author found this flap particularly useful for secondary ear reconstruction or post-traumatic reconstruction.

PARTIAL EAR RECONSTRUCTION

With far greater frequency, the reconstructive surgeon is faced with traumatic or postoperative partial ear defects. Though requiring less extensive surgery, such defects tax the ingenuity of the operator to wisely use available local tissues to full advantage. Rarely does a partial ear defect require costal cartilage grafting, as these are usually well suited for local tissue transposition, or ipsi- or contralateral conchal cartilage grafts. Some success has been reported with perichondrial or free grafts, however these techniques have not yet come into common usage.[4]

Most commonly seen is the partial helical rim loss involving skin and cartilage. For small defects, local wound closure can be obtained with normal auricular contour using scaphal and antihelical triangular excision with accessory triangles.

Extensive rim defects can be closed by advancing local tissues using the technique described by Antia and Buch[1] (Fig. 6.18) Incisions in the helical sulcus through skin and cartilage allow rim advancement after separation of cartilage from posterior auricular skin. This technique achieves closure at the small expense of vertical lobule height and has been extended by Brent through V-Y helical crus advancement. This technique is also useful in lesions involving defects of the upper third of the auricle.

More extensive upper third auricle defects may require cartilage graft covered by preauricular or banner flaps (Figs. 6.19 and 6.20). Alternatively, reconstruction may be done with a contralateral conchal graft placed beneath the hairless preauricular skin and later attached to the auricle and elevated at a separate stage. Such a graft to the auricle can be placed deep to the hair bearing scalp and be later elevated with a subcutaneous envelope to be covered with a skin graft. Finally, if local tissue proves inadequate, a complete transposition flap of ipsilateral conchal cartilage and skin can be rotated to recreate the superior portion of the auricle.[4]

Most middle third defects can be closed by techniques similar to that described above for superior third defects.

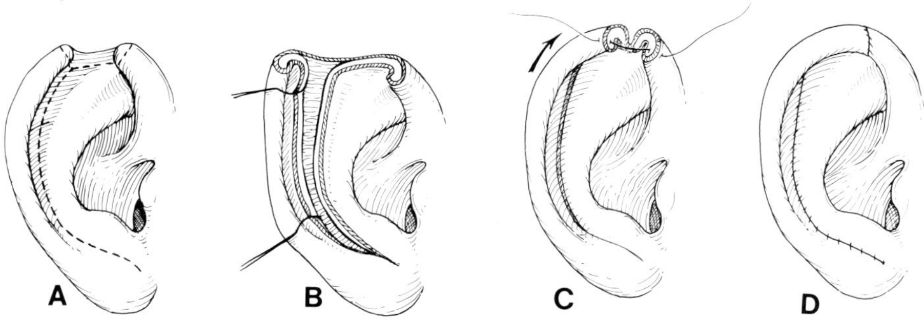

Figure 6.18 Closure of helical rim defects (*A*) can be accomplished using incisions in the helical sulcus through skin and cartilage (*B*) permitting advancement of the adjacent rim after separation from the medial or posterior auricular skin (*C*, *D*). (Reproduced with permission from N. H. Antia and V. I. Buch: *Plastic & Reconstructive Surgery*, *39*: 472, 1967.)

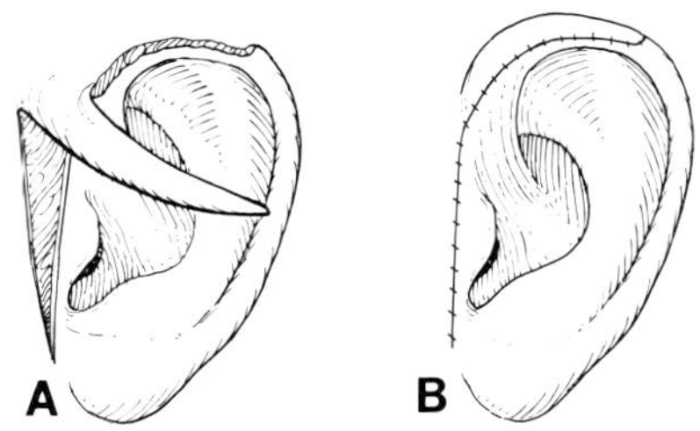

Figure 6.19 A preauricular flap can be raised to cover superior rim defects (*A*, *B*). (Reproduced with permission from B. Brent: *Plastic & Reconstructive Surgery*, *59*:475, 1977.[4])

Figure 6.20 A "banner flap" of postauricular skin can be elevated to cover extensive rim defects and rim cartilage grafts. (Reproduced with permission from B. Brent: *Plastic & Reconstructive Surgery*, *59*:475, 1977.[4])

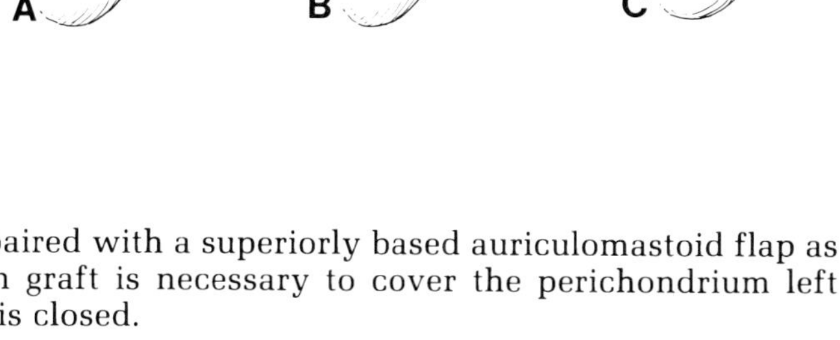

Defects of the lobule can be repaired with a superiorly based auriculomastoid flap as described by Brent. A small skin graft is necessary to cover the perichondrium left exposed after the mastoid defect is closed.

BURNED EAR DEFORMITY

Due to the exposed position of the ear and as its lack of bulk and its fragility, the auricle is particularly susceptible to thermal injury. In many ways such injuries provide deformities similar to those which the reconstructive surgeon confronts with microtia or partial ear loss. The complexity of the problem is often increased, however, by a lack of adequate soft tissue and coverage. Patients becomes a particular virtue when hypertrophic scar tissue is present. Delay for scar maturation, or thick split or full thickness skin grafting as a preliminary to reconstruction may be necessary, and lesser degrees of deformity including external auditory canal stenosis may be treated with local flaps, Z-plasty or a skin graft. Conchal cartilage (ipsi- or contalateral) may be used to supplement helical structure and, where only a helical rim defect is present, a migrated tubed cervical pedicle flap has been useful.[13] Principles of total ear reconstruction need be applied in reconstruction of the ear of the burn victim similar to the microtia patient; however, synthetic framework implantation has proven to be far less satisfactory. Dramatic extrusion rates in burn reconstruction has lead to a favoring of costal cartilage implantation. Contracture of the reformed retroauricular sulcus in such cases is particularly high, and the use of an ear conformer is particularly valuable for several weeks postoperatively.

References

1. Antia, N. H., and Buch, V. I.: Chondrocutaneous advancement flap for the marginal defect of the ear. *Plast. Reconstr. Surg.*, 39:472, 1967.
2. Brent, B.: Ear reconstruction with an expansile framework of autogenous rib cartilage. *Plast. Reconstr. Surg.*, 53:619, 1974.
3. Brent, B.: Earlobe construction with an auriculomastoid flap. *Plast. Reconstr. Surg.*, 57:389, 1976.
4. Brent, B.: The acquired auricular deformity. *Plast. Reconstr. Surg.*, 59:475, 1977.
5. Crikelair, G. F.: A method of partial ear reconstruction for avulsion of the upper portion of the ear. *Plast. Reconstr. Surg.*, 17:438, 1956.
6. Cronin, T. D., Greenberg, R. I., and Brauer, R. O.: Follow-up study of silastic framework for reconstruction of the external ear. *Plast. Reconstr. Surg.*, 42:522, 1968.
7. Cronin, T. D.: Use of a silastic frame for construction of the auricle, in *Symposium on Reconstruction of the Auricle*, p. 33, edited by R. C. Tanzer and M. T. Edgerton. C. V. Mosby, St. Louis, 1974.
8. Edgerton, M. T.: Ear reconstruction in children with congenital atresia and stenosis. *Plast. Reconstr. Surg.*, 43:373, 1969.
9. Elliot, R. A.: Otoplasty, in *Aesthetic Surgery: Trouble—How to Avoid It and How to Treat It*, p. 53, edited by E. H. Courtiss. C. V. Mosby, St. Louis, 1978.
10. Furnas, D. W.: Problems in planning reconstruction in microtia, in *Symposium on Reconstruction of the Auricle*, p. 93, edited by R. C. Tanzer and M. T. Edgerton. C. V. Mosby, St. Louis, 1974.
11. Gorney, M.: The ear as a donor site. Anatomic and technical guidelines, in *Symposium on Reconstruction of the Auricle*, p. 106, edited by R. C. Tanzer and M. T. Edgerton. C. V. Mosby, St. Louis, 1974.
12. Kaseff, L. G.: Investigation of congenital malformations of the ears with tomography. *Plast. Reconstr. Surg.*, 39:282, 1967.
13. Lynch, J. B., Bueno, R., Larson, D., and Lewis, S. R.: Reconstruction of burned ears, in *Symposium on Reconstruction of the Auricle*, p. 196, edited by R. C. Tanzer and M. T. Edgerton. C. V. Mosby, St. Louis, 1974.
14. Rogers, B. O.: Microtic, lop, cup and protruding ears. *Plast. Reconstr. Surg.*, 41:208, 1968.
15. Rogers, B. O.: Anatomy, embryology, and classification of auricular deformities, in *Symposium on Reconstruction of the Auricle*, edited by R. C. Tanzer and M. T. Edgerton. C. V. Mosby, St. Louis, 1974.
16. Steffensen, W. H.: A method of total ear reconstruction. *Plast. Reconstr. Surg.*, 36:97, 1965.
17. Stenstrom, S. J.: A natural technique for the correction of congenitally prominent ears. *Plast. Reconstr. Surg.*, 32:509, 1963.
18. Tanzer, R. C.: Total reconstruction of the external ear. *Plast. Reconstr. Surg.*, 23:1, 1959.
19. Tanzer, R. C.: Total reconstruction of the auricle. A 10 year report. *Plast. Reconstr. Surg.*, 40:547, 1967.
20. Tanzer, R. C.: The constricted (cup and lop) ear. *Plast. Reconstr. Surg.*, 55:406, 1975.
21. Tanzer, R. C., Bellucci, R. J., Converse, J. M., and Brent, B.: Deformities of the auricle, in *Reconstructive Plastic Surgery*, Ed. 2, *Vol. 3*, p. 1671, edited by J. M. Converse. W. B. Saunders, Philadelphia, 1977.
22. Tanzer, R. C.: Microtia—a long term follow-up of 44 reconstructed auricles. *Plast. Reconstr. Surg.*, 61:161, 1978.
23. Tegtmeier, R. E., Gooding, R. A.: The use of a fascial flap in ear reconstruction. *Plast. Reconstr. Surg.*, 60:406, 1977.
24. Washio, H.: Cryptotia; pathology and repair. *Plast. Reconstr. Surg.*, 52:648, 1973.

CHAPTER 7

Lip Deformities and Their Reconstruction

Malcolm A. Lesavoy, M.D., F.A.C.S.

CONGENITAL

Lip deformities can be both congenital and acquired. Of the congenital lip deformities, the most frequently seen by plastic and reconstructive surgeons are that of clefts of the lip. Occasionally, accompanying clefts of the upper lip are lip pits or lip sinuses. These lip sinuses are rare, however, they are frequently associated with clefts of the lip and palate. Patients who have clefts of the lip and lip pits have a 50% chance of having offspring with clefts of the lip and/or palate. At the present time, it is not completely understood how transmission of lip pits is accomplished genetically. Suffice it to say that lip pits are hereditary and are an important warning sign for the possibilities of clefts of the lip and/or palate in future generations. The author is presently involved with a family of Van der Hoeve's syndrome where multiple members in three generations are affected by clefts of the lip and palate and lip pits. The treatments of lip pits is that of excision. One must be aware that the actual lip pit usually is connected to a vertical tract that is lined with mucosa. One must be careful to excise the entire tract and mucosa when excising the lip pit. Most importantly, however, the patient or patient's family must realize the significance of this small (and sometimes cute) "dimple" in the lower lip. The patient and family must constantly be reminded that just because the lip pit is excised, chances for transmission for future offspring with clefts of the lip and palate are great.

It is not within the realm of this book to discuss deformities and subsequent surgical treatment of congenital clefts of the lip. Dr. D. Ralph Millard, Jr., has recently written a three-volume masterpiece that encompasses his life's work concerning clefts of the lip and palate. The reader is encouraged to read *Cleft Craft* and be stimulated by this great work.

TRAUMA

Other deformities of the lips that are acquired in nature can be traumatic or neoplastic. Of the traumatic type, the common everyday emergency room occurrence of a "split lip" of a child while falling or that of a cut lip from a belligerent fist should be understood and cared for properly. Technically, the inner border of lips are that of the firm and nongiving teeth. If a firm object subsequently strikes a direct blow to the lips, the sandwich is completed and the soft tissue between (lips) must give. For that reason, the human lip is in great jeopardy to trauma. Frequently, the lacerations of blunt trauma are not incurred by the offending object (i.e. fist, pool cue, etc.) but by the back-up of the lips, the teeth. The treating surgeon must keep in mind the tremendous bacterial content of the human mouth and understand that a cut lip must be considered a "human bite" with appropriate treatment.

If there are through and through lacerations of the lip produced by jetting teeth, total excision of the wound margins, copious irrigation, and careful closure can be accomplished under local anesthesia. The definitive closure should always maintain appropriate landmarks of the lips so that the orbicularis muscle approximation is accomplished and good skin cover is maintained. If the laceration is through and through to the buccal mucosa, frequently loose approximation or even nonclosure of the oral mucosa can be accomplished for appropriate drainage. Tetanus toxoid and penicillin is almost always appropriate in these types of cases.

If the laceration is in a vertical fashion and encompasses, not only the vermilion, but the mucocutaneous border, appropriate interrupted sutures at definitive landmarks should be placed after wound excision has been accomplished. One should not start suturing a wound of this type from either end, but first the surgeon must be absolutely certain that the *white roll* and mucocutaneous or vermilion border are perfectly alligned. One must be certain to approximate the orbicularis oris muscle so that competency of the oral stoma is maintained and splinting of the wound is accomplished. Good muscle approximation will prevent future cutaneous scar widening for lack of appropriate skin tension. Frequently, one is called to the emergency room by the uninitiated junior houseofficer who states that the lip laceration has produced missing tissue of the lip. Obviously, one must understand the function of the orbicularis oris muscle and that, if it is completely divided, contraction away from the wound will give the appearance of missing tissue. A simple maneuver of reapproximating the muscle closes the wound "miraculously." One must also keep in mind that if there truly is avulsed tissue of the upper or lower lip, one can still reapproximate and successfully join wound edges when up to 30% of the lip is missing. This accounts for the tremendous distensibility of the three elements of the lip (skin, orbicularis oris muscle, and buccal mucosa). If more than 30% of the lip tissue is missing, other reconstructive methods will have to be employed and will be discussed later in this chapter.

Electrical burns of the lip commissure are a fairly frequently observed injury. Most children affected in this manner are between the ages of 1 and 4 years. Most of these children bite the free end of a "live" extension cord. The lips, and specifically the oral commissures are wet and subsequently have decreased resistance to the electrical current. For this reason the damage is fairly localized in this area.

Immediate excision of the damaged tissue has been advocated by some, however, in general, most plastic surgeons feel that conservative therapy with topical antibiotics and tincture of time will allow the eschars to separate and the wound to demarcate. Secondary healing will occur and result in a deformity that can later be reconstructed. These patients should be hospitalized for 3 or 4 days (depending on the extent of injury). The only real difficulty will occur after 24 or 48 hours if the labial artery at the commissure is involved in the burn. Bleeding from this vessel can be both a traumatic and dangerous experience for the patient and his family if this occurs in the middle of the night in the home, and if those involved are not aware of this problem. For this reason, hospitalization for a short post-traumatic period is advisable.

NEOPLASM

Neoplastic deformities of the lips can result from leukoplakia and basal cell and squamous cell carcinomas. Leukoplakia affects the oral mucous membrane and is a premalignant lesion frequently found in cigarette smokers. Often, leukoplakia is found adjacent to areas of frank oral malignancy. It most frequently involves the lower lip and the treatment of choice is surgical excision. A "lip shave" procedure is usually performed that eliminates "most" of the leukoplakia. It is imperative that the patient be educated to eliminate tobacco, etc., and to carefully observe his lips for recurrent disease as manifested by ulceration or white plaques.

Basal cell carinomas most frequently involve the exposed areas of the body, specifically the face, and frequently the upper lip. Basal cell carcinomas vary in appearance, but are usually ulcerated at the centers with classically raised, pearly borders. In general, basal cell carcinomas do not metastasize and can be adequately excised. In general, 5–6 mm of visual normal border should be taken along with the tumor.

The lower lip is frequently involved by squamous cell carcinoma. Most squamous cell carcinomas occur in the region of the head and neck, however, the lower lip is the most frequent area of the face that squamous cell carcinomas occur. Histopathologically, squamous cell carcinomas can range from well differentiated to highly differentiated tumors, and unlike basal cell carcinomas, can metastasize to regional lymph nodes. For this reason, large squamous cell carcinomas of the lower lip (greater than 2–3 cm in diameter) should be considered for radical neck dissection accompanying the primary tumor excision. This is still a controversial point, however if clinical nodes are palpable on the ipsilateral neck, regional lymph nodes dissection is warranted.

RECONSTRUCTION

The defects of the upper and lower lips (be they created by trauma or neoplasm) should be divided into three parts: upper lip deformities, lower lip deformities, and commissure deformities. Anatomically, the lips and eyelids can be compared in that the upper lip (as is the upper eyelid) is the most important as far as contour is concerned. In eyelid reconstruction (Chapter 4) the lower eyelid is sacrificed for reconstruction of the upper eyelid. The lower eyelid is then subsequently reconstructed from local cheek skin. In the lip, one must keep in mind "the normal." The upper lip gently protrudes beyond the anterior projection of the lower lip. For this reason, the lower lip is minimally hidden by the overhanging upper lip, and is a subtle dimension that should be kept in mind. This is most important when construction or reconstruction of a commissure is attempted. The lower lip will share and give its tissue for upper lip and commissure reconstruction (specifically the vermilion), and subsequently the lower lip vermilion and fullness will be reconstructed from local buccal mucosa.

The importance of the lower lip and its contribution to the oral stoma is that, functionally, it maintains oral secretions and prevents drooling. The patient that has a magnificent looking lower lip that does not function correctly as a dam or competent portion of the oral sphincter or allows constant drooling is an unhappy patient. Therefore, cosmetically, the upper lip is most important, however, functionally, it does not have the same tremendous importance of the lower lip. Once "the normal" is appreciated, the particular defect of the lip deformity can be documented, and reconstruction can be planned.

As previously mentioned, for excision, avulsions, and incisions, of the upper or lower lips that are less than 30% of the horizontal dimension of the respective lip, direct approximation and closure can be accomplished. This must be done in layers after sharp debridement has been carried out.

If, however, the horizontal defect is greater than 30%, tissue must be added from the opposite normal lip to share this deformity. For example, if there has been a 40% loss of the upper lip, 20% of the lower lip can be used for reconstruction of the upper lip, and in this way, both lips will have less than 30% deformity. If however, there is major horizontal loss and 30% or less of the opposite normal lip will not add up to 70% (greater than 60% loss), then other distant flaps may be needed for lip reconstruction.

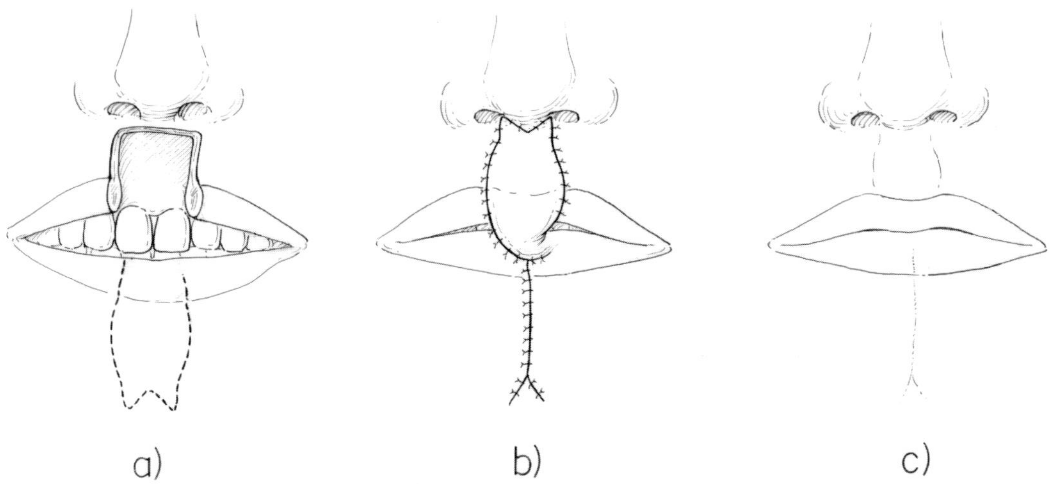

Figure 7.1 Abbé flap transposition. Shield-shaped flap is formed so that a inconspicuous blend is constructed with the base of the columella and nostril sills.

Opposing lip flaps have been well described and frequently used. Abbé in 1898 first described his lip-sharing method. This has been a tried and true reconstructive tool for adding tissue to the central philtral region of the lip from a lower lip donor area (Fig. 7.1). This flap is carried on its arterialized pedicle (the labial artery) and can subsequently be divided 7–10 days later. It has even been described as a free-composite graft from time to time, but better fullness, more pliable tissue, and a more predictable result will be achieved with a vascularized flap. The donor area is closed primarily and is insignificant. For lip flap transposition, the patient obviously must be cooperative, for constant motion of the mouth and lips will utterly destroy the reconstruction. Occasionally, Ivy loops or intermaxillary fixation on a temporary basis has allowed the flap to heal in its new position without the constant motion of an uncooperative mouth. It should also be mentioned that the labial artery runs very superficial to the oral mucosal border of the vermilion. For this reason, a very small pedicle can be designed both for comfort and ease of division and insetting 10 days after the transposition. The Abbé flap can be used for both central and lateral lip defects (Fig. 7.2) and carries with it the entire fullthickness portion of the lower lip, i.e. skin, muscle, oral mucosa, and the vermilion. For this reason, Abbé flap reconstruction allows for total continuity of the oral stoma. It has even been mentioned that the muscular portion of the Abbé flap becomes innervated by appositional nerve ingrowth (neurotization). Recently, work has been done on laboratory models, but at worst, the living muscle acts as a link in the broken chain reconstituting the competency of the oral stoma.

Reconstruction of lower lip defects can be accomplished with "lip-switch" procedures as originally described by Estlander in 1872. This also is a two-stage procedure with the donor lateral upper lip being used for sharing of tissues to reconstruct lower lip lateral defects. A secondary procedure is needed to reconstruct the obliterated commissure. The names of Estlander and Abbé are used interchangeably and incorrectly at times, but both illustrate the important principle of sharing from a normal lip for the ultimate reconstruction of missing parts of an abnormal lip. Many variations on both of these procedures can be carried out and are only limited by the imagination of the surgeon. Vermilion Abbé flaps as described by Gillies and Millard can be used for horizontal loss of vermilion both in trauma and to fill in contouring bulk in cleft lip deformities (as described recently by Kawamoto). For reconstruction of large amounts of vermilion when opposing lip vermilion cannot be shared, a mucosal apron flap as described by Gillies and Millard is very useful (Fig. 7.3). In this instance, the buccal mucosa of the opposing lip can be a donor flap based on the "normal" vermilion, and the donor defect skin grafted. Obviously, one cannot close the entire apron for a period of 7–10 days unless nasogastric feeding is accomplished. Lateral ports can be maintained and after division of the central apron, two smaller mucosal aprons can be constructed for the lateral ports (Fig. 7.4).

For massive deformities of the lower lip, bilateral lower lip and cheek advancements can be accomplished as described by Camille Bernard. This can be satisfactory in some cases, however, when competency of the lower lip is needed to prevent drooling, this operation sometimes falls short (Fig. 7.5). Karapandzic has described circular muscular advancements and tranpositions to maintain a competent oral stoma. This technique that Jabolay has recently popularized and reintroduced, is superior to the Camille Bernard reconstruction.

If both upper and lower lips have been completely destroyed, as in massive trauma, distant flaps are needed. For reconstruction of an entire mouth, it is wise to plan not only flap coverage, but also camouflage. In this vein, a temporofrontal scalp flap can be used (Fig. 7.6). A misdirected shotgun blast frequently will destroy the entire anterior portion of the face and cases such as these can illustrate graphically the essence of reconstructive surgery (Fig. 7.7 *A*). With the initial trauma, vigorous and sharp debridement must be carried out and all devitalized tissue must be discarded. Raw bone ends can be covered and saved for later reconstruction by closing oral mucosa to overlying skin (Fig. 7.7, *B* and *C*). After an appropriate period of time, swelling and edema will subside and future plans for reconstruction can be made (Figure 7.7*D*). In these types of devastating cases, the airway is of greatest importance at the initial injury and tracheostomy is almost immediately imperative.

Concern must be directed toward identifying the defect, and reconstruction of the entire upper lip must be planned. Not only are bony stabilization and reconstruction imperative, but their timing must coincide with soft tissue addition. It is not within the scope of this chapter to discuss bony reconstruction of the mandible and/or maxilla, but attention will be drawn to the upper lip. A twice delayed temporofrontal scalping flap based on the anterior branch of the superficial temporal artery can be elevated and lined with a split thickness skin graft (Fig. 7.7, *E* and *F*). Once the flap has been transposed into the upper lip position, the skin graft can be discarded if good flap coverage can be maintained for lining by turn-over adjacent "book flaps". A maxillary prosthetic obturator is important for maintenance of these lip flaps to prevent contracture (Fig. 7.7*G*). Three weeks after the inset, division and return of the temporal pedicle can be accomplished. In this way, an upper lip can be reconstructed in the male, to allow for good soft tissue augmentation and hairy camouflage of the lower lip (Fig. 7.7, *H–J*) (obviously, this is not appropriate in the female). Of interest in this patient is that the luxuriant mustache matches the moderately gray flaked scalp hair and is somewhat different in color and texture than the adjacent reddish beard. (One must wonder, what will happen 30 years from now if this patient were to develop male pattern baldness)!

In a similar case, this flap (as described by Gillies and Millard) can be used to construct a mustache even if good lip tissue is present. Camouflage is accomplished to replace skin grafts that were employed to treat burns from white phosphorus incendiary grenade. Once the flap is in place, "caterpillaring" of this flap can be used to create a central dimple (Fig. 7.8).

In many instances, tangential loss of tissue occurs from burn trauma. Because of the constant motion of the mouth and lips and the constant bathing by saliva, lip-tissue contraction and deformity frequently result. Release of this tissue and the placement of full thickness skin grafts as a cosmetic unit can be most helpful.

The production and construction of a normal commissure is frequently mandated after electrical burns of the mouth, neoplastic extirpation and second staged revision after "lip switch" transposition flaps. One must remember the principles that the upper lip cosmetically

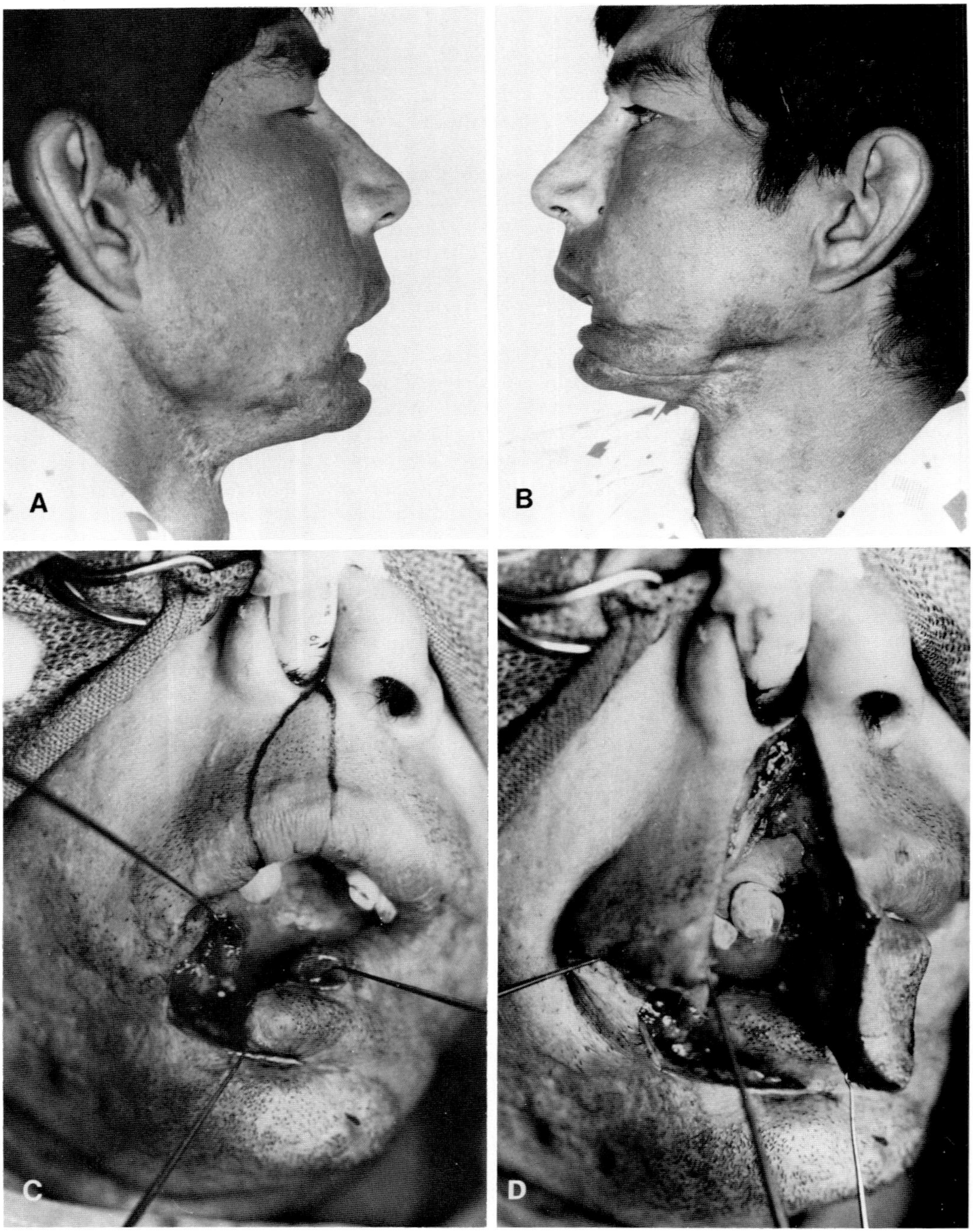

Figure 7.2 (*A*) Status post gunshot wound to lower jaw in childhood with reconstruction many years ago. Unacceptable oral commissure and contour profile. Right lateral profile. (*B*) Left lateral profile. (*C*) Oblique defect of lower lip created and upper lip transposition flap marked. (*D*) Upper lip transposition flap incised, based on labial artery.

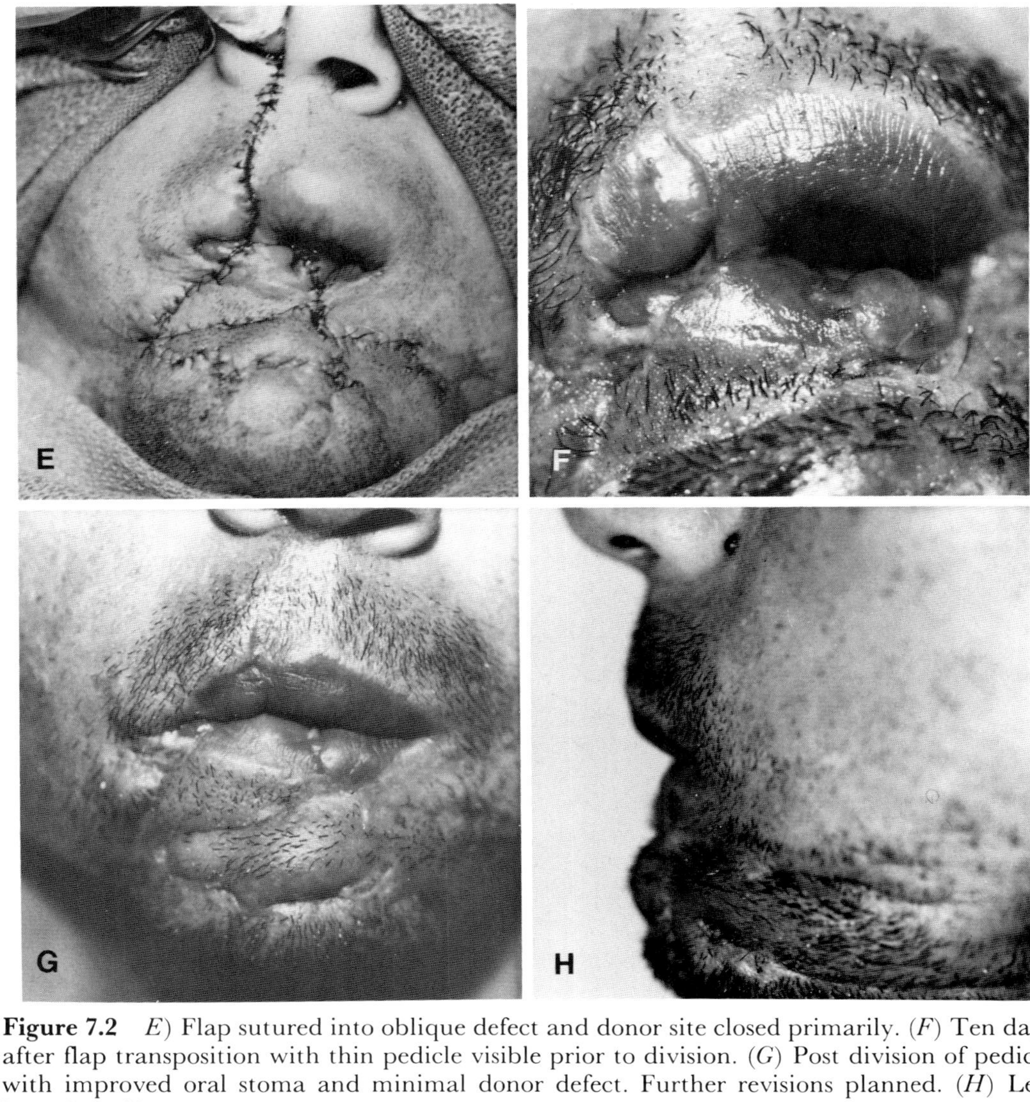

Figure 7.2 *E*) Flap sutured into oblique defect and donor site closed primarily. (*F*) Ten days after flap transposition with thin pedicle visible prior to division. (*G*) Post division of pedicle with improved oral stoma and minimal donor defect. Further revisions planned. (*H*) Left lateral profile.

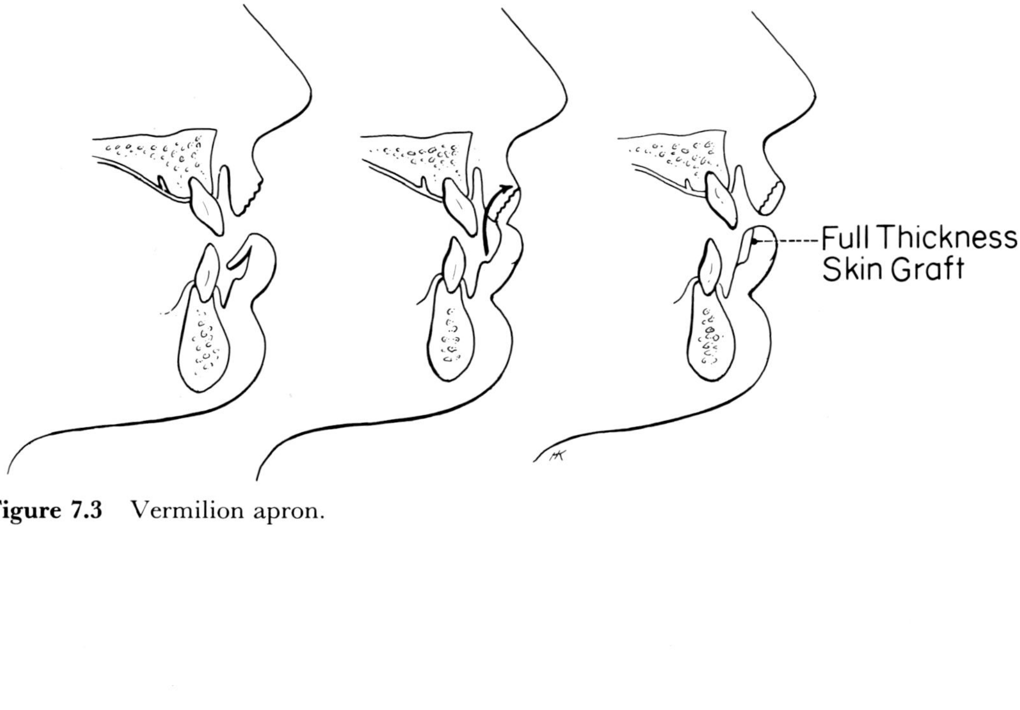

Figure 7.3 Vermilion apron.

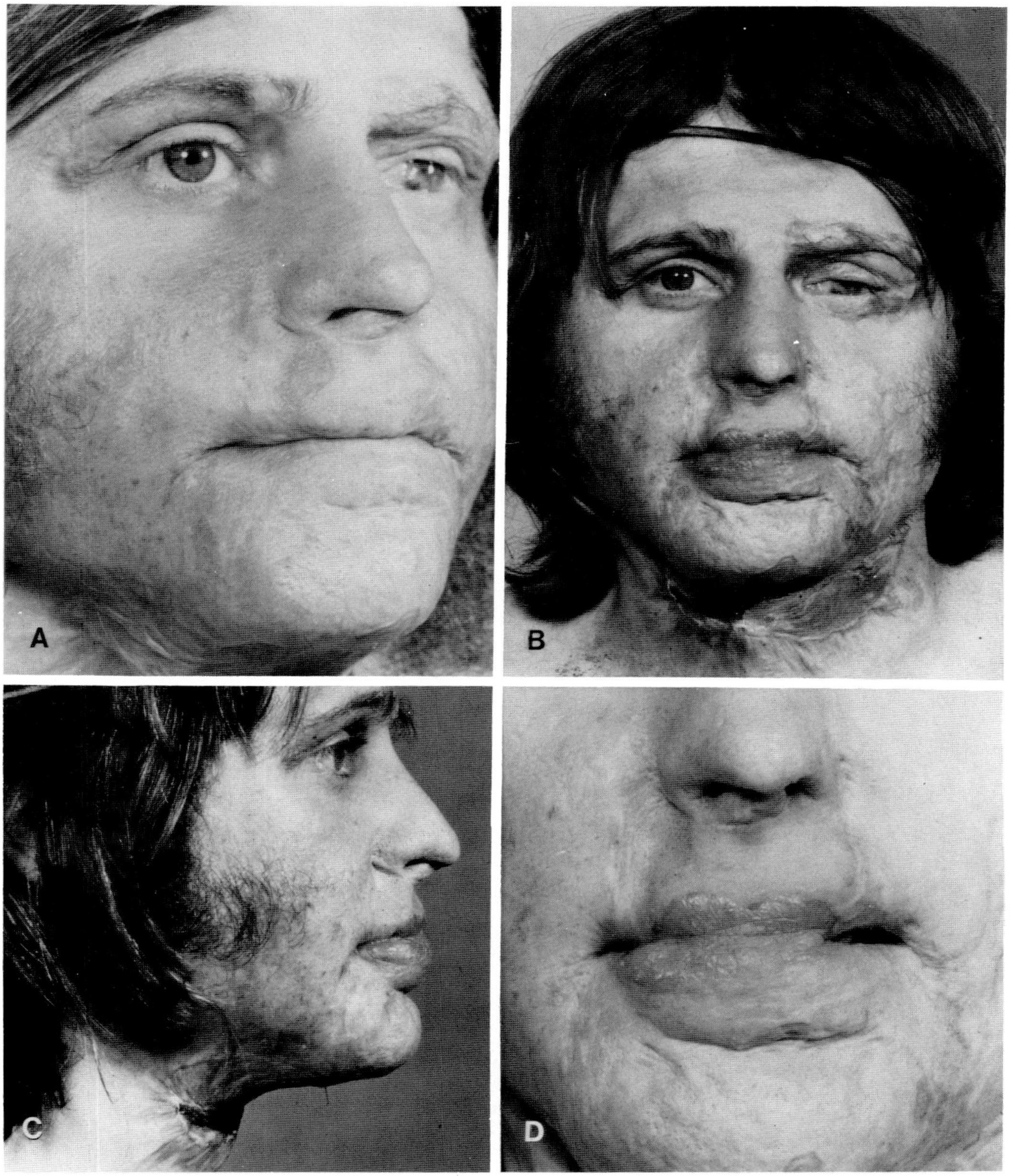

Figure 7.4 (*A*) Patient complains of dry and unacceptable "white vermilion" following severe burns. (*B*) Transposition of cupid's bow vermilion apron from lower to upper lip. Frontal view. (*C*) Right lateral view. Excised skin graft from upper lip used to cover lower lip donor site. (*D*) Prior to division of pedicle.

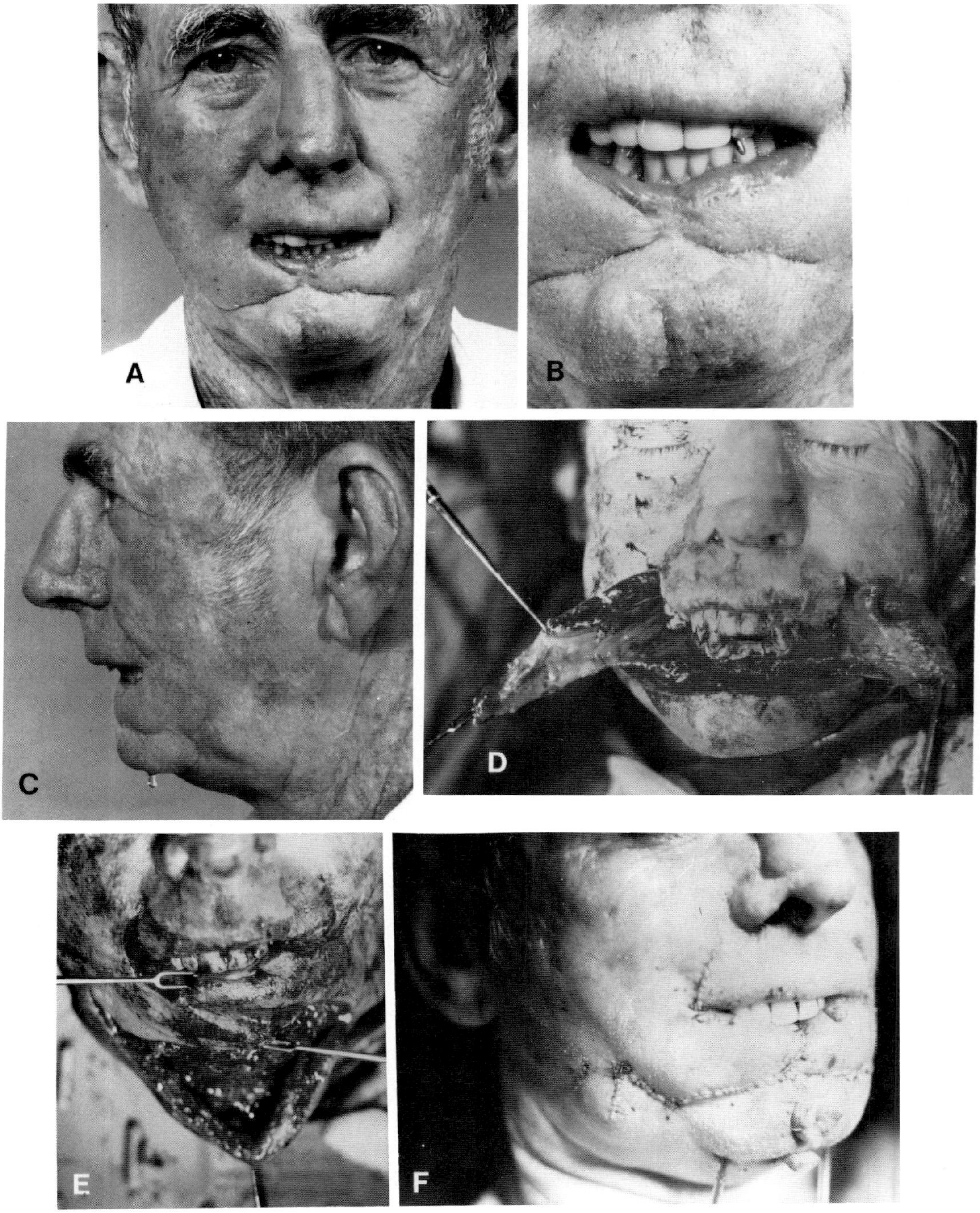

Figure 7.5 (*A*) Severe tightness and incompetent lower lip following multiple excisions for basal cell carcinoma. (*B*) Tight upper lip unacceptable as donor site. (*C*) Left lateral profile revealing drooling. (*D*) Lateral lip flaps elevated. (*E*) Chin flap elevated. (*F*) Flap sutured in place.

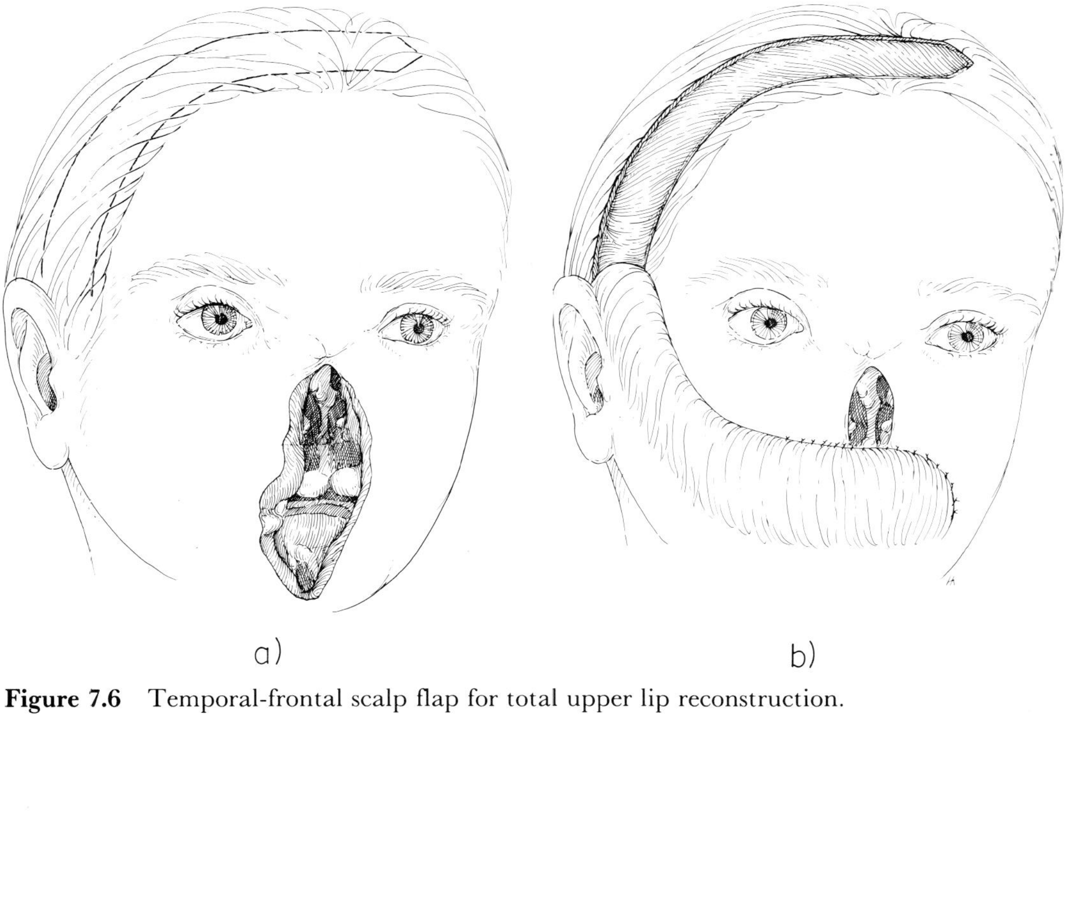

Figure 7.6 Temporal-frontal scalp flap for total upper lip reconstruction.

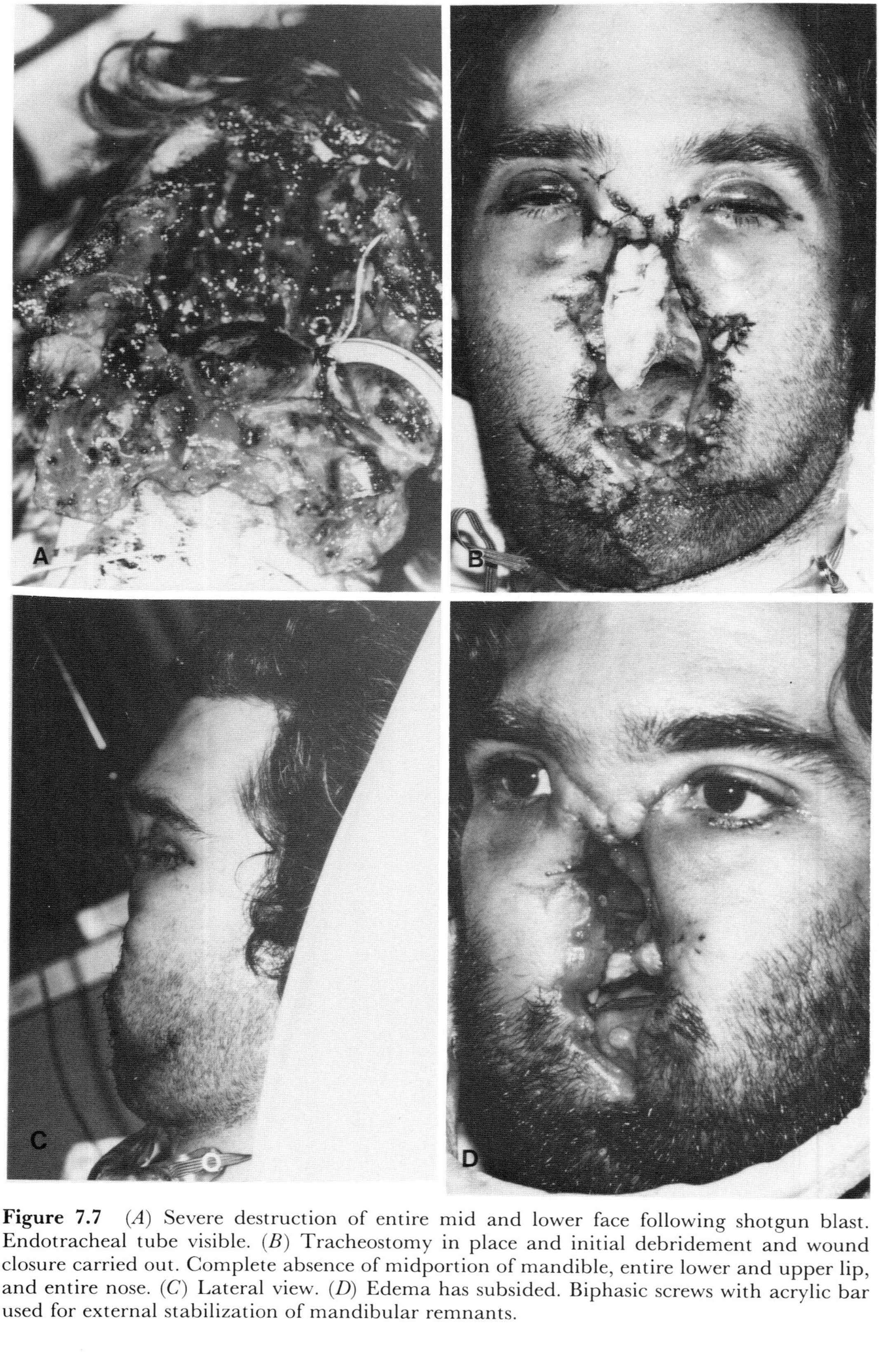

Figure 7.7 (*A*) Severe destruction of entire mid and lower face following shotgun blast. Endotracheal tube visible. (*B*) Tracheostomy in place and initial debridement and wound closure carried out. Complete absence of midportion of mandible, entire lower and upper lip, and entire nose. (*C*) Lateral view. (*D*) Edema has subsided. Biphasic screws with acrylic bar used for external stabilization of mandibular remnants.

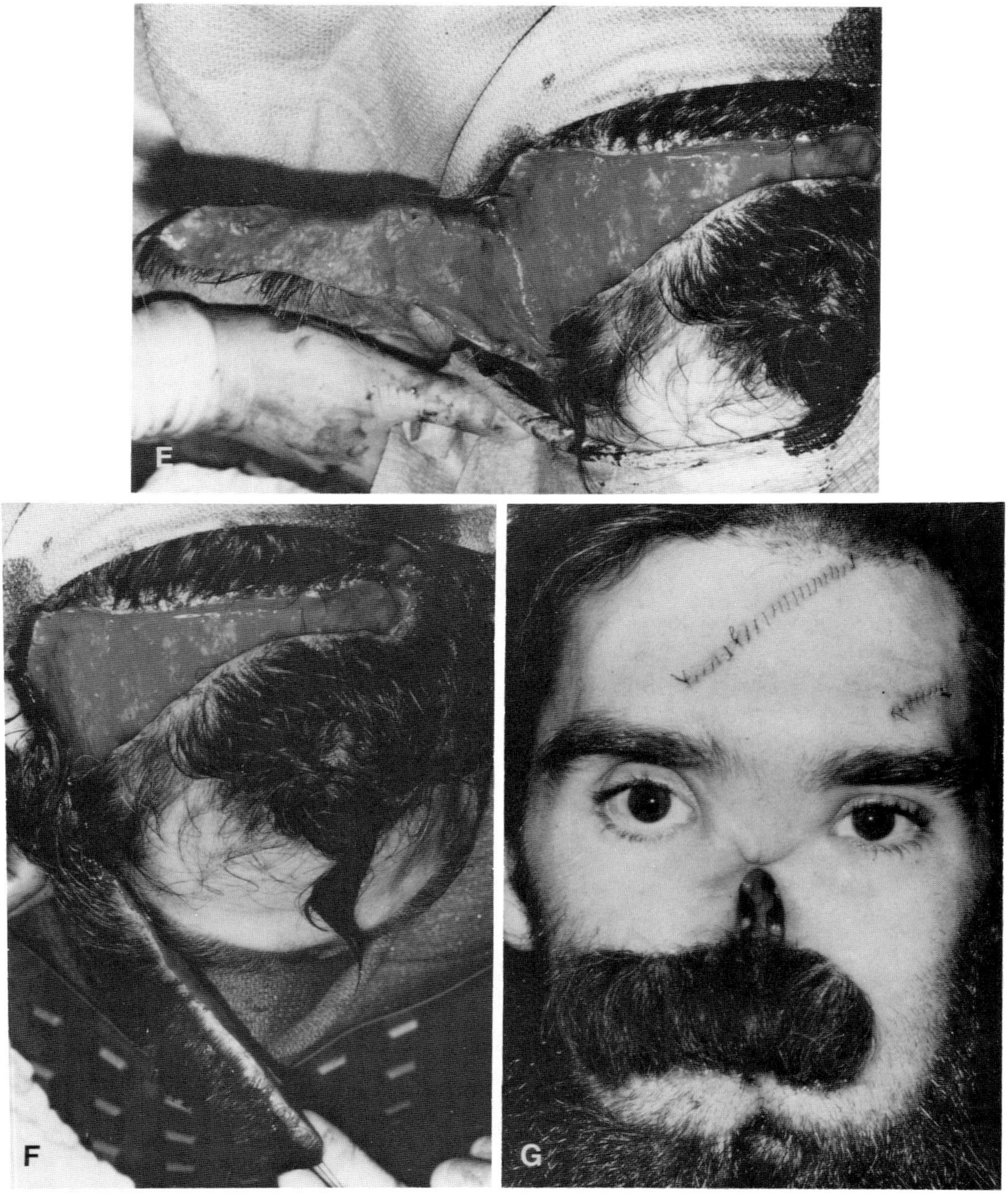

Figure 7.7 (*E*) Temporal-frontal flap elevated after two prior delays. (*F*) Transposition of flap to upper lip position. Primary closure of partial donor defect with remaining defect split thickness skin grafted. (*G*) "Upper lip" in position and delay of oblique "seagull" flap for total nasal reconstruction. Mandibular reconstruction already completed.

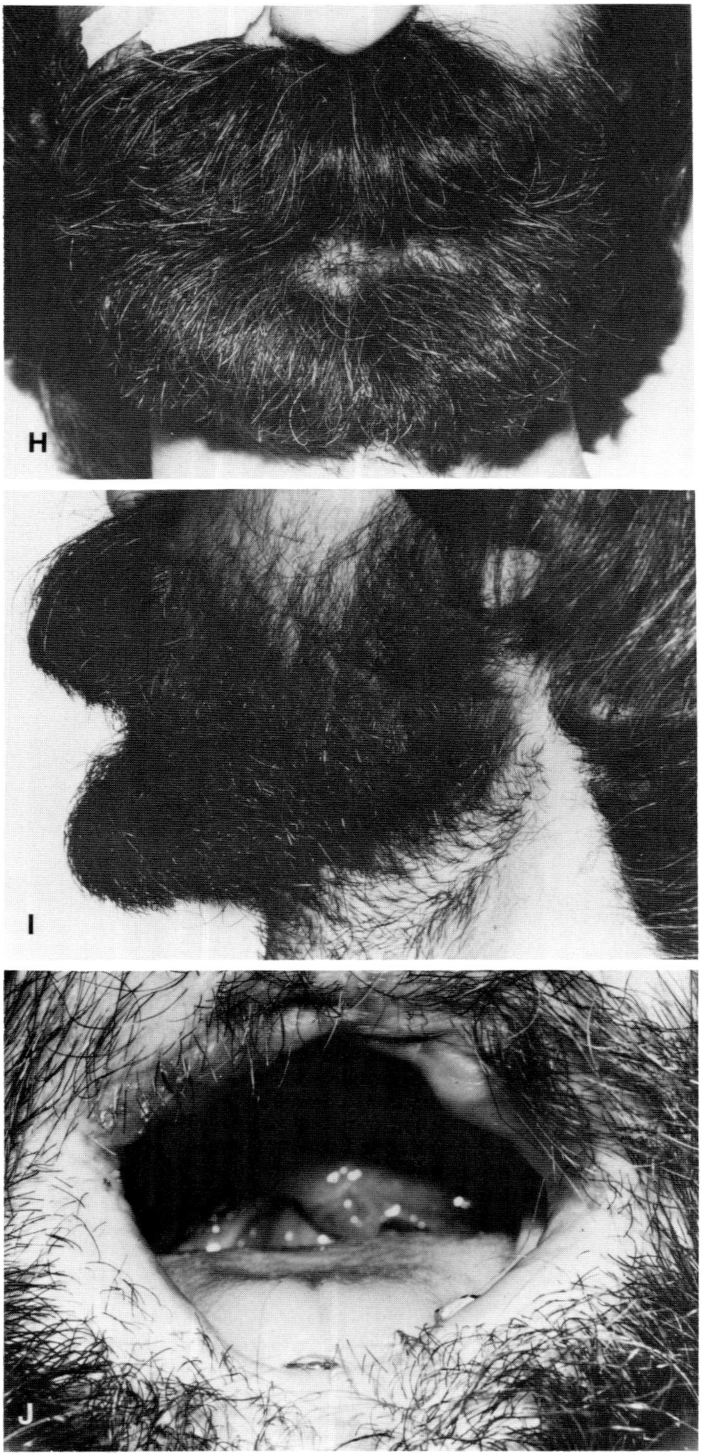

Figure 7.7 (*H*) Excellent camouflage and functional upper lip. (*I*) Left lateral profile. Mandibular reconstruction already completed. (*J*) Good functioning oral stoma.

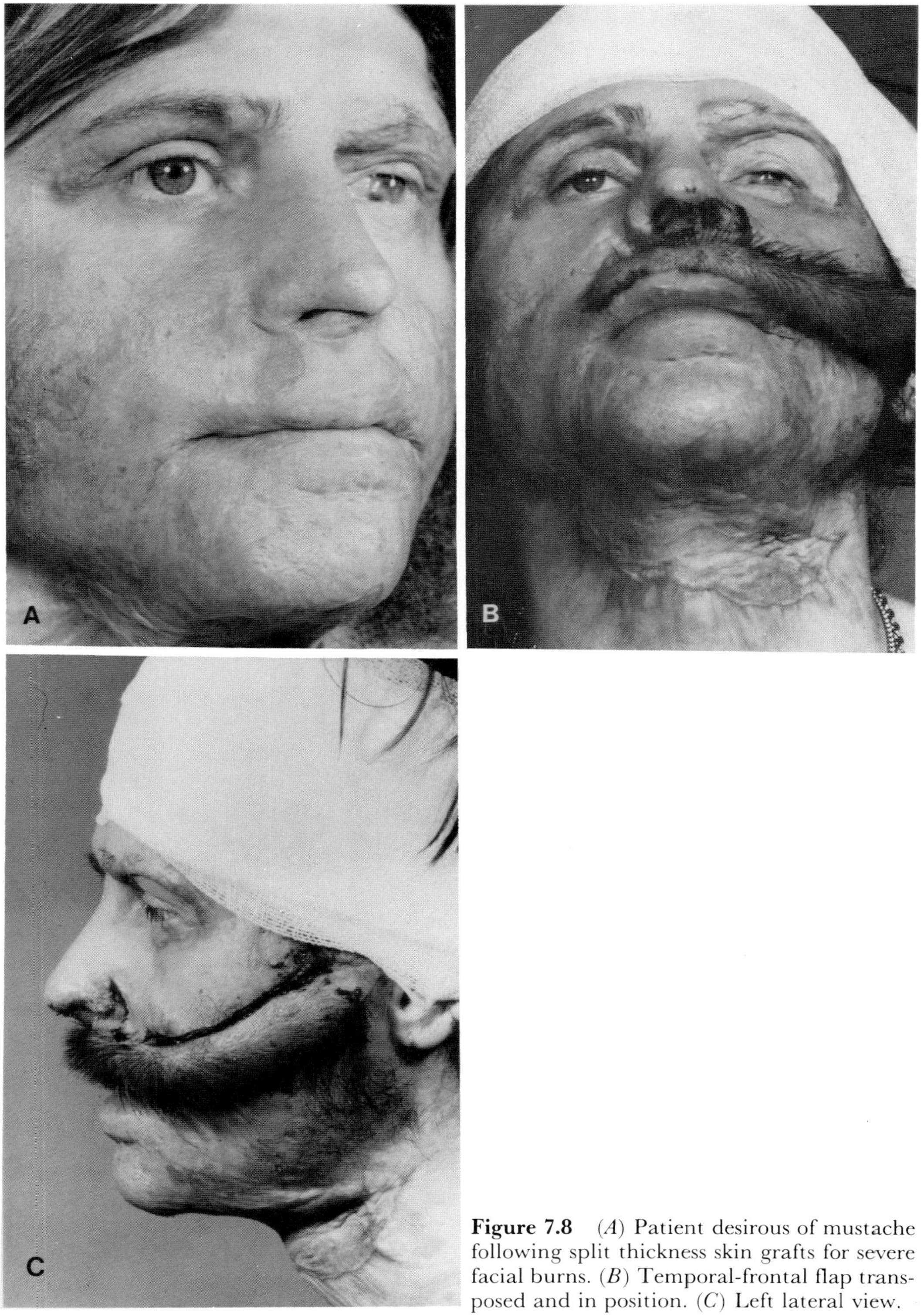

Figure 7.8 (*A*) Patient desirous of mustache following split thickness skin grafts for severe facial burns. (*B*) Temporal-frontal flap transposed and in position. (*C*) Left lateral view.

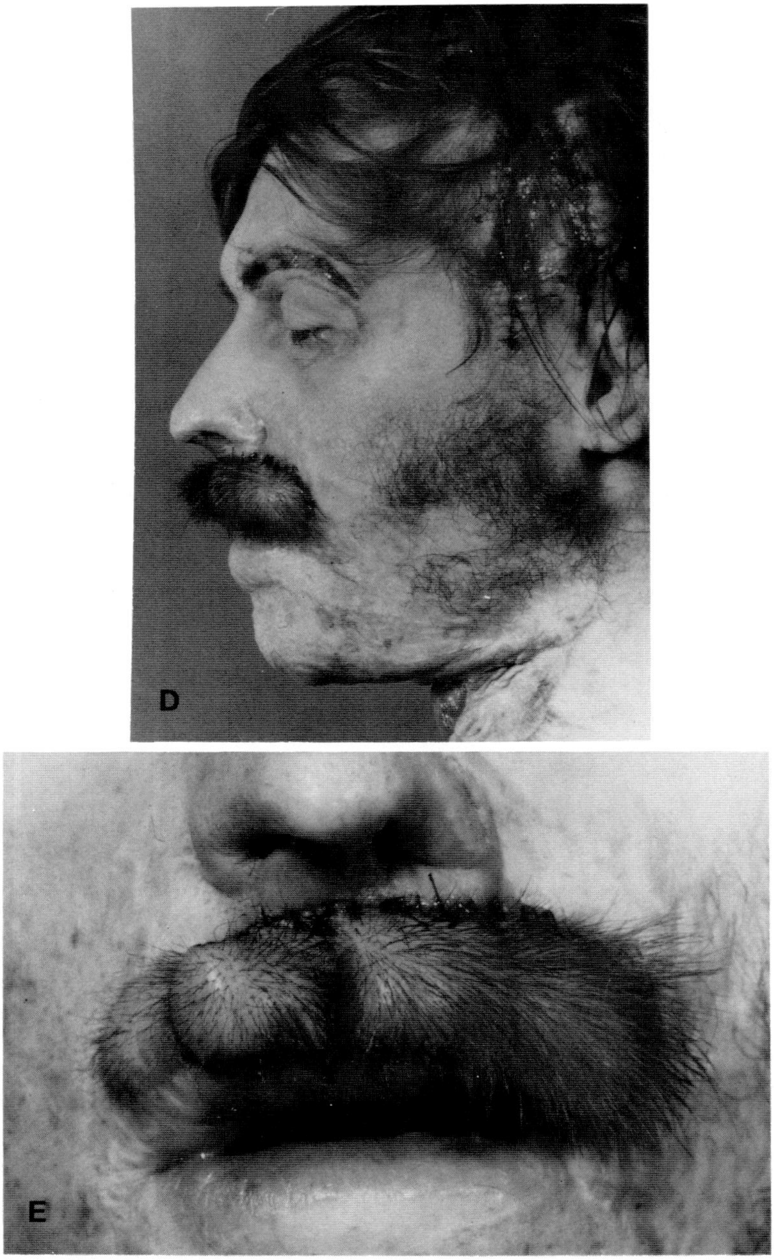

Figure 7.8 (*D*) Pedicle divided and returned to its donor site. (*E*) "Caterpillaring" of flap to produce central dimple.

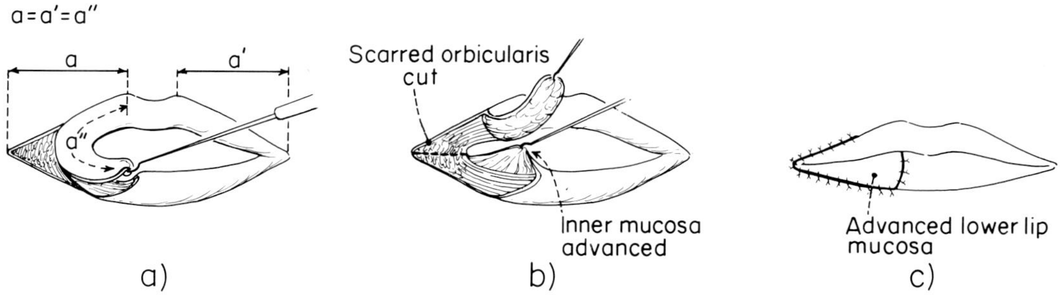

Figure 7.9 Procedure for creation of commissure (modified from Gilles and Millard (1957).

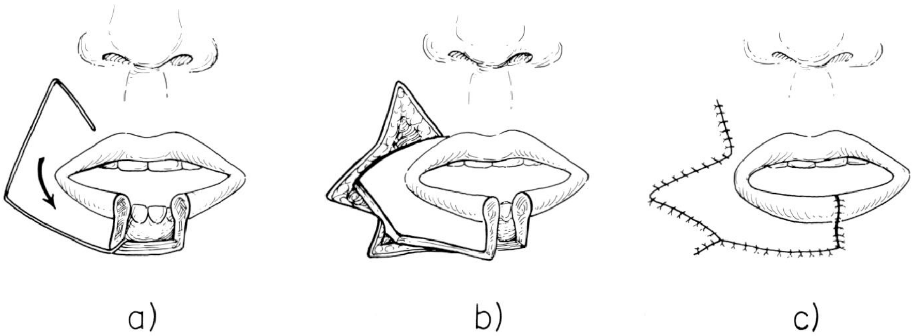

Figure 7.10 "Fan-flap" reconstruction for lower lip defect (modified from Gilles and Millard (1957).

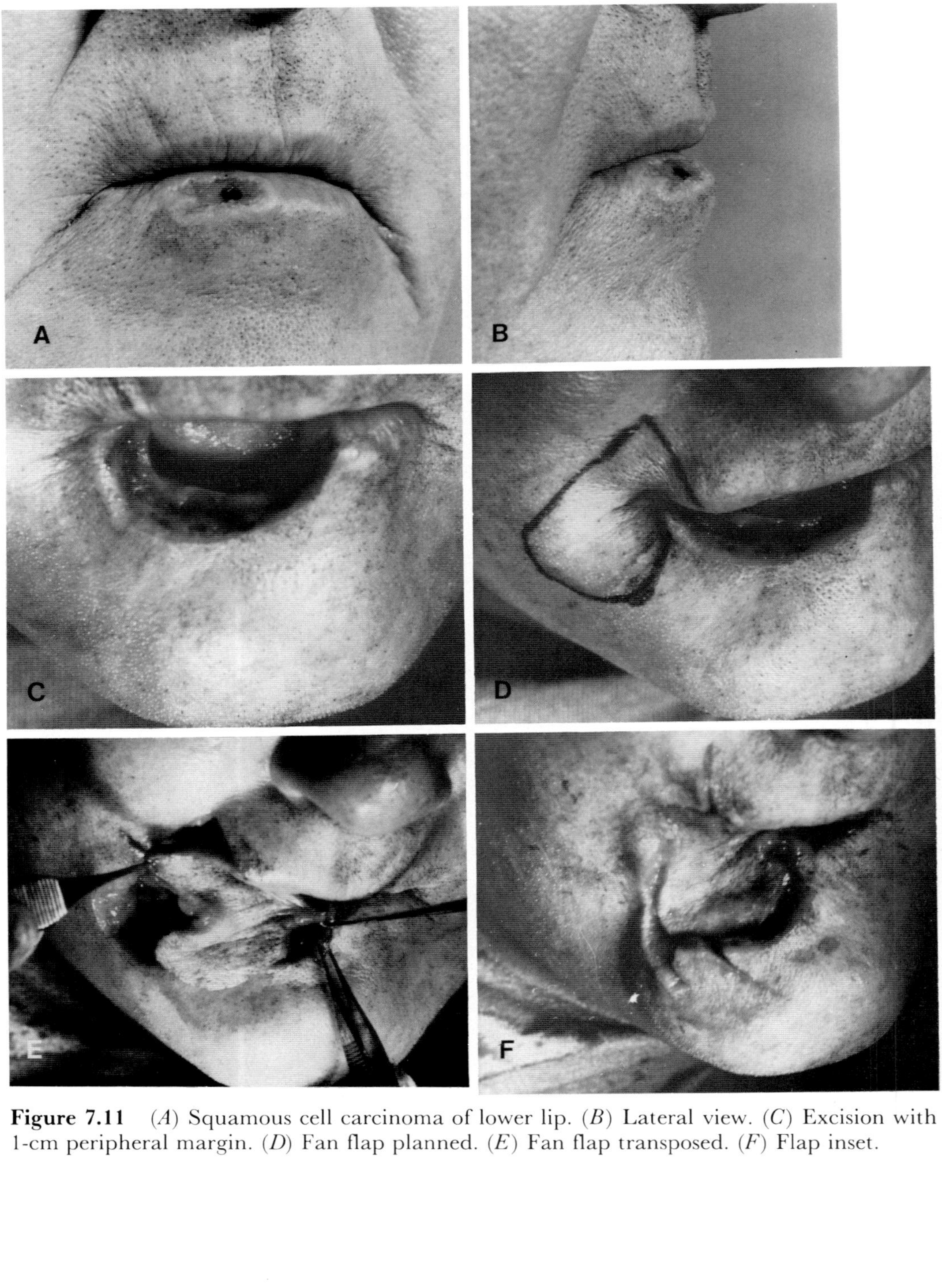

Figure 7.11 (*A*) Squamous cell carcinoma of lower lip. (*B*) Lateral view. (*C*) Excision with 1-cm peripheral margin. (*D*) Fan flap planned. (*E*) Fan flap transposed. (*F*) Flap inset.

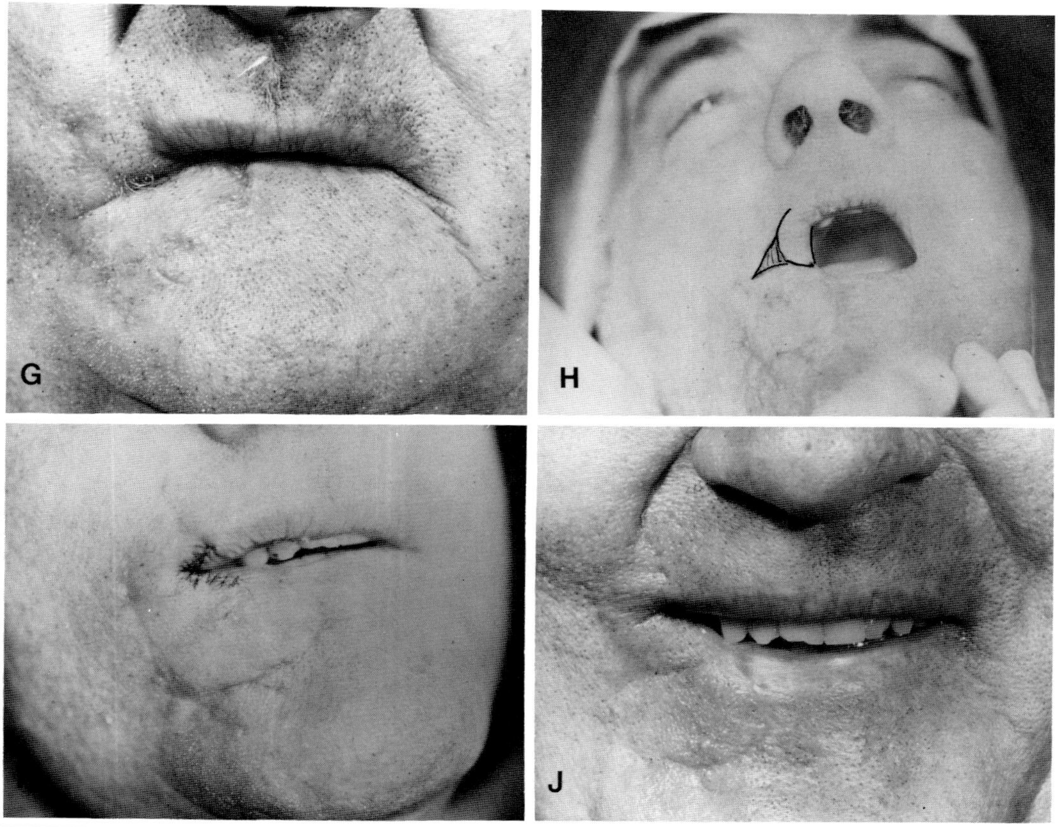

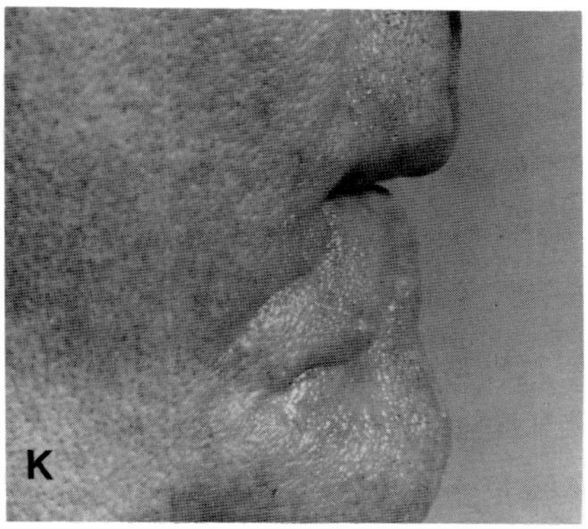

Figure 7.11 (*G*) Edema has subsided and right commissure needed. (*H*) Right oral commissure planned. (*I*) Commissureplasty. (*J*) Final result. (*K*) Right lateral view.

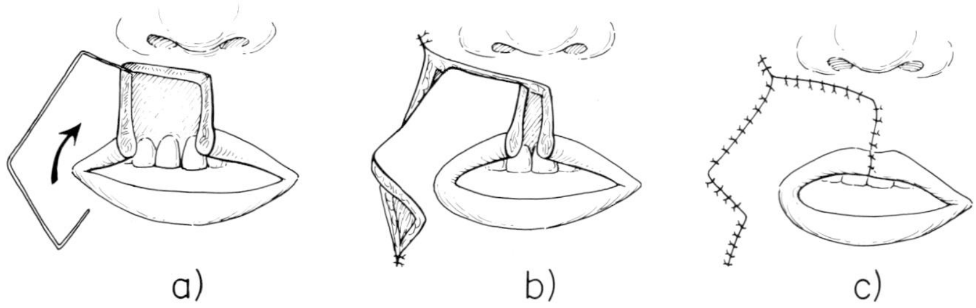

Figure 7.12 "Fan flap" for upper lip reconstruction (modified from Gilles and Millard (1957).

is more important and that sharing of the vermilion in the lower lip gives the most pleasing result. Spacial and anatomic relationships are very important and formation of a fantastic commissure in an abnormal location can look ridiculous. (This is analogous to ear reconstruction (Chapter 6). A well constructed ear in an incorrect position is not pleasing.) Careful measurement and knowledge of the "normal" is of utmost importance so that reconstruction of the commissure is placed symmetrical to the opposite normal commissure. One determines the most lateral aspect of the neocommissure (usually lies at an imaginary vertical line dropped from the midportion of the pupil). One must determine the point on this vertical line that the commissure should lie on a horizontal plane (Fig. 7.9). This can be determined on the normal side by measuring the distance from the lower eyelid to the normal commissure. The distance should then be measured from the normal commissure to the height of the normal cupid's bow and this distance tranposed from the ipsilateral cupid's bow height to the distance of the vermilion of the lower lip that corresponds. The vermilion flap is then raised from the lower lip based on the ipsilateral vermilion, the scar and orbicularis incised to the predetermined point, and the vermilion inset for reconstruction of the upper lip half of the commissure. Undermining an advancement of the adjacent lower lip buccal mucosa can then be brought up into view and sutured into the lower lip. This technique seems to offer advantages of upper lip camouflage and maintains continuity of the upper lip vermilion. It also eliminates the three mucosal flaps drawing at the angle of the mouth that subsequently tend to contract as described by others.

Defects of either the upper of lower lip can also be reconstructed by the Gillies and Millard "fan flap" (Fig. 7.10). This technique is an extension of a lip switch procedure that is given its name by the vision of an opening fan in the eventual rotation-tranposition of this flap. Primary closure of the donor defect is accomplished; however, a secondary procedure is needed to restore the angle of the mouth. This flap can be used for either lower (Fig. 7.11) or upper lip defects (Figs. 7.12 and 7.13).

Throughout the various gymnastics that one can use for reconstruction of either the upper of lower lip, the reconstructive surgeon must always keep in mind "the normal." In reconstruction of the lips, the most important "normal" is *lining*. Although one can devise various techniques of constructing a beautiful lip on the operating table, without adequate lining, this lip will contract and become diminutive as time goes on. If one plans ahead for lining, the surgeon's work will be rewarded and not detracted with time.

The oral stoma and lips are an extremely vital portion of an individual's face and personality. It provides visual contact to our fellow man and conveys feelings and emotions at a glance. When one is speaking, the listener frequently stares at one's lips. Not only are lips

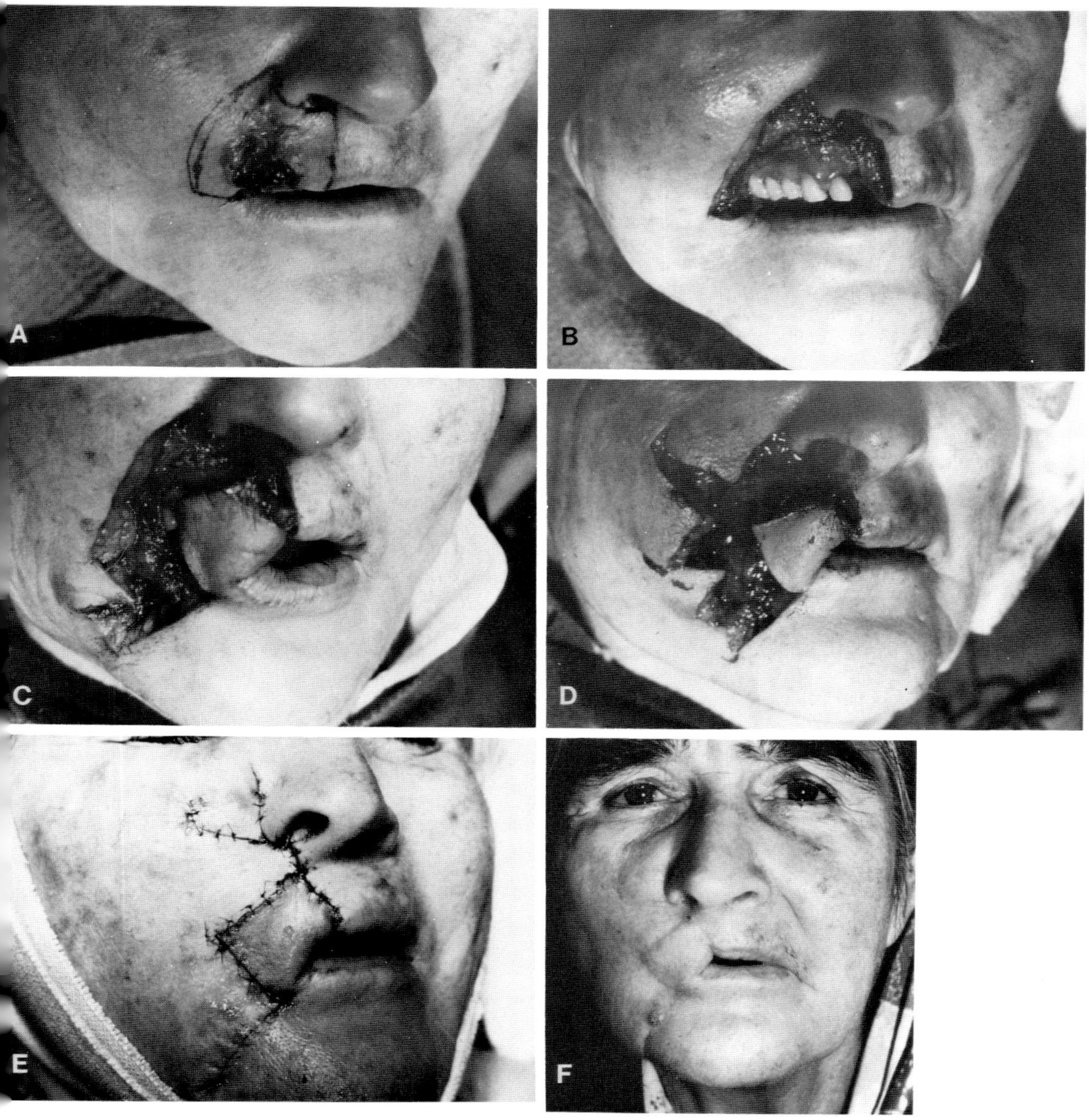

Figure 7.13 (*A*) Large squamous cell carcinoma of upper lip. (*B*) Excision of tumor with 1-cm peripheral margin including alar base and sill. (*C*) Lower lip fan flap transposed for upper lip reconstruction. (*D*) Local flap rotations for closure of donor defect. (*E*) Flap inset. (*F*) Edema has subsided and patient refused right commissureplasty.

important to the reception of speech, but they are extremely important in the formation of speech. The task of the reconstructive surgeon in maintaining this very important piece of anatomy is also encumbered by the lip function of feeding and competency of the oral stoma. At times, this can be an almost impossible task. But with ingenuity, imagination, and thought, the reconstruction of the lips can be a most rewarding and beneficial experience for all concerned.

References

1. Abbé, R.: A new plastic operation for the relief of deformity due to double harelip. The classic reprint. *Plast. Reconstr. Surg.*, *42*:481, 1968.
2. Ashley, F. L.: Reconstruction of the lower lip. *Plast. Reconstr. Surg.*, *15*:313, 1955.
3. Bakamjian, V.: Use of tongue flaps in lower lip reconstruction. *Br. J. Plast. Surg.*, *17*:76, 1964.
4. Bernard, C.: Cancer de la lèvre inférieure opéré par un procédé nouveau. *Bull. Mém. Soc. Chir. Paris*, *3*: 357, 1853.
5. Bowers, D. G.: Surgical repair of congenita—lower lip sinuses. *Plast. Reconstr. Surg.*, *49*:632, 1972.
6. Bowers, D. G., Jr.: Double cross-lip flaps for lower lip reconstruction. *Plast. Reconstr. Surg.*, *47*:209–214, 1971.
7. Cannon, B.: The use of vermilion bordered flaps in surgery about the mouth. *Surg. Gynecol. Obstet.*, *74*: 458, 1942.
8. Cervenka, J., Cerný, M., and Cisarová, E.: Heredity of fistulae to the lower lip and their relation to cleft lip and palate. *Cesk Pediatr.*, *21*:109, 1966.
9. Converse, J. M.: Technique of elongation of the oral fissure and restoration of the angle of the mouth, in *The Surgical Treatment of Facial Injuries*, edited by V. H. Kazanjian and M. M. Converse, p. 795, Williams & Wilkins, Baltimore, 1959.
10. Converse, J. M.: Orbicularis advancement flap for restoration of angle of the mouth. *Plast. Reconstr. Surg.*, *49*:99, 1972.
11. Dufourmentel, C., Mouly, R., Préaux, J., and Marchac, D.: La greffe composee libre de lèvre à lèvre. *Ann. Chir. Plast.*, *12*:119, 1967.
12. Estlander, J. A.: Classic Reprint. Eine Methode aus der Einen Lippe Substanzverluste der Anderen zu Erstetzen. (A method of reconstructing loss of substance in one lip from the other lip.) (Translated from the German by Dr. Borje Sundell.) *Arch. Klin. Chir.*, *14*:622, 1872; *Plast. Reconstr. Surg.*, *42*:360, 1968.
13. Flanagin, W. S.: Free composite grafts from lower to upper lip. *Plast. Reconstr. Surg.*, *17*:376, 1956.
14. Gillies, H. D.: *Plastic Surgery of the Face*, Oxford University Press, London, 1920.
15. Gillies, H. D., and Millard, D. R., Jr.: *Principles and Art of Plastic Surgery*, Little Brown, Boston, 1957.
16. Guerrero-Santos, J.: Use of a tongue flap in secondary correction of cleft lips. *Plast. Reconstr. Surg.*, *44*: 368–371, 1969.
17. Karapandzic, M.: Reconstruction of lip defects by local arterial flaps. *Plastic Reconstr. Surg.*, *46*:676, 1975; *Br. J. Plast. Surg.*, *27*:93, 1974.
18. Kanzanjian, V. H., and Converse, J. M.: *The Surgical Treatment of Facial Injuries*, Williams & Wilkins, Baltimore, Ed. 2, 1959; Ed. 3, 1974.
19. Kanzanjian, V. H., and Roopernian, A.: The treatment of lip deformities resulting from electric burns. *Am. J. Surg.*, *88*:884, 1954.
20. May, H.: *Plastic and Reconstructive Surgery*, Ed. 3, F. A. Davis, Philadelphia, 1971.
21. Martin, H. E., MacComb, W. S., and Blady, J. V.: Cancer of the lip. *Ann. Surg.*, *114*:226, 1941.
22. McGregor, I. A.: The tongue flap in lip surgery. *Br. J. Plast. Surg.*, *19*:253, 1966.
23. Millard, D. R.: A radical rotation in sigle harelip. *Am. J. Surg.*, *95*:318–322, 1958.
24. Millard, D. R.: Extensions of the rotation-advancement principle for wide unilateral cleft lips. *Plast. Reconstr. Surg.*, *42*:535, 1968.
25. Millard, D. R.: Closure of bilateral cleft lip and elongation of columella by two operations in infancy. *Plast. Reconstr. Surg.*, *47*:324, 1971.
26. Millard, D. R.: *Cleft Craft*, Little Brown, Boston, 1977.
27. O'Brien, B.: A muscle-skin pedicle for total reconstruction of the lower lip. *Plast. Reconstr. Surg.*, *45*:395, 1970.
28. Owens, N.: Simplified method of rotating skin and mucous membrane flaps for complete reconstruction of the lower lip. *Surgery*, *15*:196, 1944.
29. Smith, J. W.: The anatomical and physiologic acclimatization of tissue transplanted by the lip switch technique. *Plast. Reconstr. Surg.*, *26*:40, 1960.
30. Smith, J. W.: Clinical experiences with the vermilion border lip flap. *Plast. Reconstr. Surg.*, *27*:527, 1961.
31. Walker, J. C., and Sawhney, P.: Free composite lip grafts. *Plast. Reconstr. Surg.*, *50*:142, 1972.
32. Wang, M. K. H., and Macomber, W. B.: Congenital lip sinuses. *Plast. Reconstr. Surg.*, *18*:319, 1956.
33. Watson, A. C.: Innervated muco-muscular flap for correction of defects of vermilion border of lip. *Br. J. Plast. Surg.*, *26*:355, 1973.
34. Zarem, H. A., and Greer, D. M: Tongue flap for reconstruction of the lips after electrical burns. *Plast. Reconstr. Surg.*, *53*:310, 1974.

CHAPTER 8

Reconstruction of the Oral Cavity and Tongue

Harvey A. Zarem, M.D., F.A.C.S., and
John A. Perlman, M.D.

On reconstructing the oral cavity and tongue, the surgeon must carefully identify the patient's problems. Most reconstructions involving the oral cavity and tongue are complex, and there is a sparsity of literature dealing directly with problems within the oral cavity secondary to tumor ablation and radiation injury. The surgeon may be aware of various reconstructive techniques and may consider application of these techniques to the patient without the primary focus on the specific problems which the patient identifies.

DROOLING

When drooling occurs, it is the patient's primary complaint. The patients are seen with a tissue, handkerchief, or even a small towel which they keep with them at all times. They consider drooling to be a totally unacceptable problem and will often refuse to be seen in public. The drooling and associated loss of food when eating prevents them from eating in restaurants and many of these patients will refuse to eat in the presence of their immediate family. The causes of drooling are primarily an incompetent oral stoma associated with a pooling of saliva in the oral cavity. Reconstruction of the oral stoma may include excision of a portion of the lower lip in order to restore oral stoma competency.[5] However, this must not be carried to the extreme whereby the patient is unable to open the mouth adequately to use dentures or place utensils in the mouth. Reconstructing the lower or upper lip is best done with full thickness pedicle flap (skin, muscle, and mucosa) from the adjacent lip, the opposing lip, or the adjacent cheek.[11] Priority must be given to the lower lip when both lips are involved. Reconstructing the lower lip with remote tissues that do not include muscle and mucosa is sometimes necessary. When the lower lip is reconstructed with a skin pedicle flap such as the popular deltopectoral flap, the lip must have significant height and must have a good vertical attachment to avoid laxity and resultant drooling. Efforts to establish support of the lower lip with fascia lata sling are usually a failure.[24] In order to support the lower lip adequately with the fascia lata sling, the opening of the oral stoma is often reduced to the point where it is impractical. However, fascia lata sling support is sometimes the only straightforward approach

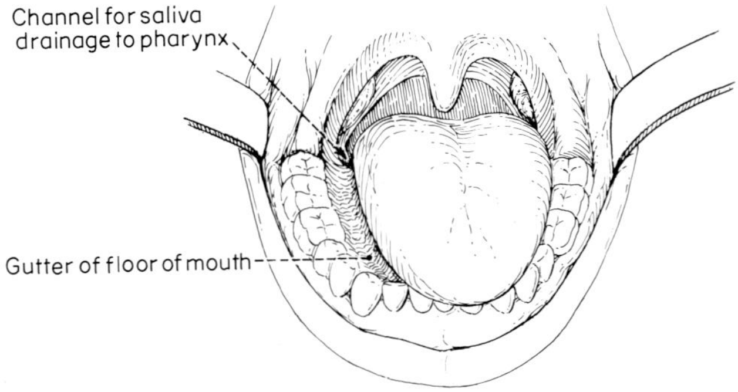

Figure 8.1

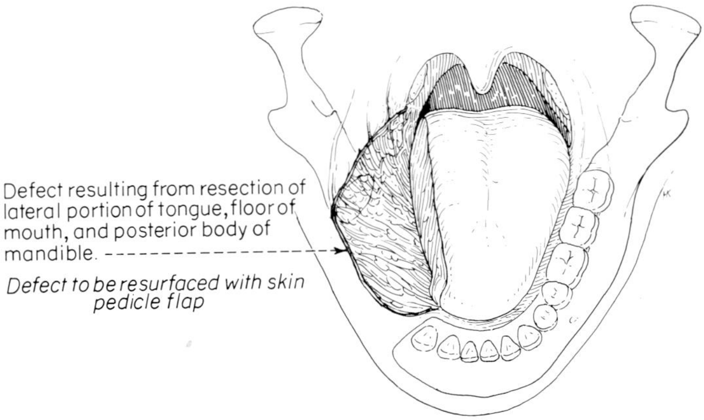

Figure 8.2

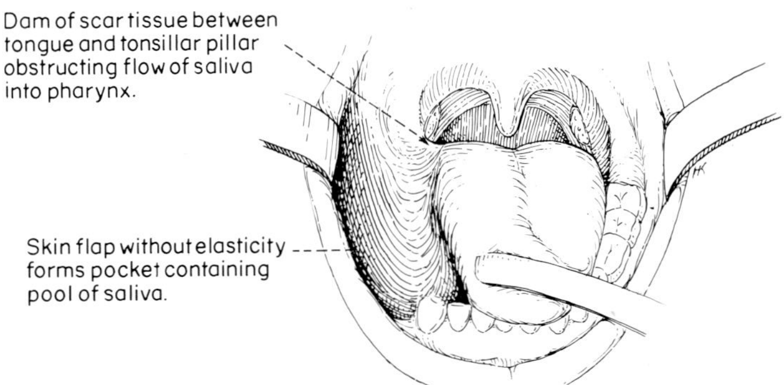

Figure 8.3

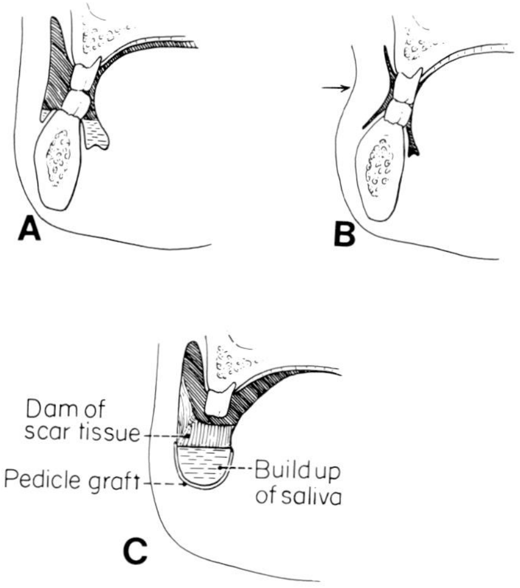

Figure 8.4

to supporting the lip. When the lower lip is intact, reconstruction of the upper lip is usually successful and drooling is not a primary problem.

Pooling of saliva in the anterior oral cavity or in the lateral oral cavity is another factor in drooling. Normally saliva is produced by the parotid glands and minor salivary glands and collects in the gingivo-buccal sulcus. On swallowing, the buccinator muscles squeeze the saliva posteriorally along the gutter into the pharynx[22] (Fig. 8.1). If the buccinator muscle is paralyzed or absent, pooling of saliva in the lateral sulcus can result in drooling (Fig. 8.4, *A* and *B*), but it is more likely to occur if there is in addition disruption of the oral stoma. Since buccal and floor of mouth mucosa has an inherent elasticity, it is often necessary in reconstructing the oral cavity with pedicle flap tissue to add additional skin as a compromise between the removed mucosa in a relaxed state versus a stretched state (Fig. 8.2). This excess tissue which is necessary to allow mobility of the tongue or adequate opening of the oral cavity can result in an exaggerated gutter anteriorly or laterally and as such cause drooling (Fig. 8.3). When this occurs, and everything possible has been done to restore the oral stoma competency, then it may be necessary to reach a compromise between tongue mobility and opening of the mouth versus reduction of the gutter and diminution of the drooling. Commonly drooling is exaggerated by a scar between the base of the tongue and the tonsillar region causing a dam to interfere with the passage of the saliva into the hypopharynx (Figs. 8.3 and 8.4*C*). When this dam occurs, and it has been common in my experience, correction with either Z-plasties or additional soft tissue between the base of the tongue and the tonsillar region can dramatically improve the problem of drooling.[25]

Since the tongue functions to squeeze the saliva from the floor of the mouth, abnormalities of the tongue and immobilization of the tongue with scar tissue can exaggerate the problem of drooling. Rarely does drooling occur simply as a consequence of a tongue abnormality when the remaining oral cavity and oral stoma are intact.

Correction of drooling can be frustrating. Restoration of the oral stoma is the most direct and necessary approach when possible to correct drooling. Using adjacent lip or cheek for skin, muscle, and mucosa for pedicle flaps appear to be the most effective means. It is controversial as to whether this muscle becomes functional or whether it simply has the necessary elasticity to allow adjacent muscles to function effectively. The fact, however, that functionally adjacent skin, muscle, and mucosa is more effective than remote skin pedicle flaps turned onto themselves in restoring the lower lip is quite clear. Reducing any deep gutters[18] and correcting a posterior dam between the base of the tongue and the tonsillar regions will further improve the problem of drooling.

When all of the above anatomic corrections have been accomplished to the best of the ability of the reconstructive surgeon, and when drooling persists as a problem, it may be necessary to consider reduction of saliva production.[10, 23] Most of the saliva produced in the mouth comes from the parotid and the submandibular glands. There are of course the sublingual glands and other minor salivary glands throughout the oral cavity. Experience has demonstrated, primarily through the work of Wilkie, that removal of the submandibular glands and the posterior diversion of the parotid glands into the hypopharynx can sufficiently reduce the saliva in the oral cavity to correct drooling. This experience was primarily on the basis of children with neuromuscular dysfunction. However, the concept has been applied successfully to patients following head and neck cancer ablation. Several comments must be made, however, about the reduction of saliva production. Many of these patients have been irradiated and the reduction of saliva in the oral cavity can be quite discomforting. The lack of saliva can result in serious damage to intact teeth. Furthermore, the symptoms of xerostomia can be quite disconcerting. Patients who have x-ray mucositis have further difficulties from the xerostomia.

Since many patients following cancer ablation of the head and neck region have already had removal of one or both submandibular glands or sublingual glands, it is reasonable to approach the reduction of saliva stepwise with diversion of the parotid glands alone or diversion of one parotid gland on the side of the disrupted anatomy. This conservative approach may sufficiently reduce the problem of drooling without extending oneself into the essentially irreversible problems of xerostomia.

SWALLOWING

The versatility of the swallowing mechanism is remarkable. At the very worst, a patient is able to maintain an open gullet and simply feed food from the oral cavity into the hypopharynx and into the esophagus if the hypopharynx and esophagus are not stenotic. However, the complicated anatomic physiology of swallowing is often symptomatic in the individual who expects to eat normally. Opening of the oral stoma to allow placement of food is often not as demanding as the ability to open the mouth adequately for dentures. However, oral stomal stenosis due to lack of tissue or severe scarring can be a problem and generally the oral stoma can be opened adequately. However, the surgeon must judge in opening the stoma to avoid weakening the oral stomal competency and thereby change the problem of limited oral stomal opening to one of incompetency and drooling. Generally the stoma should be enlarged by widening the oral commissures.[24] Numerous techniques have been described for opening the oral commissures and each technique requires some experience and finesse on the part of the surgeon. One principle that has become apparent is the need to reconstruct the oral commissure by maintaining the normal mucosa on either the upper or the lower lip and then resurfacing the opposite lip with the advanced mucosa. Dividing the existing lip mucosa between the upper and lower lip and then adding additional mucosa for both the upper and lower lip has resulted in small scars which reduce the elasticity of the normal mucosa. Another factor in disruption of the swallowing mechanism is the immobilization of the tongue. When the tongue is partially paralyzed, the mobility of the tongue in speech and swallowing is remarkably good. However, if the tongue is bound by scar to the mandible or adjacent cheek, the remaining muscle function is greatly limited. Although there are instances where it is necessary at the time of the original operative resection to suture the tongue to the gingiva or to the cheek and thereby significantly limit the tongue mobility, these instances should be minimized to situations where a flap either could not be done or had not been adequately anticipated prior to the resection. With those exceptions, any time a significant amount of floor of mouth is removed, it should be a part of the operative procedure to restore that lining in order to maintain tongue mobility.[1, 4, 6, 8, 9, 13–15] If restoration had not been done at the time of the original procedure, the tongue mobility can be regained by either recreating the defect and using skin grafts or by adding pedicle flap tissue. Skin grafting the defect in the floor of mouth or cheek area is effective[6] as long as recreating the defect does not expose the mandible, especially an irradiated mandible. In those instances pedicle flap tissue seems mandatory. Rarely can tongue mobility be restored without additional tissue in the form of a skin graft or a pedicle flap. When skin grafts are deemed inappropriate, the most commonly used pedicle flaps within the mouth are the forehead flap[14, 15] and the nasolabial flap.[4, 8, 9, 25] Extensive tissue can be brought into the mouth to restore tongue mobility with musculocutaneous flaps[1] such as the Barron flap which is basically usage of neck skin that is brought into the oral cavity with the platysma muscle as the vascular supply of the pedicle. Once tongue mobility has been restored, swallowing and speech will be greatly improved.

All patients who complain of difficulty in swallowing following treatment for carcinoma of the oral cavity should have direct endoscopic examination and cine-fluorographic studies with particular attention to the hypopharynx and upper esophagus.[5, 17, 19] Of course the first consideration is to search for the possibility of additional tumor and secondly to establish that there is not an anatomic stenosis or area of dysfunction. If there indeed is an anatomic stenosis, then the correction would be obvious. Some authors have suggested release of the cricopharyngeous muscle by a transcutaneous myotomy with improvement in swallowing in patients that have had extensive operative procedures and/or irradiation for cancers of the oral cavity.[17] Although experience with this procedure is limited and in fact difficult to assess, the concept of simply relaxing any neuromuscular dysfunction, spasm, or stenosis of the hypopharynx seems valid and when performed properly is a safe operative procedure. It has been interesting to observe that patients that have nasogastric, orogastric, or feeding esophagostomies frequently have difficulty in swallowing and in maintaining their own nourishment.[11, 12, 20] These tubes are placed because of swallowing difficulties but then it appears that they perpetuate the problem. It is often appropriate to remove the tube empirically to allow the patient to swallow without the tube with the understanding that it may need to be replaced. If the hypopharynx and esophagus are patent, the patient should be able to swallow as an open gullet and it should be safe to remove any tubes which seem (because of muscle spasm or discomfort) to interfere with the swallowing mechanism. A simple esophagostomy can be done at the time of a major head and neck procedure by a transcutaneous placement of a feeding tube through the neck skin into the esophagus. This tube is relatively symptom-free and can be insignificant to the patient as far as recovery time is concerned.

PAIN

Patients who have undergone treatment of cancers of the oral cavity and who subsequently have pain present a major problem. Any persistent pain related to cancer of the oral cavity must be considered to be additional cancer until categorically ruled out. Usually recurrent or persistent cancer is apparent within the oral cavity itself but in the tongue it can be deceptive. Pain in the tongue in these patients must be considered to be persistent cancer and multiple biopsies in search for areas of erosion or induration, especially in the base of the tongue, must be exhaustive. Once any anatomic areas of abnormality have been removed and pain persists, it is often related to irradiation and radiation osteonecrosis. Thorough x-ray examination of the bones around the oral cavity must then be carried out with the search for osteoradionecrosis. Any area of persistent pain and "radionecrosis" within the oral cavity must be considered as cancer. We have too often seen patients who have had persistent pain and "radionecrosis" of bone or soft tissues which ultimately prove to include aggressive recurrent cancer. An area of radionecrosis within the oral cavity must be excised if it persists for more than 4–8 weeks. It is rare for chronic radionecrosis to correct itself and a large percentage of these patients will indeed have radionecrosis with associated cancer. After all of these possibilities have been eliminated, it is rarely necessary to seek pain relief such as by neurotomy or other neurosurgical approaches to pain in the head and neck region.

OPENING OF THE ORAL STOMA

The problem of opening the mouth presents itself primarily when the patient wishes to use dentures. Feeding requires less of an oral stoma. The management of the soft tissues is usually related to stenosis of the oral stoma but limitation of opening the mouth can be secondary to temporomandibular ankylosis. It is remarkable following partial resection of the mandible how well the mandible maintains function. Unless the remaining temporomandibular joint has been anatomically disrupted or has been involved with disease, opening of the mandible is usually effective. Contracture of the cheek is rarely a cause of the difficulty unless a through and through defect including skin, muscle, and mucosa has been created. When it is due to contracture of the buccal mucosal area alone or to skin alone, correction is usually straightforward. However, full thickness defects of the cheek can be underestimated and can create significant problems including limitation of opening the mandible. Full thickness defects require extensive tissue to replace. Pedicle flap tissue that has been brought in to replace full thickness defects does not have the normal elasticity of the cheeks and as such the surface area replacement must be greater than the collapsed surface area resected. This applies particularly in assessing the defect within the oral cavity such as the buccal mucosa. It is important to recreate the defect and to have in the operative plan of reconstruction the ability to bring in pedicle flap tissue that is excessive compared to the preoperative judgment as to how much tissue will be necessary.[1, 2, 7, 11, 13–15, 21, 25]

SPEECH

The requisite for effective speech is an intact larynx. Despite distortion of the tongue and oral cavity, effective speech for communication is usually present. Prior to any treatment for cancer of the oral cavity and tongue, patients are quite anxious about the ability to communicate by speech. Unless the larynx is removed, it is usually safe to assure the patients that they will be able to communicate with speech but distortion of the speech is to be expected. Speech interference is usually an accompaniment of extensive resections of tumors in the oral cavity and tongue. Inability to open the mouth adequately can result in some speech impairment which is most noticeable on the telephone. Patients with facial nerve palsy will have some blurring of speech which is most exaggerated on the telephone. Simply statically retracting the side of the mouth and cheek with a sling will often be an effective improvement in speech. Tongue mobility is a significant factor in adequate speech. Any release of the tongue from the mandible or cheek will usually result in some improvement of speech and is appreciated by the patient. A speech pathologist is often useful in assessing the specific pathophysiology of speech impairment and will give the patient confidence in his ability to communicate.

CHEWING

The limitation of a patient's ability to eat following treatment of cancers of the oral cavity and tongue can be due to inadequate opening of the oral stoma, inability to wear a denture, lack of tongue mobility to move the food into the dental occlusal plane (chewing), or interference with the swallowing mechanism. The anatomic requirements to allow a patient to wear a denture are an adequate oral stoma to place the denture in the mouth and an adequate alveolar ridge of the mandible to allow retention of the denture. Patients who have had mandibular reconstruction can anticipate the ability to wear a denture although the soft tissue over the reconstructed jaw must be sufficient to prevent erosion from the denture and there must be some vestibule between the gingiva and the labial or buccal mucosa. Frequently minor operative procedures consisting of Z-plasties or full thickness skin grafts are necessary to restore the vestibule for denture wearing.[6, 18] On planning one's goals in this regard, it is usually safe for the surgeon to anticipate the ability to wear a denture for cosmetic purposes but it is usually unrealistic to expect effective denture wearing for chewing. There are some patients who can, under optimal circumstances and with careful dental prosthetic construction, chew with a denture following oral cavity and tongue resection, even when jaw has been resected. However, these are not the rule and most patients will have to accept the fact that dentures can be worn primarily for cosmetic purposes but without any expectation that they will be able to chew difficult foods.

APPEARANCE

The role of appearance in the mind of the patient that has had resection of a tumor for carcinoma of the oral cavity or tongue is quite variable.[11, 16] Usually patients place appearance in a low priority in relation to the above problems such as drooling, chewing and pain. However, some patients will place appearance in a priority and it is for this reason that the surgeon must carefully assess the individual and identify the problems that the patient sees as his/her primary difficulty. The greatest deformity associated with treatment of carcinoma of the oral cavity results from the need to resect major soft tissues such as the lip or cheek and from resection of the mandible, most importantly the anterior body of the mandible. When the anterior body of the mandible must be resected, the recessed chin and the lack of support of the chin and the lower lip result in significant deformity, edema of the lip, and drooling. It is these patients in whom jaw reconstruction becomes most important.[3] Usually functional restoration of the soft tissues and jaw results in the most effective restoration of appearance. When the optimal functional restoration has been accomplished, patients are especially grateful to the surgeon who is willing to proceed with additional operative procedures when necessary to improve their appearance. It is common for the treating physician to feel that the patient's deformities are so great that minor procedures to improve appearance such as improvement of a scar would not be of any use. To the contrary, patients who have had extensive problems express gratitude for any help and interest in their plight. It is important to encourage patients in the early post-treatment stage that the scars and appearance of the tissues will improve dramatically, and in due time (usually a minimum of 4–6 months) further minor operative procedures to improve the appearance of the scars and tissues can be accomplished. In this period of time there will be significant improvement and the patient will also accept their problems more readily than in the early post-treatment phase. Because the airway can be a difficult problem in these patients, procedures to improve the appearance can often be done under local anesthesia and as outpatient procedures. In decades past any reconstructive and cosmetic surgery necessitated extensive hospitalizations and life-threatening operative procedures. For this reason many physicians are reluctant to encourage patients to undergo secondary reconstructive procedures. On the other hand, with improved techniques of anesthesia and with the ability to undertake many reconstructive and cosmetic procedures under local anesthesia, these procedures should not be withheld from the patient who desires them. At this point it is important to remind the physician that our primary goal is to relieve pain and discomfort and in so doing we must consider the patient with extensive cancer of the oval cavity or tongue as a patient who can be relieved of some discomfort or mental anguish with improvement by esthetic surgery. Improvement in the patient's morale by relatively minor procedures to improve their appearance has always been gratifying to the patient and to the treating surgeon.

References

1. Ariyan, S.: One-stage reconstruction for defects of the mouth using a sternomastoid myocutaneous flap. *Plast. Reconstr. Surg., 63:*618, 1989.
2. Chambers, R. G., Jacques, D. A., and Mahoney, W. D.: Tongue flaps for intraoral reconstruction. *Am. J. Surg., 118:*783, 1969.
3. Boyne, P. J., and Zarem, H. A.: *Am. J. Surg., 132:*49, 1976.
4. Cohen, I. K., and Edgerton, M. T.: Transbuccal flaps for reconstruction of the floor of the mouth. *Plast. Reconstr. Surg., 48:*8, 1971.
5. Dingman, D. L.: Postoperative management of the severe oral cripple. *Plast. Reconstr. Surg., 45:*263, 1970.
6. Edgerton, M. T.: Replacement of lining to oral cavity following surgery. *Cancer, 4:*110, 1951.
7. Edgerton, M. T.: Role of immediate reconstruction in treatment of head and neck cancer, in *Symposium on Malignancies of the Head and Neck*, p. 169, edited by R. Anderson and J. E. Hoopes, C. V. Mosby, St. Louis, 1975.
8. Elliott, R. A., Jr.: Use of nasolabial skin flap to cover intraoral defects. *Plast. Reconstr. Surg., 58:*201, 1976.
9. Gewirtz, H. S., Frederick, R. E., and Zarem, H. A.: Use of the nasolabial flap for reconstruction of the floor of the mouth. *Am. J. Surg., 136:*508, 1978.
10. Glass, L. W., Nobel, G. L., and Vecchione, T. R.: Treatment of uncontrolled drooling by bilateral excision of submaxillary glands and parotid duct ligations. *Plast. Reconstr. Surg., 62:*523, 1978.
11. Jabaley, M. E.: Reconstruction of patients with oral and pharyngeal cancer. *Curr. Probl. Surg., 14:*12, 1977.
12. Ketcham, A. S., and Smith, R. R.: Elective esophagostomy. *Am. J. Surg., 104:*682, 1962.
13. Leeb, D. C., Ben-Hur, N., and Mazzarella, L.: Reconstruction of the floor of the mouth with a free dorsalis pedis flap. *Plast. Reconstr. Surg., 59:*379, 1977.
14. Lewis, M. B., and Remensnyder, J. P.: Forehead flap for reconstruction after ablative surgery for oral and oropharyngeal malignancy. *Plast. Reconstr. Surg., 62:*59–65, 1978.
15. McGregor, I. A.: The temporal flap in intraoral cancer; its use in repairing the post-excisional defect. *Br. J. Plast. Surg., 16:*318, 1963.
16. Marchetta, F. C.: Function and appearance following surgery for intraoral cancer. *Clin. Plast. Surg., 3:*471, 1976.
17. Mladick, R. A., Horton, C. E., and Adamson, J. E.: Immediate cricopharyngeal myotomy. *Plast. Reconstr. Surg., 47:*6, 1971.
18. Morgan, L. R., Gallegos, L. T., and Frileck, S. P.: Mandibular vestibuloplasty with a free graft of the mucoperiosteal layer from the hard palate. *Plast. Reconstr. Surg., 51:*359, 1973.
19. Rappaport, I., Shramek, J., and Brummett, S.: Functional aspects of cancer of the base of the tongue. *Am. J. Surg., 114:*489, 1967.
20. Royster, H. P., Noone, R. B., Graham, W. P., and Theogaraj, S. D.: Cervical pharyngostomy for feeding after maxillofacial surgery. *Am. J. Surg., 116:*610, 1968.
21. Sharzer, L. A., et al.: Intraoral reconstruction in head and neck cancer. *Clin. Plast. Surg., 3:*495, 1976.
22. Shedd, D. P., Scatliff, J. H., and Kirchner, J. A.: The buccopharyngeal propulsive mechanism in human deglutition. *Surgery, 48:*846, 1960.
23. Wilkie, T. F., and Brody, G. S.: The surgical treatment of drooling—a ten-year review. *Plast. Reconstr. Surg., 59:*791, 1977.
24. Wustrack, K. O., and Silsby, J. J.: Reconstruction of incompetent oral commissures with dermal-muscle flaps from the lips. *Plast. Reconstr. Surg., 62:*118, 1978.
25. Zarem, H. A.: Current concepts in reconstructive surgery in patients with cancer of the head and neck. *Surg. Clin. North Am., 51:*149, 1971.

CHAPTER 9

Surgery of the Jaws

Henry K. Kawamoto, Jr., M.D., D.D.S.

The functional and aesthetic importance of the orofacial structures cannot be overstated. Fundamental activities of mastication, deglutition, and speech are dependent on the soundness of the area. The jaws provide the skeletal support for these physiologic needs and strongly influence the form of the major portion of the face.

Concentrated within a space of a small cube with 10-cm sides, the jaws must meet the difficult demand of balancing form, function, and aesthetics. Any deformity of the mandible and the maxilla can, therefore, have a profound effect on basic bodily activities and facial appearance.

TYPES OF DEFORMITY

Based on etiology, malformations of the jaws can be divided into three main categories: (1) acquired, (2) congenital, and (3) developmental deformities.

Acquired Deformities

By far the most common cause of acquired jaw deformities is trauma. No region of the craniofacial skeleton is spared. The resulting disfigurement and disruption of orofacial function can be severe. Equally devastating defects are created following ablative procedures for treatment of neoplasms.

Congenital Deformities

A wide variety of congenital malformations of the jaws exists. The deformity can be subtle and overlooked on casual examination at the time of birth. When the involvement is unilateral in nature, the discrepancy becomes magnified with growth.

Other birth defects of the jaw are immediately apparent. They can be unilateral or bilateral in occurrence. Common examples are the deformities associated with cleft lip and palate, craniofacial microsomia (first and second branchial arch syndrome), Pierre Robin anomaly, and mandibulofacial dysostosis (Treacher Collins syndrome). The list is long.

The treatment of congenital orofacial malformations is reviewed in Chapter 15. However, the principles discussed in this chapter to manage developmental and acquired jaw deformities are equally applicable.

Developmental Deformities

Developmental jaw deformities are accentuated with the passage of time. Facial distortion progresses as the child matures. They can be primary or secondary in nature.

Primary malformations are commonly seen. They have no obvious cause. In the early years, the child has a normal facial appearance. In late adolescence, the distortion in harmony is magnified as the face assumes its adult form. A partial list of representative deformities includes a receded chin, mandibular prognathism, maxillary hypoplasia, or excessive protrusion of the teeth.

Secondary malformations are the result of abnormalities of the adjacent structures or systemic disease. The earlier the insult, the greater will be the aftereffects. In total number,. their frequency is less. Examples include maldevelopment due to facial paralysis, faulty tongue habits, regional infections or soft tissue growths such as a hemangioma, and mandibular prognathism associated with acromegaly.

Regardless of the cause of the jaw deformity and the complexity of the problem, a knowledge of the regional anatomy is essential.

BASIC ANATOMY

The mandible and the maxilla are derivatives of the first branchial arch. The cranial nerve that is associated with this arch is the trigeminal nerve. The internal maxillary artery provides the main blood supply to the area.

Nerve Supply

The two roots of the trigeminal nerve join to form the trigeminal (semilunar) ganglion. From this ganglion three divisions are formed: the ophthalmic nerve (first division), the maxillary nerve (second division), and the mandibular nerve (third division). All three divisions carry sensory fibers, but only the mandibular nerve contains motor fibers.

MAXILLARY NERVE

Sensibility of the maxillary structure is provided by the maxillary nerve. As the nerve leaves the trigeminal ganglion it passes through the foramen rotundum to enter the pterygopalatine fossa. Traversing the fossa, the nerve enters the orbit through the inferior orbital fissure and courses along the floor of the orbit in the infraorbital groove and canal. It exits the infraorbital foramen to emerge into the overlying soft tissues of the face.

In the pterygoid fossa the maxillary nerve sends branches to the sphenopalatine ganglion and also gives off branches of the posterior superior alveolar nerves. The greater and lesser palatine nerves descend from the ganglion and pass through the pterygopalatine canal to

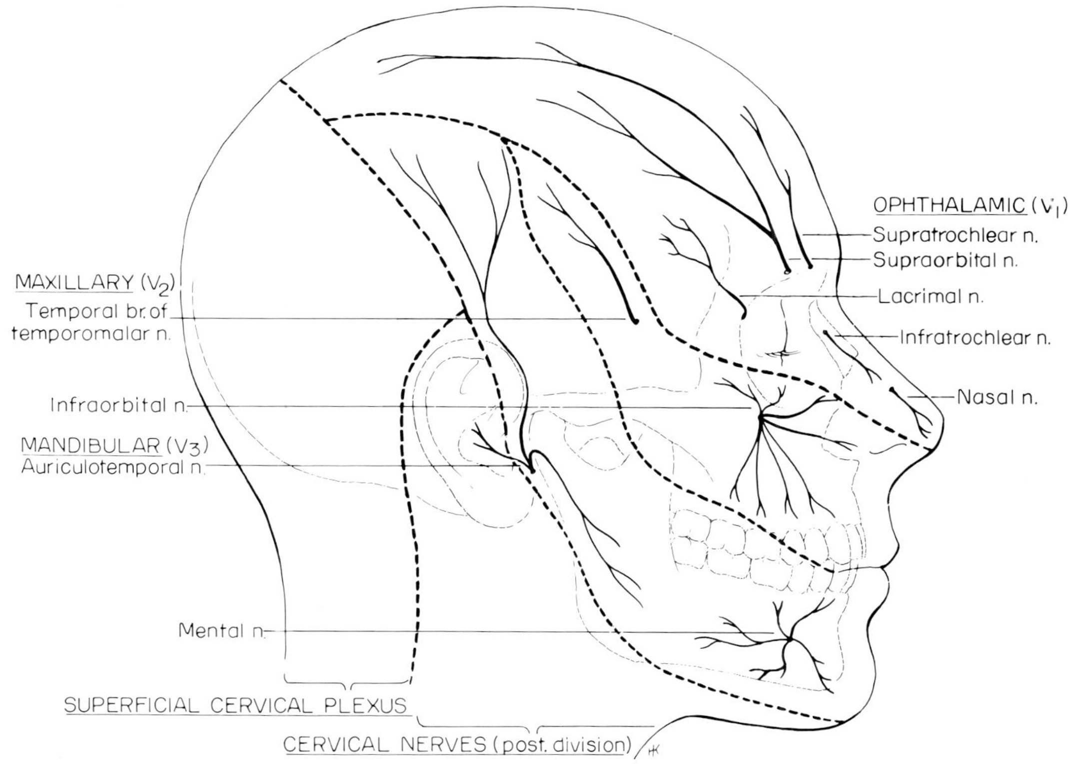

Figure 9.1 Sensory nerve supply to the head and neck. Face and anterior two-thirds of scalp are supplied by three main branches of trigeminal nerve: ophthalmic (V_1), maxillary (V_2), and mandibular (V_3) divisions. Cervical nerves provide sensibility to remainder of scalp, major portion of external ear, and neck.

provide sensory branches to the hard and soft palate, respectively. The posterior superior alveolar nerves penetrate the infratemporal surface of the maxilla to innervate the molars.

In the infraorbital canal, the middle superior alveolar nerves are given off to run through the lateral wall of the maxilla to supply the premolars. Coursing through the anterior wall of the maxilla are the anterior superior alveolar nerves which are directed toward the canine (cuspid) and the incisors. Considerable territorial overlap between the superior alveolar nerves is present as they supply the teeth and the adjacent gingiva.

On the face, the terminal branches of the maxillary nerve provide sensibility to the infraorbital region and the upper lip (Fig. 9.1).

MANDIBULAR NERVE

The largest branch of the trigeminal nerve is the mandibular nerve. It leaves the middle cranial fossa through the foramen ovale. Once in the infratemporal space, the nerve sends motor branches to the muscles of mastication (medial and lateral pterygoids, masseter, and temporalis) and the tensor tympani and the tensor veli palatini. Just prior to entering the mandibular foramen, the mylohyoid nerve is given off to innervate the mylohyoideus and the anterior belly of the digastricus.

The sensory component of the mandibular nerve provides sensibility to the preauricular and temporal area (auriculotemporal nerve), skin and mucous membrane of the cheek and adjacent mandibular gingiva (buccal nerve), and the tongue (lingual nerve) (Fig. 9.1). The nerve enters the mandibular foramen on the medial aspect of the ramus and is renamed as the inferior alveolar nerve. Branches to the molar and premolar are sent as the nerve courses through the mandibular canal. At the mental foramen it bifurcates to terminate as the incisive branch and the mental nerve. The incisive branch is the intraosseous continuation of the inferior alveolar nerve and supplies sensory fibers to the canine and incisors. The mental nerve exits the mental foramen to be distributed to the region of the labial gingiva, lower lip and chin.

Blood Supply

Branching off the external carotid artery, the internal maxillary artery provides the main blood supply to the deep structures of the jaws. The artery can be conveniently divided into three portions (Fig. 9.2).

The first or mandibular portion of the artery has several branches, but the main branch to the jaw is the inferior alveolar artery. It is the principle blood supply of the mandible and it also sends a branch to the mylohyoideus.

The pterygoid portion is the middle segment. The muscles of mastication obtain their blood supply from branches of this second portion of the internal maxillary artery.

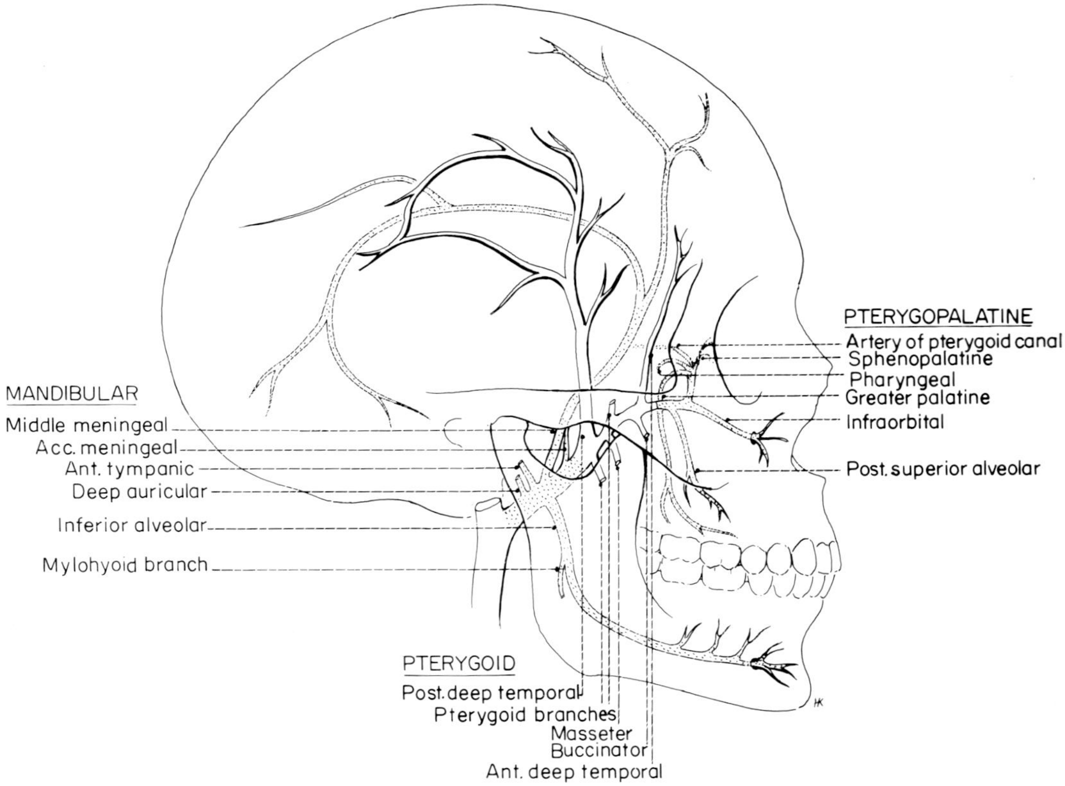

Figure 9.2 Three major divisions of internal maxillary artery. Mandibular segment (*shaded*) provides the major blood supply to lower jaw. Pterygoid portion (*unshaded*), supplies muscles of mastication. Distal portion, pterygopalatine division, is the principle vessel of maxilla.

The final third or the pterygopalatine portion is the principle blood supply to the maxilla, the hard and soft palate, and the infraorbital region. The distribution of the branches is similar to that of the maxillary division of the trigeminal nerve.

The Skeleton

The jaws function as a highly coordinated unit. Yet, structurally the principle bones of the system are remarkably dissimilar.

The mandible is the only bone of the craniofacial skeleton, besides the ossicles of the middle ear, that is capable of undergoing any significant movement. It is a solid horseshoe-shaped structure that can withstand the tremendous forces generated by the muscles of mastication.

In direct contrast is the maxilla. It must play a somewhat passive role since it is a stationary object that is subjected to the same might of the forces of mastication. However, unlike the dense bony mass of the mandible, the maxilla is a light weight structure that has thin walls and is surrounded by air spaces and cavities. Only the strategic placement of bony buttresses by nature prevents the collapse of this delicate frame as it endures gigantic physiologic stresses.

The mandible is a single solid structure that can be conveniently subdivided into regions: condyle, subcondylar neck, coronoid process, ramus, angle, body, symphysis, and alveolar process (Fig. 9.3). The condyle, together with a fibrocartilaginous meniscus, the glenoid fossa of the temporal bone, and the surrounding capsular ligament, forms the temporomandibular

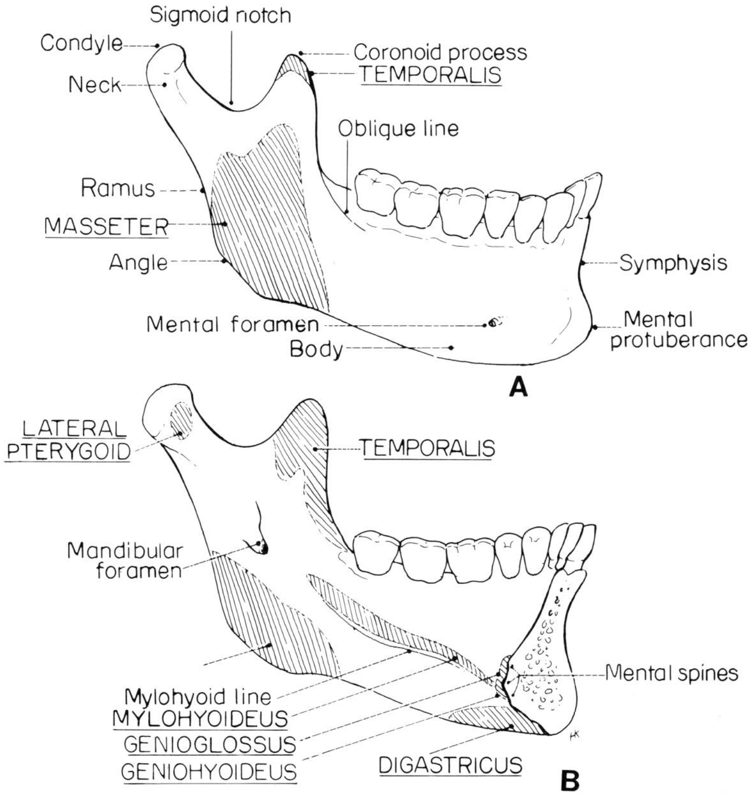

Figure 9.3 Regions of mandible and attachment of muscles. Major muscles are underlined and shaded areas indicate sites of their attachment. (*A*) Lateral view, (*B*) medial view.

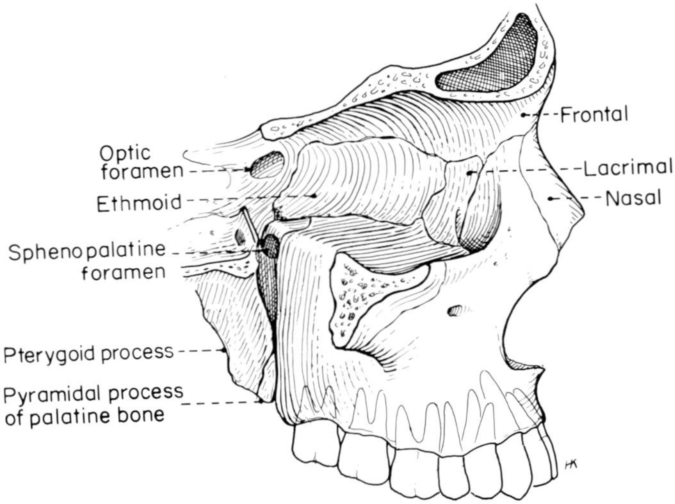

Figure 9.4 Lateral view of maxilla. Zygoma is removed to show relationship of maxilla with bony structures of orbit and infratemporal fossa.

joint. With this modified ball and socket joint, the mandible meets the functional demands of moving through a complicated multidirectional range of motion.

The vertical component (ramus and condyle) of the mandible is primarily concerned with the movement. The joint and the insertion of all the muscles of mastication are located in this region. The horizontal portion (body and symphysis) furnishes the foundation for the working surface. This base is composed mainly of dense, compact bone similar to the vertical part. On this solid foundation rests the alveolar process which contains a greater portion of cancellous bone into which the roots of the teeth are embedded.

The inferior alveolar neurovascular bundle enters the lower jaw through the mandibular foramen on the medial aspect of the midportion of the ramus. It courses through the ramus in an oblique caudal and anterior direction. As it passes the region of the mandibular angle, it assumes a path that is nearly parallel with the inferior border of the body. The bundle exits through the mental foramen which is located on the lateral surface of the body near the root apex of the second premolar.

The architecture and interrelationships of the maxilla are more complex. This bone is a paired structure which articulates superiorly with the nasal, frontal, lacrimal, and ethmoidal bones (Fig. 9.4). Posteriorly, it is separated from the perpendicular plate of the sphenoid bone by the palatine bone. The two maxillary bones meet in the midline to form the palate.

The maxilla occupies a strategic location that is surrounded by cavities. Medially is the nasal cavity. Cephalad is the floor of the orbital cavity. Caudal and laterally it is exposed to the oral cavity. The delicate walls of the maxilla surround the maxillary sinus. Thickening of the bone in the region of the pyriform aperture, frontal process, and the zygomatic buttress enables this, otherwise fragile structure, to withstand the forces of mastication.

The alveolar process is similar in bony character to that of the mandible and provides the support of the dentition.

The Dentition

The mandible and the maxilla have an identical number of deciduous and permanent teeth. The 20 deciduous teeth are exfoliated between the ages of 6–12 years. A slight variation in time is present as the deciduous incisors (8), cuspids (4), and the molars (8) are replaced by the permanent incisors (8), cuspids (4), and premolars (8), respectively. The permanent molars (12) erupt posterior to the deciduous arch to bring the total number of adult teeth to 32.

Deciduous Teeth	maxillary	4 incisors	2 cuspids	4 molars	0	Total 20 Teeth
	mandibular	4 incisors	2 cuspids	4 molars	0	
Permanent Teeth	maxillary	4 incisors	2 cuspids	4 premolars	6 molars	Total 32 Teeth
	mandibular	4 incisors	2 cuspids	4 premolars	6 molars	

In dental terminology, the tooth surface nearest to the apex (anterior portion) of the dental arch is called *mesial* (Fig. 9.5). The surface nearest to the posterior end of the arch is termed *distal*. The surface of the tooth that is closest to the tongue is designated as being *lingual*. The outer facial surface of the incisors and cuspids is named the *labial* surface and in the premolar and molar regions it is called the *buccal* surface because of the respective juxtaposition of the lips and cheeks. The working surface of mastication in the anterior segment of the dental arch (incisors and cuspids) is known as the *incisal* edge. In the premolar and molar regions the term *occlusal* surface is used.

The mandibular arch is slightly shorter in length and smaller in width than that of the maxilla. Thus, the mandibular teeth are located slightly anterior and lingual to their counterpart in the maxilla.

In a set of dentition with an ideal occlusion (Class I relationship) the mesiobuccal groove of the maxillary first molar occludes with the buccal groove of the mandibular first molar (Fig. 9.6).[1] Departures from this model relationship are common. When the mandibular first molar is located in a more *distal* (posterior) location a Class II malocclusion is created. The term Class III malocclusion is used when the mandibular first molar is positioned more *mesial* (anterior).

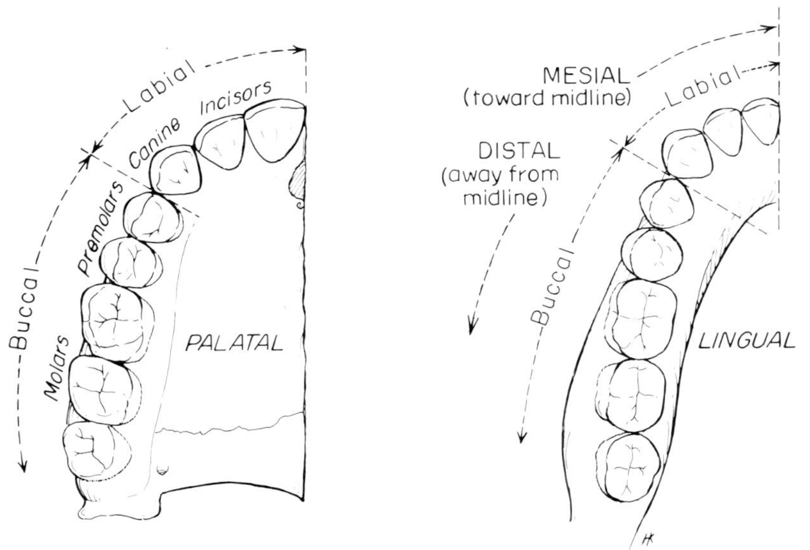

Figure 9.5 Nomenclature related to maxilla and mandible. (*Left*) Occlusal view of maxilla, (*right*) occlusal view of mandible.

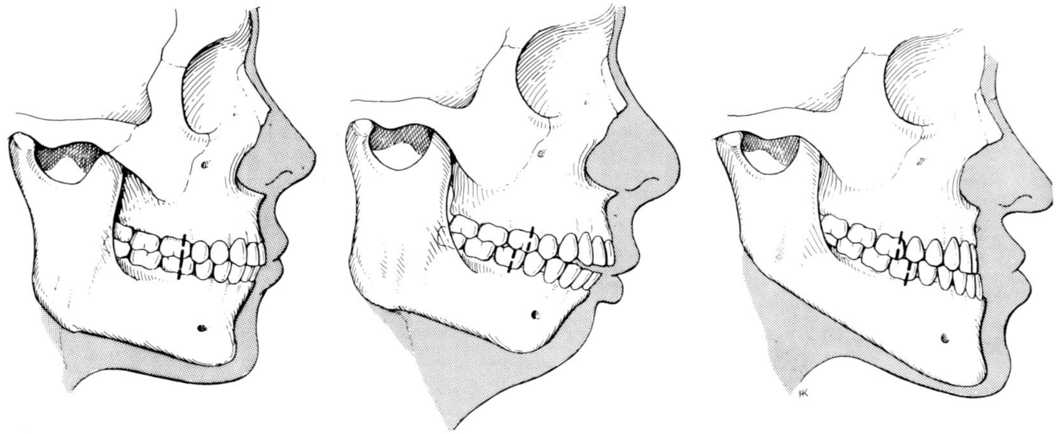

Figure 9.6 Relationship of facial profile and Angle classification of malocclusion. Ideal molar relationship shown by alignment of molar in Class I. Facial appearance reflects underlying dental and skeletal deformities.

The relationship of the dental arches to one another has a direct bearing on the facial profile. People who have a Class I occlusion tend to have a balanced, more harmonious profile. Those with a Class I malocclusion frequently have a receded appearance of the lower jaw. The bird-face deformity ("Andy Gump") is an extreme example. The opposite tendency is often seen in patients with a Class III malocclusion; the mandible appears to be excessively strong in its prognathic position.

The Musculature

The maxilla can be quickly dispensed with in any discussion concerning muscles that influence the movement of the jaws: it is devoid of any important muscular attachments that are involved in moving the mandible. It does, however, provide sites of origin for many of the delicate muscles that animate the face.

The mandible is the only facial bone that is designed for movement. The range of movement is extremely complex. In overly simplistic terms, the primary path of movement of the mandible is to open and close like a hinge. Little work is required to open the mandible. Thus, gravity plus the contraction of the weak muscles attached to the horizontal portion of the mandible is all that is needed. To close the mandible is a different matter. To chew efficiently, strong forces must be generated by the muscles of mastication that are attached to the vertical segment of the mandible. Because of a design fault by nature, additional requirements for strength are imposed on this posterior group of muscles.

In terms of bioengineering, nature chose a poor plan for the mandible. An inefficient Class III lever system was installed with the temporomandibular joint acting at one end of the fulcrum and the load being placed on the teeth at the other end (Fig. 9.7). The power supply (the muscles of mastication) is placed in the middle. A Class III lever system is designed to produce a long arc of movement at the end opposite the fulcrum. However, the power requirements are high. Efficient mechanical breakdown of food requires the teeth to be moved through small arcs with sufficient grinding power. Mandibular excursions of great distance are not needed.

The muscles that control mandibular movement can be conveniently divided into a powerful posterior group (muscles of mastication) attached to the vertical portion of the mandible and a weak anterior set of muscles associated with the horizontal branch of the mandible.

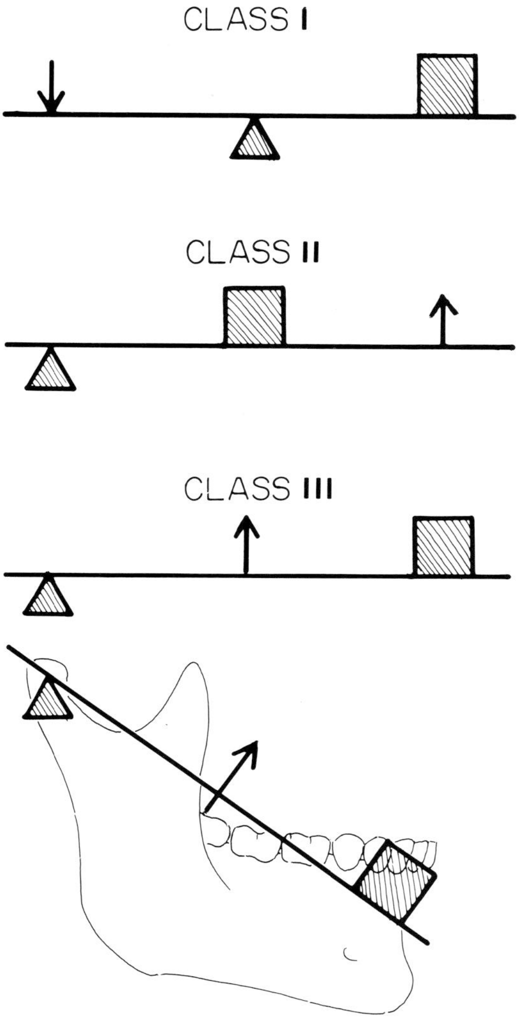

Figure 9.7 Diagramatic representation of Class III lever system imposed upon the mandible. Fulcrum point represented by *triangle* is located in temporomandibular joint. Direction of vector of muscular forces depicted by *arrow*. The load (area of mastication) is shown as a *square*.

POSTERIOR GROUP

The muscles of mastication are four in number: masseter, temporalis, medial (internal) and lateral (external) pterygoids. They act to elevate and protrude the mandible.

Temporalis (Fig. 9.8). Arising from the whole of the temporal fossa and the deep surface of the temporal fascia, the fibers of this fan-shape muscle converge to insert on the coronoid process and along the anterior border of the ramus. Its primary action is to close the mandible. The posterior fibers also serve to retract the lower jaw.

Masseter (Fig. 9.8). The body and the arch of the zygoma provide the origin of this bulky, rectangular shaped muscle. Superficial fibers are directed downward and backward and the deep portion is oriented in a more vertical direction. The muscle inserts on the lateral surface of the ramus and the region of the mandibular angle. Its primary function is to elevate the mandible.

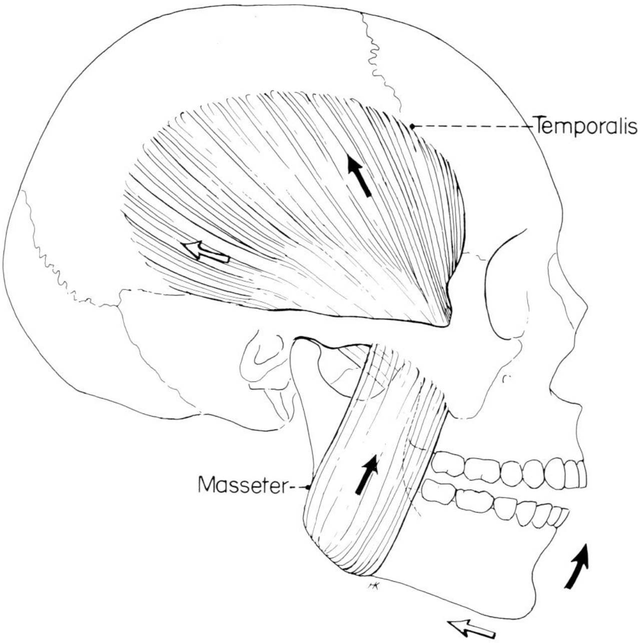

Figure 9.8 Masseter and temporalis. *Solid arrows* indicate direction of muscular pull and resulting movement of mandible. *Clear arrows* show posterior horizontal fibers of temporalis responsible for retropositioning of mandible.

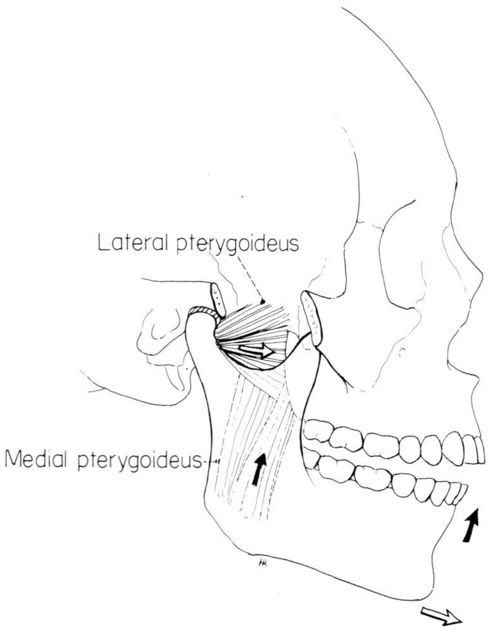

Figure 9.9 Medial and lateral pterygoideus. *Solid arrows* represent direction of pull of medial pterygoideus and resultant movement of mandible. *Clear arrows* indicate protrusion of mandible caused by contraction of lateral pterygoideus. Zygomatic arch is omitted for clarity.

Medial (Internal) Pterygoid (Fig. 9.9). This muscle is similar to that of the masseter in size, shape and orientation. It arises from the medial surface of the pterygoid plate of the sphenoid bone and the pyramidal process of the palatine bone. Passing downward, backward, and laterally it inserts onto the medial aspect of the ramus below the mandibular foramen. It elevates the mandible and also exerts a medial force.

Lateral (External) Pterygoid (Fig. 9.9). This short fan-shaped muscle arises by two heads; the upper from the infratemporal surface of the greater wing of the sphenoid bone and the lower from the lateral surface of the lateral pterygoid plate. Its fibers converge as they pass backward and laterally in a horizontal manner. The major portion inserts onto the anterior surface of the neck of the condyle. A small slip attaches into the articular disk of the temporomandibular joint. The mandible is protruded as the muscle pulls the condylar neck forward, medially, and downward.

ANTERIOR GROUP

The muscles used in opening the jaws are often called the *anterior* or *depressor* group. They are the digastricus, the geniohyoideus, and the mylohyoideus (Fig. 9.10). Acting on a stabilized hyoid bone, they pull in a caudal and posterior direction to open the mandible.

Digastricus. The two fleshy bellies of the digastricus are joined to one another by an intermediate tendon that is attached to the hyoid bone. The anterior belly arises from the inner surface of the lower border of the symphysis and is innervated by a branch of the mandibular nerve. The posterior belly originates from the mastoid notch and receives branches of the facial nerve.

Geniohyoideus. The muscle arises from the inferior mental spine of the symphysis and inserts onto the body of the hyoid bone. Innervation is provided by branches of the first cervical nerve.

Myohyoideus. Arising from the myohyoid line, the myohyoideus extends from behind the last molar to the symphysis. The paired muscles meet in the midline to form the muscular floor of the mouth and are inserted into the hyoid bone. The myohyoideus is innervated by

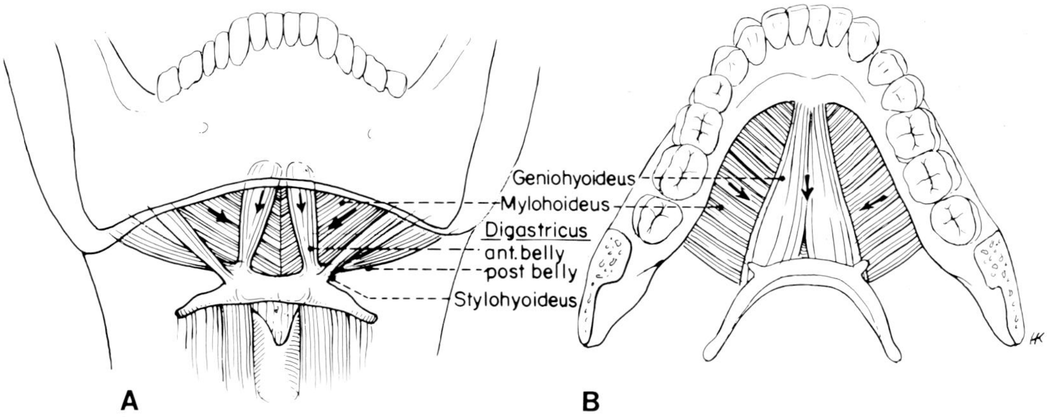

Figure 9.10 Anterior muscle group of mandible. (*A*) Submental view showing attachments to mandible and hyoid bone. (*B*) Intraoral view of floor of mouth. *Arrows* depict direction of force exerted on mandible when hyoid bone is stabilized.

fibers from the mandibular division of the trigeminal nerve. The primary function of the muscle is to elevate the tongue and the hyoid bone.

ACQUIRED DEFORMITIES

Trauma and ablative procedures for neoplasms are the principle causes of acquired deformities of the jaws. To restore form and function (1) the displaced parts must be returned to the normal position, (2) stabilization of the skeletal segment during healing is required for bony consolidation, and (3) missing components (e.g., soft tissue coverage, skeletal support, and lining) need replacement.

The correction of deformities such as facial fractures caused by civilian injuries is generally straight forward. Restoring alignment and providing a method of fixation is usually all that is required.

In contrast, war and gunshot wounds and defects produced by irradication of neoplastic disease are inclined to pose a greater challenge. The third element of treatment is added; namely, the need to replace soft and hard tissues that have been destroyed.

Facial Fractures

GENERAL CONSIDERATIONS

The vast majority of facial fractures are the results of motor vehicular accidents and fist fights. Active adults account for most of the fractures. Children under the age of 12 are less prone because of their sheltered life and their resilient bones. Approximately 5% of the facial fractures are sustained by this young age group.[2–5]

The exact incidence of facial fractures varies from study to study. However, it is generally accepted that the number and magnitude of facial fractures have been diminished by the imposition of lower automobile speed limits and the greater use of passenger restraint systems. Regardless of the cause and the severity of injury, priorities have been well established for the treatment of facial fractures. Reduction of the fracture is not considered an emergency. Establishment of an airway takes precedence. The oropharynx must be inspected and cleared of secretions and foreign bodies that would interfere with the exchange of air. The simple placement of the victim in a prone position is often beneficial. In a face down position, the effects of gravity are advantageously employed. Oral secretion and blood are free to drain. The tongue falls to a dependent position away from the posterior pharyngeal wall; keeping the oropharynx open.

In the past, considerable stress was placed on the use of a tracheotomy. However, valuable time can be lost in performing this operation. In an emergency room setting, the passage of an oroendotracheal tube can be accomplished much quicker and with greater safety except in patients with associated injuries to the cervical spine. Improvements in the endotracheal tubes and their management has made it possible to keep the patient intubated for several days with little risk. Conversion to a nasotracheal tube can be made at the time of the reduction of the facial fractures.

Once the airway is secured, attention should be directed toward the control of hemorrhage. Following this, a thorough evaluation of the entire body must be made to rule out unseen life threatening injuries. Actual reduction of the facial fractures can be deferred several days until the patients condition is well stabilized.

The clinical diagnosis of a facial fracture often can be made by inspection and palpation.

Disturbance in occlusion and intraoral ecchymosis provide valuable clues as to the site of the fractures. Palpation of the outlines of the orbital rims, zygomatic arches, and the inferior border of the mandible should also be performed. In addition, abnormal movement of the jaws can be discovered by bimanual manipulation of the maxilla and the mandible.

Paresthesia of the lower lip and the infraorbital region is often present. If the fracture traverses the inferior alveolar canal, numbness of the ipsilateral lower lip is commonly seen. Similarly, disruption of the maxilla involving the infraorbital canal can produce paresthesias of the ipsilateral upper lip and cheek. Pain and tenderness over the area of fracture can be expected.

As soon as the patient's condition permits, confirmatory roentgenograms should be obtained. A basic series would include a posteroanterior and lateral view of the skull, a mandibular series, a Waters' projection, submental vertex view, and a panoramic roentgenogram. The panoramic roentgenogram requires a special dental apparatus that is not readily available in most hospitals. Therefore, in addition to the standard mandibular series, a reverse Towne's view can be ordered to provide greater detail of the condylar and subcondylar neck region.

Furthermore, in automobile accidents, injuries to the neck and cervical spine should be suspected.[6] A cervical spine series is required to rule out a potentially fatal injury.

When indicated, the prophylactic antibiotic of choice is penicillin. Compound fractures that disrupt the overlying mucosa to communicate with the oral cavity are candidates for coverage. Similarly, consideration should be given for fractures involving a socket of a tooth.

It is advisable to preserve intact teeth found in the path of a fracture. In many instances, partially extruded teeth or teeth with fractured crowns can be retained. Reimplantation of a totally avulsed permanent tooth is feasible especially in young children who still have large openings in the apex of the roots. The prognosis of older teeth with fully developed roots is less favorable but they still can be salvaged with endodontic therapy. However, when the root itself is severed, the tooth is doomed for extraction. As a general rule, an involved tooth should not be removed if fixation of the fracture is compromised.

FRACTURES OF THE MANDIBLE

Approximately half of the facial fractures involve the mandible.[7,8] The majority of the fractures occur in areas of thinness (subcondylar neck and mandibular angle) and weakness (mandibular foramen).[9] Because of its horseshoe shape, any unilateral fracture should be regarded with suspicion. A careful search for a fracture on the contralateral side is warranted.

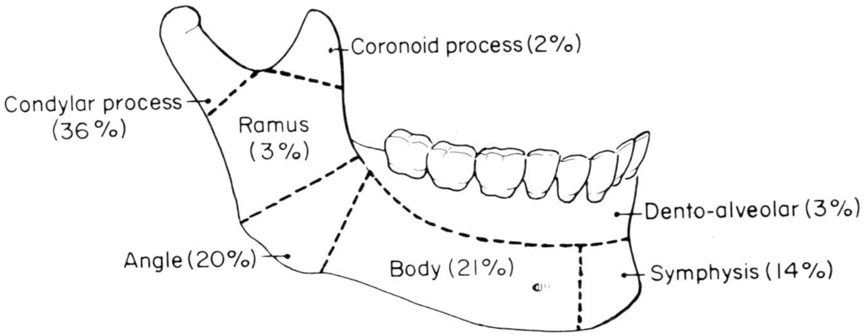

Figure 9.11 Regional distribution of mandibular fractures. (After Dingman and Natvig.[9])

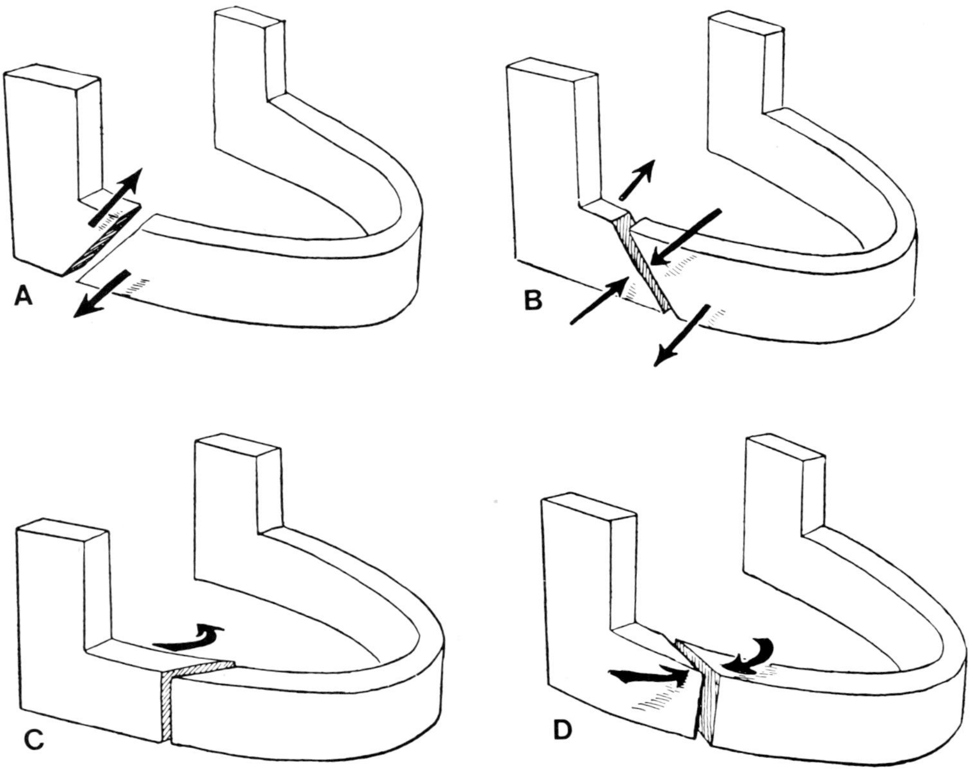

Figure 9.12 Influence of muscle pull on mandibular fractures. Arrows indicate direction of movement caused by muscular contraction. (*A, C*). Unfavorable fractures due to distraction of fragments by muscular pull. (*B, D*) Favorable fractures where muscular forces tend to coapt the fragments. (Reproduced with permission from V. H. Kazanjian and J. M. Converse: *The Surgical Treatment of Facial Injuries,* Ed. 3. Williams & Wilkins, Baltimore.[3])

Classification. Several classification schemes are applicable to fractures of the mandible. The separation can be made as to *severity* (simple versus compound) and to *type* (greenstick, complex, comminuted, impacted, and depressed). More specific are those systems based on *direction* of the fracture and the influence of muscular forces (*favorable* versus *unfavorable*), *presence or absence of teeth*, and *region* of involvement.

A fracture is said to be favorable when the pull of the muscles tend to coapt the segments. A common example is the fracture through the mandibular angle. The fracture extending anteriorly and inferiorly from the retromolar region (Fig. 9.12*A*) would be *favorable* in direction; the vectors of force of the powerful muscles of mastication favors the approximation of the fragments. Conversely, an angle fracture directed posteriorly and inferiorly would be characterized as being *unfavorable* since the pull of the muscles would distract the segments (Fig. 9.12*B*). Both the vertical (Fig. 9.12, *A* and *B*) and the horizontal (Fig. 9.12, *C* and *D*) obliquity of the fracture must also be considered.

The *presence* or *absence* of teeth has been used by Kazanjian and Converse as a guide to treatment.[10] The classification has practical implications. The teeth serve as a source of anchorage for the various fixation devices. Therefore, their number and location have an important bearing on the choice of the method of stabilization. The classification is as follows:

Class I. Teeth present on both sides of the fracture line.
Class II. Teeth present on only one side of the fracture line.
Class III. Fragments are edentulous.

Dingman and Natvig favor the catagorization of mandibular fractures into *regions*: alveolar process, symphysis, body, angle, ramus, coronoid process, and condylar process (Fig. 9.11). Each zone is unique and tends to behave in a characteristic manner following bony disruption.

Approaching problems with these classification systems in mind helps to clarify needs and simplify management.

Treatment. Most mandibular fractures can be treated by closed reduction. However, each fracture initially should be approached as a candidate for an open reduction. A systematic search can then be made to rule out this possibility to avoid errors of omission.

Alveolar Process. Fractures of the alveolar process are usually confined to a segment of the dental arch. Even when the disruption is severe, the fragments can be salvaged if a bridge of mucosa remains to supply circulation from the adjacent tissues.

When sound teeth are present on each side of the fragment, stabilization is achieved by ligating the teeth to an arch bar. If anchorage is absent at one end, an acrylic splint can be fabricated to the buccal and/or lingual surface of the teeth. The teeth are ligated to the splint to prevent drift of the fragment. Intermaxillary fixation is not required.

Fixation is maintained for 3–6 weeks depending on the severity of the disruption.

Symphysis. Uncomplicated nondisplaced symphyseal fractures can be managed by applications of arch bars and intermaxillary fixation for 5–6 weeks. However, on occasion, the lateral pull of the muscles of mastication will tend to distract the inferior border of the symphysis. Should this occur, open reduction with the placement of an interosseous wire along the inferior border is recommended. The conventional degloving technique[3] or an external incision in the submental region can be used.

A relative indication for an open reduction would be the association of a subcondylar neck fracture. This combination is frequently seen. Early mobilization is desired to minimize the possibilities of ankylosis. Greater stability of the symphyseal fracture is achieved by open reduction and direct interosseous fixation.

Body. When teeth are present on both sides of the fracture, closed reduction with intermaxillary fixation for 5–6 weeks is adequate. A body fracture with an unfavorable angulation and the absence of teeth in the distal fragment is best managed by an open reduction and internal fixation plus intermaxillary fixation for 5–6 weeks.

Angle. Anatomically a weak point, fractures of the angle are common. Because of the absence of teeth in the posterior fragment (Class II fracture), the direction of the fracture line is of paramount importance in determining the method of treatment. The powerful muscles of mastication will pull the proximal segment cephalad. Therefore, when the line of disruption extends inferiorly and *anteriorly*, a favorable relationship exists (Fig. 9.12). Conversely, a fracture traversing inferiorly and *posteriorly* is unfavorable in direction since the muscular forces will distract the fragments.

Favorable fractures are managed by closed reduction. An open reduction is required for unfavorable fractures to furnish additional internal stabilization. An intraoral approach can be used to place an interosseous wire across the superior portion of the fracture. An external approach is equally effective. An incision is made 1.5–2 cm below the angle following a natural crease in the skin (Risdon approach).[11] Care must be exercised to avoid injury to the marginal mandibular branch of the facial nerve which is deep to the platysma muscle.

Whether the fracture is favorable or unfavorable in nature, intermaxillary fixation for 5–6 weeks is required.

Ramus. Fractures of the ramal regions are infrequent. A muscular sling, composed of the masseter on the lateral surface and the internal pterygoid medially, serves to splint the fracture. Closed reduction with internal fixation for 5–6 weeks is usually adequate.

Coronoid Process. Little functional dearrangement is incurred by fractures of the coronoid process. They are the least common of the mandibular fractures and require no treatment.

Condylar Process. Fractures of the condylar region can be divided by their relationship to the insertion of the lateral pterygoid muscle. Fractures above this insertion are confined mainly to the capsular portion. Treatment consists of maintaining the patient on a soft diet.

Fractures below the insertion of the lateral pterygoid muscle (subcondylar neck fractures) present a greater problem. The condylar fragment is displaced medially and anteriorly by the pull of the lateral pterygoid muscle. Undisplaced and subluxated fractures can be best managed by closed reduction and intermaxillary fixation.[12] Difficulty in management arises when the condylar fragment is dislocated out of the glenoid fossa.

It is usually futile to attempt manual manipulation of the fragment in hopes of returning it to a more favorable position in the glenoid fossa. The strong pull of the lateral pterygoid muscle is not easily neutralized under these circumstances. Thus, one is left with two directly opposite methods of treatment: closed versus open reduction.

Advocates of the closed method of management feel that intermaxillary fixation alone is sufficient. The deep location of the medially dislocated condylar fragment and the close proximity of the facial nerve are cited as hazards against an open reduction. Satisfactory results can be achieved in most instances by the spontaneous gradual return of the fragment to the glenoid fossa[13] or by resorption and remodeling to restore the joint to a preinjury facsimile.[14, 15]

Proponents for an open reduction believe that spontaneous restoration of a functional joint is unlikely when the condylar fragment is driven out of the joint. Dislocation of this magnitude shortens the ramal height causing premature tooth contact on the ipsilateral side and an anterior open bite. The chin deviates to the affected side. A particularly troublesome situation is faced by totally edentulous adults with bilateral subcondylar fractures. Alterations in intermaxillary arch alignment can pose a serious problem for the prosthodontist when an attempt is made to construct functional dentures.

A special dilemma is encountered when a dislocated fracture is sustained by a growing child. Added to the problems of a malocclusion is the possibility of growth disturbances. At one end of the spectrum there are those who favor treatment consisting only of a soft diet and no fixation at all.[16] Long term bite and growth disturbances are reported not to be a problem. Balancing this extreme are those who feel that the dangers of maldevelopment are real and open reduction should be performed.[9, 17]

If an open reduction is elected, the joint can be approached through a preauricular, retromandibular, or a Risdon incision. Anatomical reduction is not necessary since remodeling will restore a functional joint. The jaws are immobilized for 3–4 weeks; a period similar to that used when treatment consists of only closed reduction. Early movement is desirable to minimize the danger of ankylosis.

FRACTURES OF THE MAXILLA

Fractures of the maxilla tend to behave differently from those of the mandible. The differences can be explained on the basis of the muscular attachments and the underlying unique skeletal support.

Unlike the mandible, the maxilla is free of attachments of any strong muscle groups. Only the lateral pterygoid, acting directly through its origin on the sphenoid bone, has any appreciable effect on the maxilla Consequently, the major displacement of the maxilla is incurred at the time of initial injury and not by continued distracting muscular forces.

Despite its delicate walls, the maxilla is able to withstand considerable abuse. The force of trauma is absorbed by the unique architectural arrangements of the sturdy bony buttresses. However, when the tolerance of the skeletal framework is exceeded, the maxilla tends to crumble along predictable lines.

Classification. Because of the anatomical differences, the classification of maxillary fractures differs from those of the maxilla. Only fractures of the alveolar process mimic those of the lower jaw and are treated in a like manner. The similarity ends here.

The foundation for categorizing fractures of the maxilla date back to 1901 and the classical investigations of Le Fort. Inflicting violent blows with a wooden club to the midface of fresh cadavers, he noted distinct patterns of separation of the maxilla from the remainder of the craniofacial skeleton (Figs. 9.13–9.15).

Le Fort I Fracture. The Le Fort I fracture is often called a horizontal fracture of the maxilla (Fig. 9.13). The line of fracture extends transversely above the apices of the teeth cutting across the maxillary sinus and the nasal septum. In addition, the path of the fracture continues posteriorly across the pyramidal process of the palatine bone and the perpendicular plate of the sphenoid bone.

In effect, the maxilla and the two bones neighboring its posterior surface are separated from the remainder of the midfacial skeleton.

Le Fort II Fracture. Because of its shape, the Le Fort II fracture is also known as the pryamidal midfacial fracture (Fig. 9.14). In the posterior region, the separation is similar to that of the Le Fort I. However, as one progresses anteriorly, the line of fracture rises obliquely into the medial portion of the orbital cavity and across the nasal bones.

The nasal complex is now included with the maxilla in being detached from the remainder of the midface. The main portions of the zygoma remain undisturbed.

Le Fort III Fracture. Separation of the entire midface from the cranium characterizes this fracture (Fig. 9.15). The breach occurs along the frontozygomatic suture line and continues through the orbit coursing along the lateral, inferior, and medial orbital walls and across the

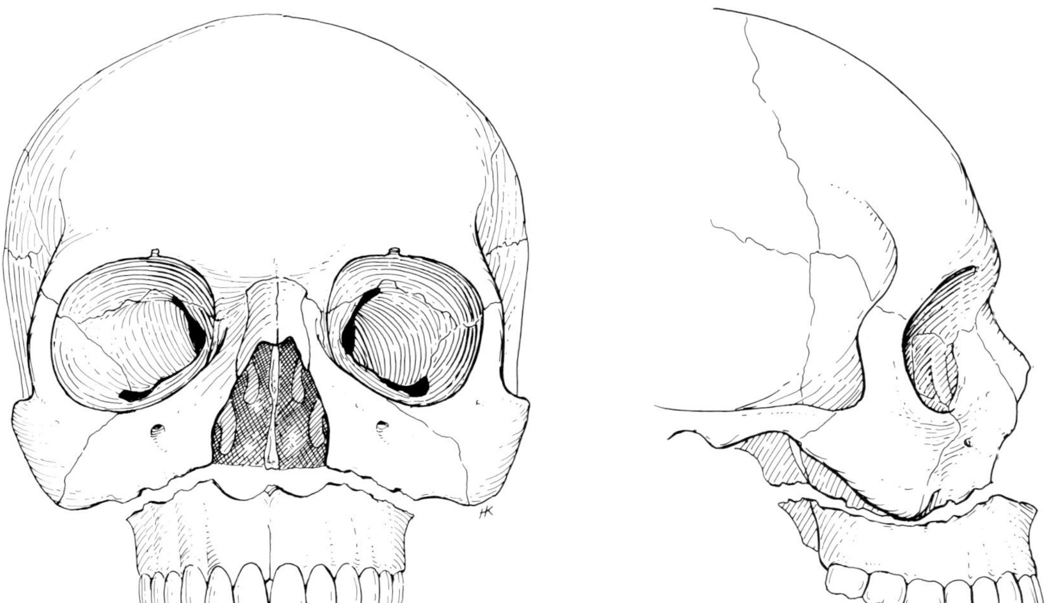

Figure 9.13 Le Fort I fracture. Separation of the inferior portion of maxilla from remainder of facial skeleton.

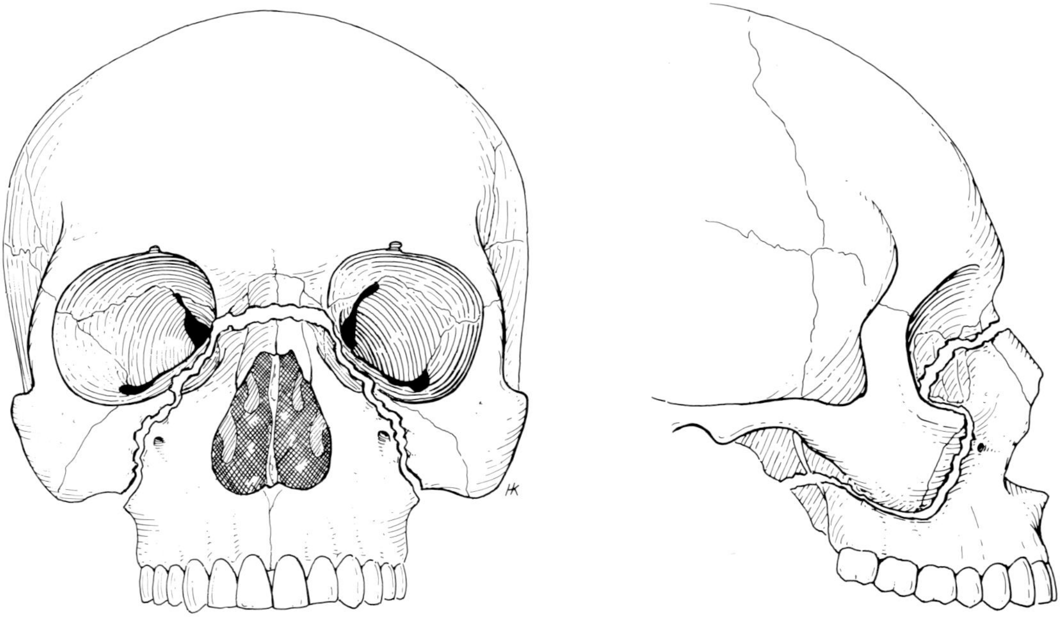

Figure 9.14 Le Fort II fracture. Maxilla and nose are detached from facial skeleton. Fracture extends into orbit and across nasal bones.

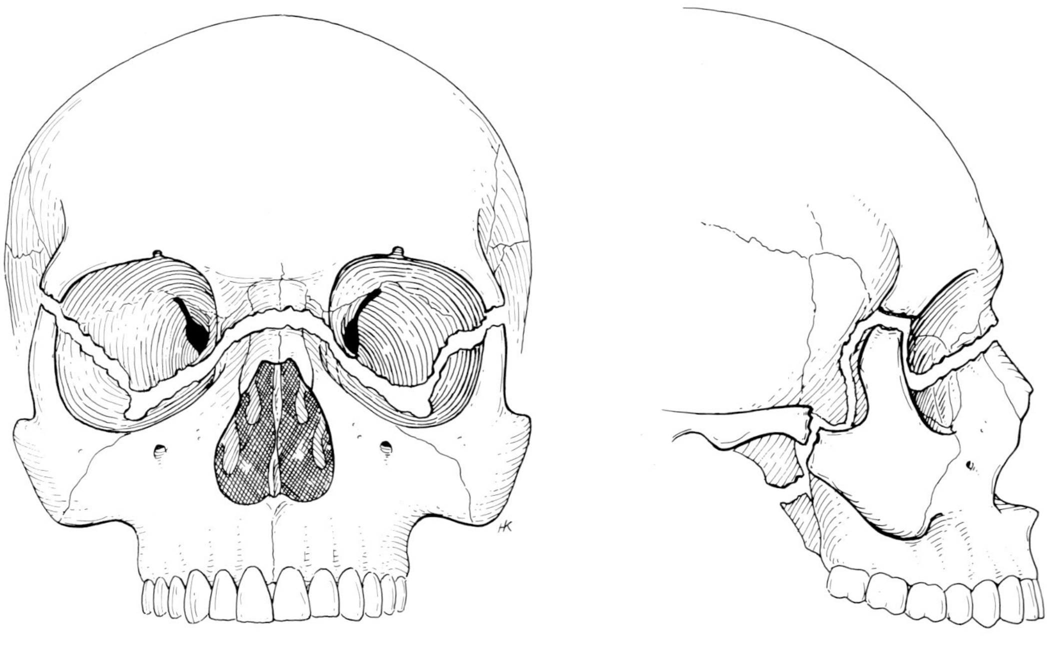

Figure 9.15 Le Fort III fracture. Craniofacial dysfunction. Entire midfacial mass is separated from its cranial attachments.

nasal bones. Posteriorly, the separation is completed by the fracture of the zygomatic arch and the perpendicular plates of the sphenoid bone.

Although the midfacial fractures are described in their pure form, it should be understood that they are often found in combination with one another. The pattern is variable and the separation is unlikely to be as clean as those depicted by the artist of the textbook illustrations. For example, the thin delicate bony framework of the naso-orbital regions are particularly prone to be comminuted. Nevertheless, an understanding of the basic patterns of midfacial fractures is helpful in their treatment.

Treatment. As with any fracture, the basic principle of stabilizing the displaced segment to the nearest intact bone holds true for fractures of the maxilla. Inferiorly the mandible is used to immobilize the maxilla with intermaxillary appliances. Depending upon the level of the midfacial fractures, the points of cephalad fixation and suspension will vary.[19]

Alveolar Fractures. Treatment of alveolar fractures of the maxilla are similar to those of the mandible. If the dentoalveolar complex on each side of the displaced segment is intact, simple stabilization with an arch bar is all that is required. When a neighboring stable segment is not present, intermaxillary fixation with or without an acrylic splint may be required for orientation purposes.

The period of fixation is generally 3 weeks but may be extended if the extent of disruption is extensive.

Le Fort I (Fig. 9.16). Horizontal fractures of the maxilla are treated by closed reduction. The displaced fragment is returned to its normal position with the use of disimpaction forceps and intermaxillary fixation is applied.

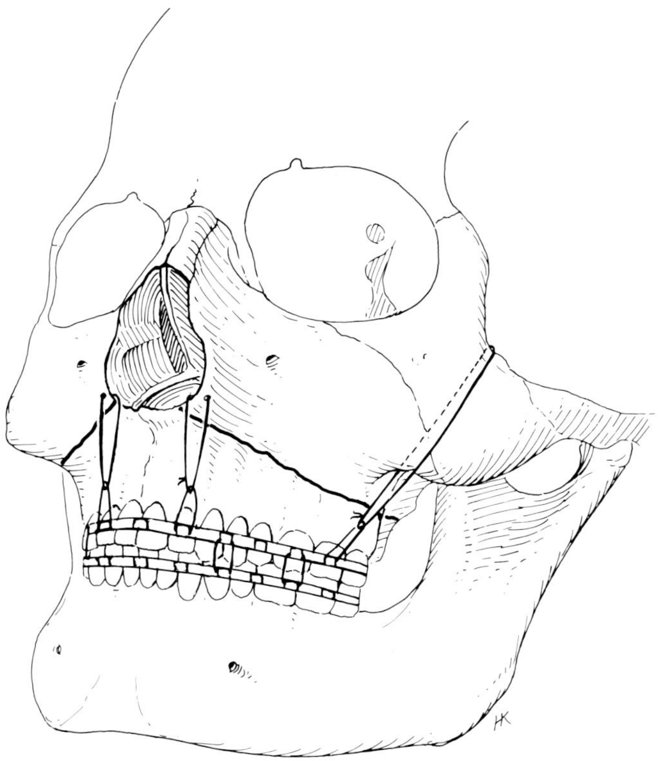

Figure 9.16 Fixation of Le Fort I fracture. Arch bars and intermaxillary wires stabilize maxillary to mandible. Suspension wires prevent caudal displacement of maxilla. Either circumzygomatic loops or suspension wires through pyriform rim can be used.

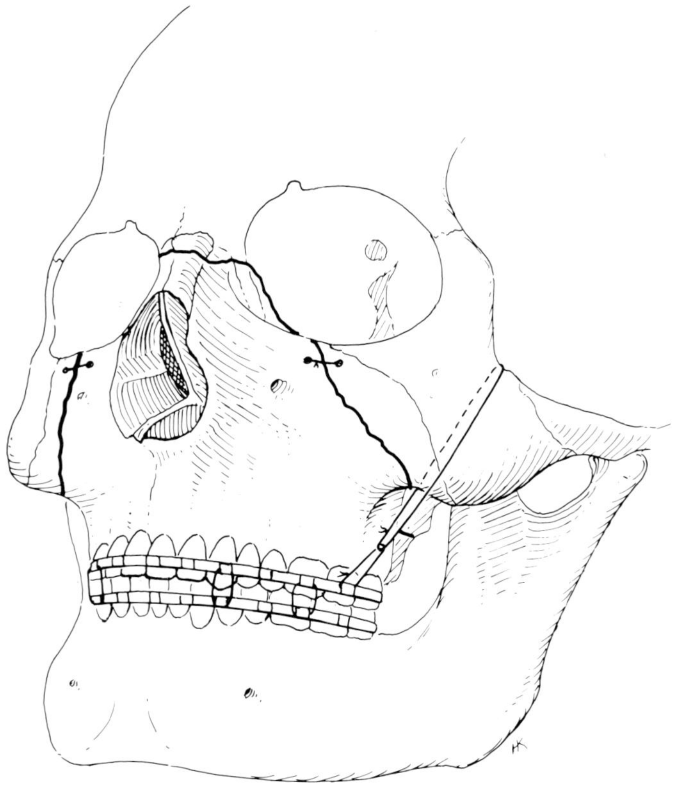

Figure 9.17 Fixation of Le Fort II fracture. Arch bars and intermaxillary wires relate the maxillary fragment to mandible. Interosseous wires through inferior orbital rim realigns the orbit. Circumzygomatic suspension wires are used to neutralize caudal distraction forces.

A suspension wire is generally passed around the zygomatic arches and is attached to the arch bars. A wire can also be passed through a drill hole in the pyriform rim or the inferior orbital rim and dropped down to the arch bar. It is wise to incorporate an auxillary loop of wire between the main suspension wire and the arch bar. During intermaxillary fixation, any tightening of the suspension system is performed through the auxillary loop. The main suspension loop should not be used for adjustment. Metal fatigue can weaken the wire and its breakage would destroy the suspension system. However, breakage of the auxillary loop would not pose a problem since a new wire can easily be substituted between the main loop and the arch bar.

Fibrous union takes place quite quickly with fractures of the maxilla. The fixation period can be as short as three to four weeks. The period of immobilization is extended if clinical mobility is present at that end of this time.

Alternatives to the circumzygomatic suspension wires are drop wires passed through the inferior orbital rim or through the rim of the pyriform aperture above the line of fracture.

Le Fort II (Fig. 9.17). Displaced pyramidal fractures are repositioned with a disimpaction forceps. Intermaxillary fixation is established with the mandible to restore occlusion. The fracture of the inferior orbital rim is reduced by an interosseous wire placed through a lower eyelid incision. Suspension wires can be passed around the zygomatic arch down to the arch bar. A fixation period of 4–6 weeks is usually sufficient.

Le Fort III (Fig. 9.18). The superior fixation point for these craniofacial separation fractures is at the frontozygomatic suture line. Interosseous wire fixation is required to reapproximate the segments. A common approach to the region is that of a lateral brow incision. One must be careful to bevel the incision in such a manner as to avoid the hair follicles. If this precaution is not heeded, a noticeable scar in the eyebrow will result due to the loss of hair.

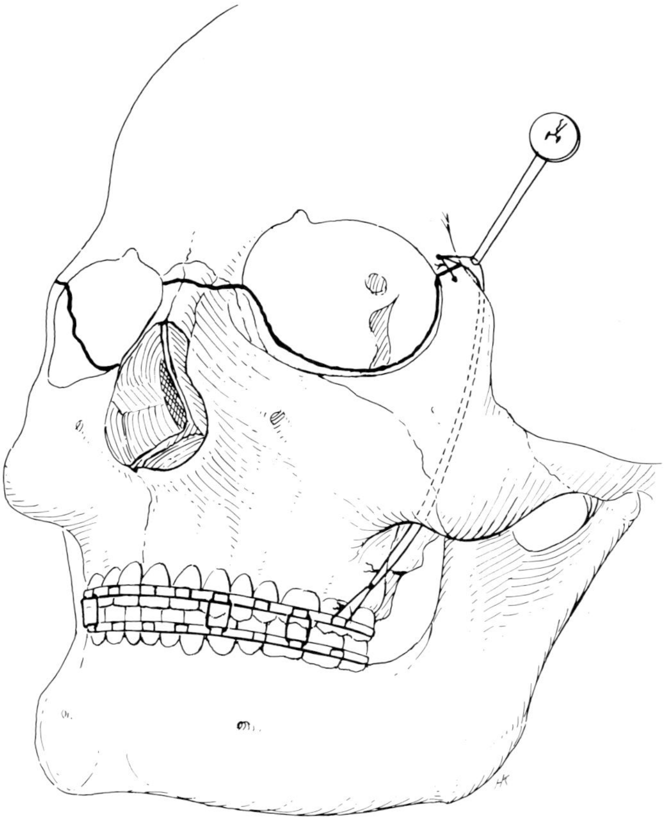

Figure 9.18 Fixation of Le Fort III fracture. Arch bars and intermaxillary wires restore proper relationship of midfacial skeleton to mandible. Interosseous wires used to reduce frontozygomatic separation. Cranial suspension wire is passed through drill hole in stable zygomatic process of frontal bone. Pull out wire is brought out skin in temporal area and tied over a button.

In the author's opinion, it is safer to use the lateral portion of an upper blepharoplasty incision to expose the frontozygomatic suture. The skin is quite mobile and access to the nearby fracture site is excellent through such an incision. If one follows the natural crease lines, the scar is practically invisible and the danger of injuring hair follicles is avoided.

Inferiorly, stabilization is again provided by intermaxillary fixation to the mandible.

The zygomatic arch and the infraorbital rims can no longer be used as suspension points since these areas are involved in the fracture. Consequently, the intact zygomatic process of the frontal bone is used as a cranial fixation point for the suspension wire. A pull-out wire is looped through the suspension wire and brought out near the frontotemporal hairline to be tied over a button. A 4–6-week period of fixation is usually required.

As mentioned earlier, any combination of midface fractures can be found. Isolated fractures of the orbital floor (blow-out), naso-orbital complex, and zygoma are also seen. Discussion of these fractures is deleted from this chapter since they are outside the anatomic confines of the jaws.

ACQUIRED DEFORMITIES WITH ABSENCE OF PARTS

The degree of difficulty in reconstructing a jaw becomes compounded multifold when there is an actual loss of tissues. To reestablish normal alignment, additional materials must be introduced to compensate for the loss of parts. In civilian life, ablative procedures for cancers of the head and neck account for the major number of these deformities. Gunshot injuries are another source and are apt to be more devastating since the disruptive force is uncontrolled.

To succeed in restoring a jaw toward normlacy, the following elements must be provided: (1) soft tissue covering, (2) supporting framework, and (3) lining. The principles and techniques of providing soft tissue covering and lining are similar to those of oncologic surgery. The task of providing a replacement for the lost skeletal support will be discussed in this section.

Before one embarks on a treatment plan to reconstruct a jaw, the question must be asked, "Is it necessary?" In many instances, especially those associated with loss of the maxilla, the surgeon's ability to match the results of a skilled maxillofacial prosthodontist is indeed challenged. Facial form and function can be restored to the maxilla by a prosthesis. When there is a skeletal defect in the horseshoe shape of the mandible, functional derangements can be serious especially when the symphyseal region is involved. However, even with an entire half of the mandible absent, many patients can accommodate well and be left with little functional impairment. The main complaint is apt to be the residual facial asymmetry.

Therefore, before considering the reconstruction of a jaw, the patient's complaint should be well heard. The functional and aesthetic demands must be balanced.

REPLACEMENT MATERIALS

The materials used to replace the skeletal defect can be divided into four main groups: (1) alloplastic materials, (2) heterologous bone, (3) homologous bone, and (4) autologous bone.

The obvious attraction to be able to replace human tissue with an alloplastic material has generated numerous articles. Everything from ivory to sophisticated space age metals and plastics has been used. In almost every instance the newly discovered alloplastic material generates a flurry of enthusiastic reports. With time and experience the enthusiasm is dampened and the material in question quietly fades from vogue because of the lack of long term success.

Many of the currently available alloplastic materials are well tolerated by the body. The main stumbling block that prevents their widespread use is located at the interface between the alloplastic material and the host tissue. The soft tissue and bony ingrowths are limited. In spite of the use of all manners of fixation devices, with time and use, the interface between the material and the host bone breaks down. Once the cohesion problem is solved, a significant step will have been made.

Heterologous and homologous bone have also been used.[21, 22] Various processes have been used to alter their antigenicity in hopes of reducing the rejection rate. Again, the lack of long term success has discouraged their widespread use and failed to sustain their initial popularity.

Autologous bone remains the material of choice in restoring the framework of the mandible. Favored donor sites are the rib cage and the ilium. In most instances, cancellous bone fares better than cortical bone.[23] Thus, the ilium with its higher percentage of cancellous bone remains a favored donor site. Cases that require a condyle-ramus reconstruction are an exception. In these instances, a rib graft, using the costal cartilage junction to replace the condyle, is a popular method.[24] An alternative would be to use a metatarsal complex from the foot.

The size of the mandibular skeletal defect influences the method used in the reconstruction. For defects caused by benign disease, an entire half of the mandible can be successfully replaced.[25] The quality of the surrounding soft tissues is much more favorable in these instances as compared to those defects caused by ablative surgery for malignant disease. Moderate sized defects in either case can be corrected by the insertion of a carved block of ilium.

Larger defects produced by ablative cancer operations and gunshot wounds pose additional problems. The skeletal defect is apt to involve more than one anatomical unit of the mandible (e.g., body plus symphysis). In addition to the bulk requirement to fill the defect, the graft must be altered to follow the normal contours of the mandible. The technique of using cancellous bone chips overpacked into a meshed titanium tray has been shown to provide satisfactory results.[26] The advantages of this technique are the rapid vascularization of the cancellous bone chips, the ability to shape the tray to reproduce normal mandibular contours, and possible elimination of the need for intermaxillary fixation or other stabilization devices due to the rigidity incorporated in the tray. A relative contraindication in using this technique is the presence of irradiated soft tissues. The failure rate is apt to be high unless soft tissue damaged by irradiation is replaced.[27]

The entire concept of reconstruction of the mandible will undergo dramatic change in the years to come. The foundations of microsurgical techniques have been well established and are being applied. In addition, musculocutaneous transfer of soft and hard tissues is also beginning to show exciting applications. The capability to simultaneously transfer in a safe manner overlying soft tissue, skeletal support, and lining is indeed attractive.

DEVELOPMENTAL DEFORMITIES

The treatment considerations demanded by developmental malformations differs from those required by acquired deformities. Thought processes must be reorganized.

With acquired deformities, the surgeon's goal is to return distorted structures back to their norm, i.e., their pre-existing state. The aim is to *re*construct destroyed parts toward their pre-insult condition. In contrast, patients with developmental malformations fall short of ever achieving normal form and function. The surgical challenge, therefore, is changed from one of *re*construction to that of *con*struction: normal relationships must be built from malformed parts.

With developmental malformations, the basic elements of size and position are distorted. Deformation takes place in three dimensions and is exaggerated when the defect is unilateral in nature. The deformities become more pronounced with growth. Treatment is, thus, generally deferred until the final adolescent growth spurt has passed.

Diagnosis

To establish a diagnosis on clinical examination alone can be hazardous when dealing with developmental jaw deformities. A sense of facial proportion is helpful but the soft tissue relationships that one sees may not accurately reflect the underlying problem. To complement the clinical assessment, it is necessary to obtain photographs, dental casts, and roentgenograms.

Properly oriented black and white photographs of the face are indispensible. On profile, the Frankfort line should be parallel to the floor. A proper frontal view would find the midline of the face perpendicular to the floor and an absence of rotation of the head. The clinical impressions of facial proportion can be confirmed or modified. If necessary, the photographs can also be sectioned in an attempt to roughly visualize the desired results.

A detailed study of the occlusal relationship is provided by the dental casts. Spacial manipulation of the casts can be used to forecast the changes in occlusion of an en bloc movement of either jaw. If necessary, the casts can be sectioned to mock the surgical procedure. An appreciation of the amount of movement and the location of the necessary osteotomies is achieved. The casts are also used to fabricate splints in those cases that require them.

Intraoral and panoramic roentgenograms, as in the case of acquired deformities, provide useful information. The most valuable diagnostic roentgenogram for developmental deformities is, however, the cephalogram. A special unit is required that places the patient's head in fixed positions and 60 inches from the energy source. Because of the standard distance and positions, films taken at different intervals can be compared. From the lateral cephalogram, a pencil tracing of the skeleton and the soft tissue profile is made on an acetate sheet. Using anthropometric skeletal points on the tracing, orthodontists have established normal values for various distances and angles of a well balanced face. The patient's findings can be compared with the normative data to gain further insight into the deformity.

The role of the orthodontist cannot be overly stressed. His clinical assessment of the patient and analysis of the cephalogram will provide valuable information for the development of a treatment plan. Several schools of cephalometric analysis exist. Each orthodontist has has favorite system. It would be naive for the surgeon to assume he possesses a similar working knowledge of the nuances of the various analysis systems. It is, therefore, imperative that the surgeon seek the cooperation of the orthodontist, review the findings with him, and agree upon an appropriate treatment plan.

It is important to distinguish between deformities that are primarily dentoalveolar in nature from those that are primarily confined to the underlying supporting skeleton (Fig. 9.19). The dentoalveolar complex consists of the teeth and the pliable alveolar bone that surrounds their roots. Cancellous bone is a major component of the alveolus. It is covered by a thin layer of cortical bone. Because of this configuration, the dentoalveolar portion of the jaws respond well to orthodontic forces. On the other hand, the basilar skeleton on which the dentoalveolar structure rests is composed of a greater proportion of cortical bone and is resistant to orthodontic forces.

For the most part, orthodontic treatment alone can be used to correct dentoalveolar malrelationships. When the underlying skeletal malformation is minor, sufficient compensation can be achieved by the orthodontist. However, the greater the participation of the skeleton in

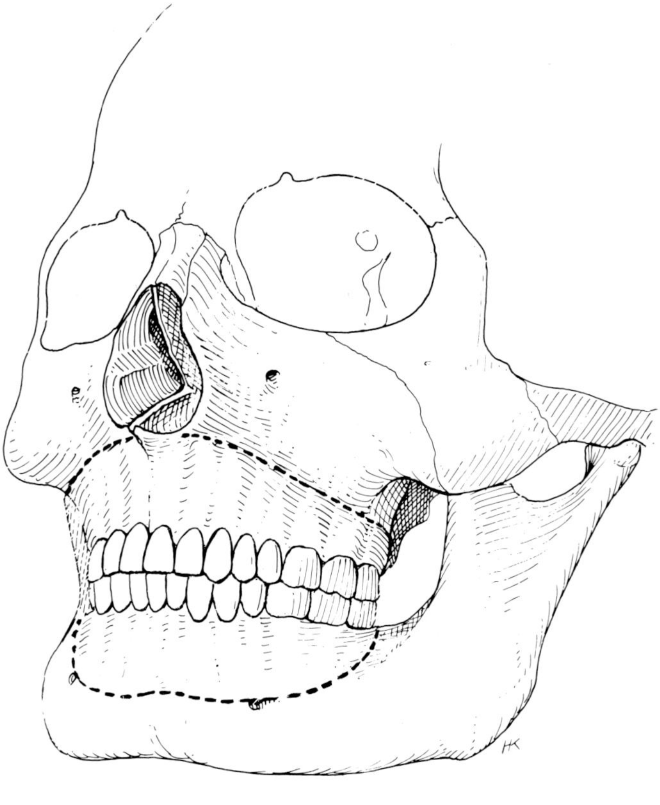

Figure 9.19 Dentoalveolar complex. *Dash lines* indicate junction between the dentoalveolar structures and remainder of mandible and maxilla.

the deformity, the greater will be the need for surgical intervention. Furthermore, in adults with dentoalveolar deformities, a combined orthodontic-surgical approach is often considered to decrease the amount of treatment time.

Types of Developmental Jaw Deformities

Jaw deformities are categorized on the basis of three-dimensional relationships. The position of the various components are compared to one another and to the cranial base. Anteroposterior, vertical, and lateral spacial relationships must be taken into consideration.

MANDIBLE

A mandible that is underdeveloped assumes a retruded postion. The terms mandibular *retrognathia* or *micrognathia* are used interchangeably. However, a subtle difference exists. Technically speaking both are located posteriorly but a retrognathic mandible is normal in size and a micrognathic jaw is smaller than normal. A Class II malocclusion is associated with the deformity.

In contrast, overdevelopment is a feature of mandibular *prognathism.* An absolute increase in the dimension of the jaw causes it to jut out to disrupt the normal profile. The term *pseudo*mandibular prognathism is used when the mandible is normal in size but clinically appears to be prognathic because of an underdevelopment of the maxilla. In either instance, the accompanying malocclusion is of the Class III type.

Lateral deviation of the mandible is seen when the deformity is unilateral in nature. Thus, in cases of unilateral condylar overgrowth, the chin is deflected to the contralateral side. The opposite effect is seen when arrest in normal condylar growth occurs; the chin deviates to the ipsilateral side.

CHIN

It is important to consider the chin as a separate entity. All mandibular deformities mentioned above can be mimicked by alterations of the size of the chin. Thus, the mandible and occlusion can be normal in every way and the facial harmony be destroyed because of a malformation of the chin. *Microgenia* and *macrogenia* are at opposite ends of the spectrum. In microgenia, the chin is usually small in all dimensions. With macrogenia, the direction of enlargement can be anteroposterior (e.g., witch's chin), vertical, or both. Lateral deviations are also seen.

MAXILLA

The most common upper jaw deformity to be called to the surgeon's attention is that of maxillary *hypoplasia.* The patient has a "dish face" appearance. The lower jaw, which is normal in size, takes on a pseudoprognathic silhouette.

When a major discrepancy occurs in a vertical direction, the result is a *short* or *long face syndrome.* In a short face syndrome deformity, there is a disproportional decrease in vertical dimension of the lower third of the face. The facial configuration is square. The mandible appears overclosed and the corners of the mouth take a downward slant. The teeth are barely visible, if at all, when the patient smiles.

Conversely, patients with the long face syndrome have an unusually elongated lower half of the face. With the lips in repose, there is an excessive exposure of teeth. To span the excess distance, the lips must strain to meet one another. On laughter, a "gummy smile" is seen because of the unflattering display of teeth and gingiva.

MANDIBULAR AND MAXILLARY PROTRUSION

In contrast to the forementioned malformations, protrusion deformities are dentoalveolar in nature. The size and location of the skeletal bases are within normal limits. The anterior teeth protrude excessively to produce a full appearance of the lips. When the deformity is confined mainly to the maxilla, the term "buck teeth" is often teasingly applied.

Mild amounts of bimaxillary protrusion is a normal racial feature in blacks and orientals.

OPEN BITE (APERTOGNATHIA)

The teeth normally contact their counterpart of the opposing jaw. An open bite is produced when the teeth fail to meet due to a vertical discrepancy. This can occur in the incisor-canine region (anterior open bite), premolar-molar region (posterior open bite), or in both areas simultaneously with contact only of the posterior most teeth (total open bite).

Treatment

The operation, per se, is but a small part of the total treatment. To achieve the most stable results, orthodontic preoperative setup and postoperative detailing of occlusion must be provided. The amount of presurgical orthodontic treatment will depend upon the philosophy of the orthodontic-surgical team.

The surgeon and the orthodontist must sit down and review the initial treatment plan and make any necessary alterations prior to surgery. If the dental arch is to be moved in several segments, a mock operation on the dental casts will give the surgeon an idea about the amount of displacement that will be required. Whether or not to use a splint and its design should be discussed. Modification of the orthodontic appliance may also be necessary so that they can be used for the intermaxillary fixation. Arch bars used in the treatment of fractures are crude and far less hygienic when compared to the orthodontic appliance. Therefore, whenever possible the orthodontic appliances should be used for the fixation.

Blood loss during mandibular operations is usually not excessive. In major maxillary osteotomies, one can, however, encounter a fair amount of bleeding. In these cases, it is wise to draw a unit of autologous blood a few weeks prior to the operation. The blood loss can be kept at a minimum by injecting a solution containing a vasoconstrictor into the operative site and by the use of hypotensive anesthetic technique.

Tracheal intubation is through the nose. A tracheotomy is not required.

Prophylactic antibiotic therapy is begun preoperatively and continued postoperatively.

Following the fixation period, orthodontic treatment can be immediately reinstituted. The surgeon can hope to bring the jaws within tenths of a millimeter of the preoperative goals. If this is accomplished, the operation is a success. However, the orthodontist must work within far finer tolerances as he applies the finishing detail movements of the teeth.

MANDIBULAR PROGNATHISM

In 1895, Jaboulay[28] performed bilateral condylectomies to correct mandibular prognathism. Since that time, practically every region of the mandible has been sectioned in every conceivable manner to treat the deformity. Two techniques have survived the evolutionary process: the vertical (oblique) ramal osteotomy and the sagittal splitting osteotomy of the ramus.

Vertical (Oblique) Osteotomy. In 1954, Caldwell and Letterman[29] described the vertical section of the ramus from the sigmoid notch to a point just anterior to the mandibular angle.

A slight variation of the theme was introduced a few years later by Robinson[30] (1956) and Hinds[31] (1957) who favored an oblique osteotomy that started at the sigmoid notch and ended at a point just posterior to the mandibular angle. Initially, an external approach was used. Refinements of technique and instrumentation have made it possible to perform the procedure through an intraoral approach.

Extraoral Approach. A 3-cm Risdon incision is made in a skin crease below the mandibular angle (Fig. 9.20). Once the platysma muscle is divided, care must be exercised not to injure the marginal mandibular branch of the facial nerve. The periosteum is divided along the inferior border of the mandible and the masseter muscle is reflected from the ramus by blunt dissection.

The sigmoid notch is identified. A reciprocating power saw or a high speed drill is used to section the ramus in a vertical or oblique direction. The cut should be beveled in an anterior to posterior manner. This will increase the surface contact of the cancellous bone, carry the cut further away from the mandibular foramen, and help maintain the proximal (condylar) fragment lateral to the distal fragment.

The attachment of the medial pterygoid is stripped of the proximal fragment. After the same steps are followed on the contralateral side, the mandible can be recessed to the desired position and held in place by intermaxillary fixation. A final check is made to see that the proximal fragment is well seated in the glenoid fossa and overlaps onto the lateral surface of the ramus. Interosseous fixation of the fragment is not required. A layer closure of the wound completes the procedure.

Intraoral Approach. The same operation can be performed through an intraoral route. An incision is made along the anterior border of the ramus and follows the oblique line to the region of the molars (Fig. 9.21). A subperiosteal plane is followed to reflect the masseter off the ramus. The soft tissues are freed from the posterior border of the ramus and the mandibular angle with a pterygomandibular stripper. The masseter is retracted laterally and a vertical or oblique osteotomy is made with an angulated oscillating saw. The attachment of the medial pterygoid is separated from the proximal fragment which is allowed to rest on the lateral surface of the distal fragment.

The contralateral side is treated in a similar manner. The mandible is repositioned to correct the prognathism and intermaxillary fixation is established. The incision is closed in a single layer.

Both the extraoral and intraoral approaches are widely practiced. The extraoral approach provides excellent exposure, requires little in the way of special instruments, and is simple to learn. Its disadvantages are the external incision and the risk of injuring the marginal mandibular nerve. Even with specially designed instruments the exposure is limited in the intraoral technique. However, a visible scar is avoided and the marginal mandibular nerve is not put at risk. Working through the mouth theoretically increases the possibility of infection but this complication is rarely seen when antibiotic coverage is used.

The difference between the vertical and oblique osteotomies is not significant. In theory, bony union is encouraged by using the vertical osteotomy since greater bony contact is provided. But, regardless of the direction of the cut, nonunion is exceptionally rare. In either case, intermaxillary fixation is maintained for 6 weeks. With the oblique osteotomy, the

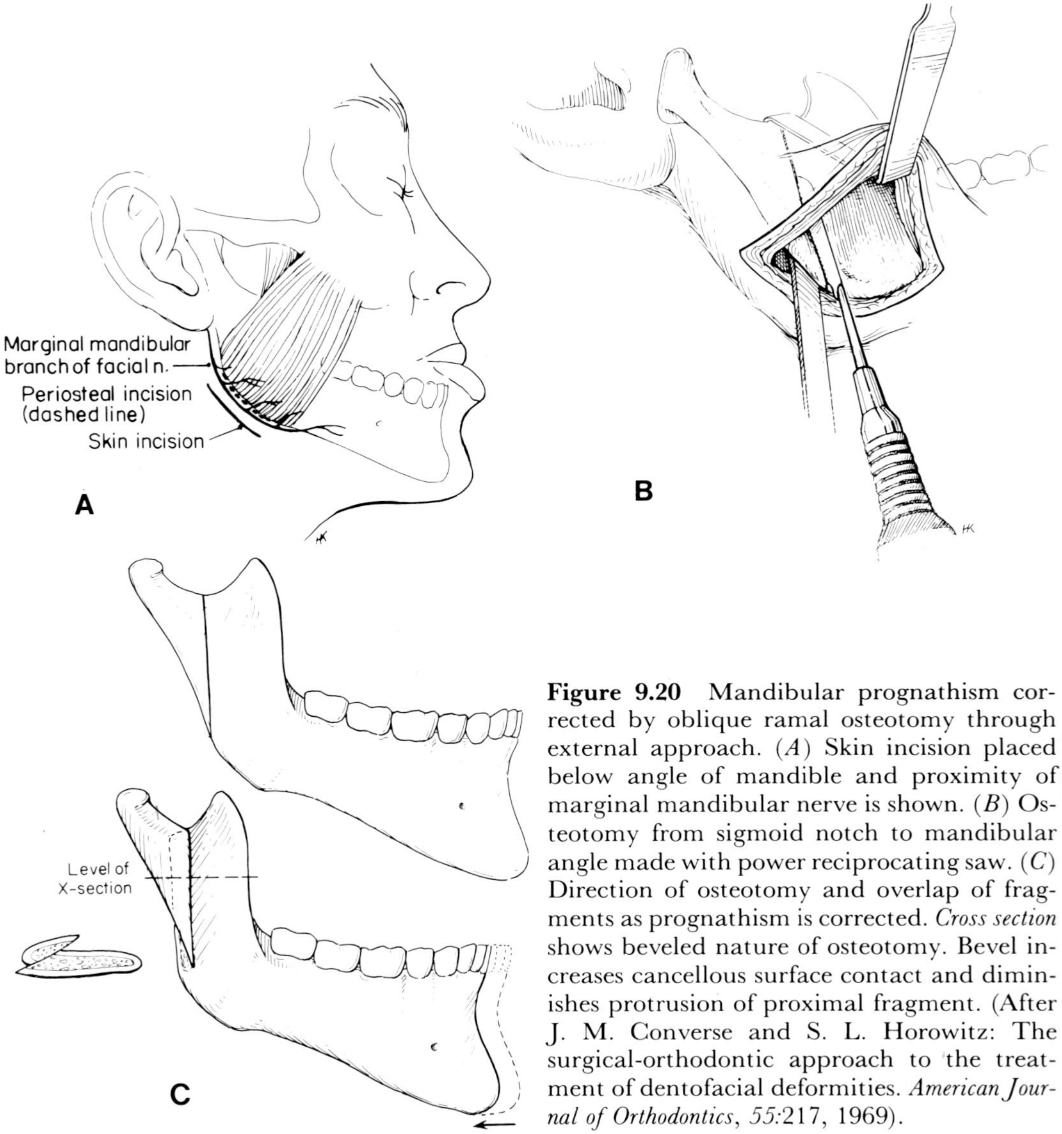

Figure 9.20 Mandibular prognathism corrected by oblique ramal osteotomy through external approach. (*A*) Skin incision placed below angle of mandible and proximity of marginal mandibular nerve is shown. (*B*) Osteotomy from sigmoid notch to mandibular angle made with power reciprocating saw. (*C*) Direction of osteotomy and overlap of fragments as prognathism is corrected. *Cross section* shows beveled nature of osteotomy. Bevel increases cancellous surface contact and diminishes protrusion of proximal fragment. (After J. M. Converse and S. L. Horowitz: The surgical-orthodontic approach to the treatment of dentofacial deformities. *American Journal of Orthodontics*, *55:*217, 1969).

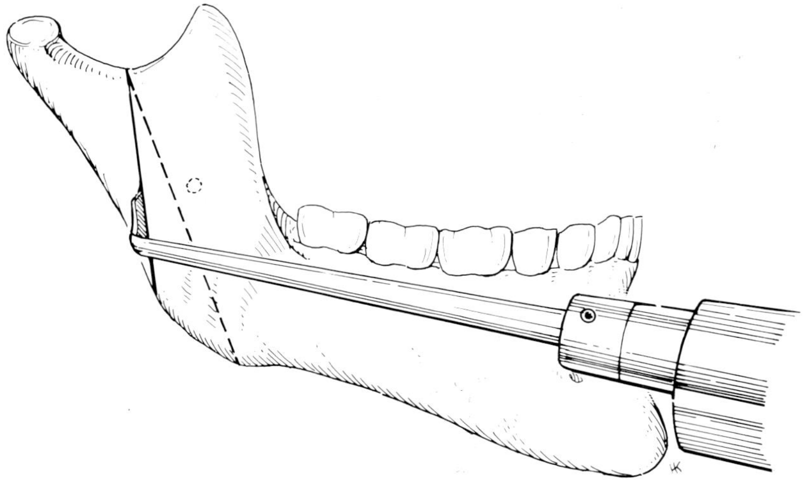

Figure 9.21 Intraoral ramal osteotomy. Angulated powered oscillating saw used for oblique sectioning of ramus. Dash lines indicate direction of vertical osteotomy. Mandibular foramen on medial surface represented by dotted circle.

likelihood of injuring the mandibular nerve is less since the cut is made slightly more posterior to the mandibular foramen.

Sagittal splitting osteotomy. Another popular method of sectioning the mandible is the sagittal splitting osteotomy of the ramus. The basic technique was developed by Obwegeser[32] and modified by Dal Pont.[33] The versatility of the procedure has led to its wide acceptance.

The ramus is approached through an intraoral incision similar to that used in the vertical osteotomy (Fig. 9.22). The inferior portion of the masseter is reflected off the ramus and the subperiosteal dissection is continued anteriorly to the molar region. On the medial surface the soft tissues above the mandibular foramen are separated in a subperiosteal plane. Specially designed channel retractors are inserted to protect the overlying soft tissues and the mandibular neurovascular bundle.

A series of burrs is used to outline the osteotomy. Care must be exercised to penetrate only through the cortical surface. On the medial aspect of the ramus, the osteotomy is directed horizontally and approximately 1 cm cephalad to the mandibular foramen. It is only necessary to carry this cut just posterior to the mandibular foramen.[34] The osteotomy is continued along the anterior border of the ramus following the oblique line. In the region of the second molar, the direction is changed to a vertical one to end the osteotomy at the inferior border of the mandibular body.

In the original technique, a large wide osteotome was used to split the ramus in a sagittal plane. Because of its width, the osteotome delivers a wedging force which causes the ramus to split along its weakest point, i.e., through the cancellous bone and mandibular canal. The neurovascular bundle is thus exposed and subject to injury. To minimize this possibility, Dautrey[35] advocated the use of fine, thin osteotomes. Hugging the inner surface of the lateral cortical plate the split is made lateral to the mandibular canal by a cutting, rather than a wedging, action.

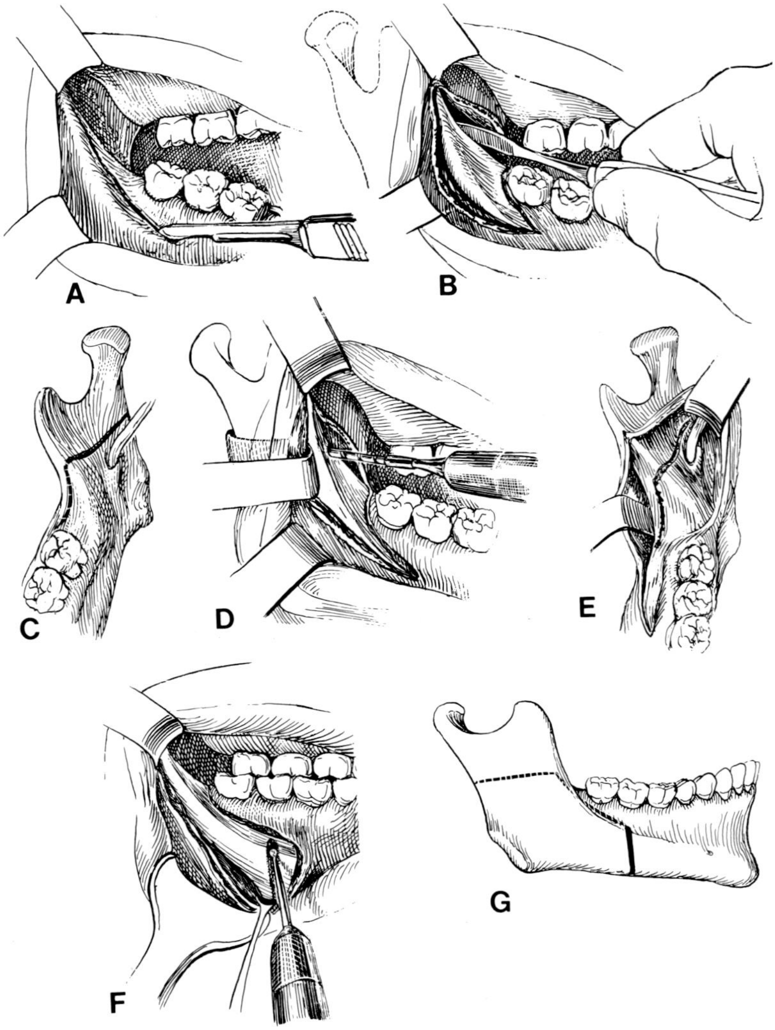

Figure 9.22 Sagittal splitting of ramus (Obwegeser-Dal Pont technique). (*A*) Mucosal incision following anterior border of ramus and oblique line. (*B*) Subperiosteal reflection of mucosa and muscle. (*C*) Path of osteotomy along medial aspect of ramus above mandibular foramen and neurovascular bundle. (*D*) Lindemann burr creating medial horizontal cut. (*E*) Cut through cortical bone of medial surface and anterior border of ramus. (*F*) Vertical cut with burr through lateral cortex of body in molar region. (*G*) Overall view of osteotomy. *Dotted line* represents medial horizontal and anterior ramal cuts. (*H*) Osteotome beginning the sagittal splitting. (*I*) Cross section of ramus showing path of cleavage through cancellous bone and mandibular canal. (*J*) Medial view of proximal fragment after split. (*K*) Lateral view of proximal fragment. (*L*) Lateral view of distal fragment. Intact neurovascular bundle coursing through canal. (*M*) Amount of overlap produced by retropositioning of prognathic mandible and area to be resected is shaded. (*N*) Circumferential wire to approximate fragments. (Reproduced with permission from J. M. Converse, H. K. Kawamoto, D. Wood-Smith, P. J. Cocarro, and J. G. McCarthy: Deformities of the jaws, in *Reconstructive Plastic Surgery*, Ed. 2, edited by J. M. Converse. W. B. Saunders, Philadelphia, 1977).

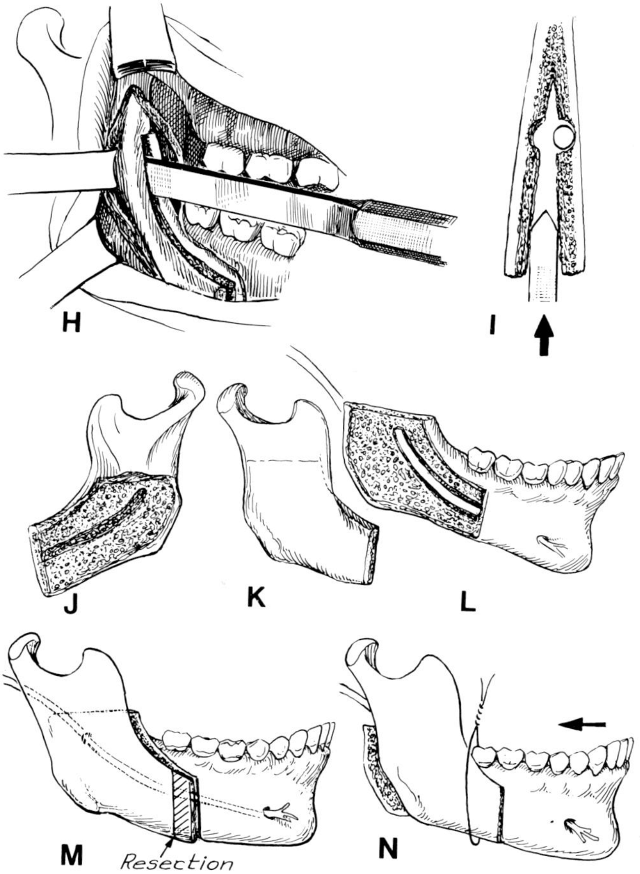

Figure 9.22 *(H–N)*

The steps are repeated on the opposite side to free the tooth-bearing distal fragment. The mandible is now repositioned to correct the prognathism and intermaxillary fixation is established. The excess bone along the vertical osteotomy of the body is trimmed off the proximal fragment. Interosseous wire fixation is used to stabilize the proximal fragment after the condyle is well seated in the glenoid fossa. The intraoral incisions are closed and intermaxillary fixation is maintained for 5–6 weeks.

The principle advantage of the sagittal splitting procedure is that it provides a broad surface of contact between the fragments. Since the opposing surfaces are cancellous in nature, consolidation is rapid. In addition, the mandible can be rotated to close anterior open bites and also advance to correct mandibular retrusion without losing bony contact.

The major drawback of the sagittal splitting osteotomy is the high incidence of injury to the inferior alveolar nerve. Careful long term studies have shown that hypesthesia of the lower lip

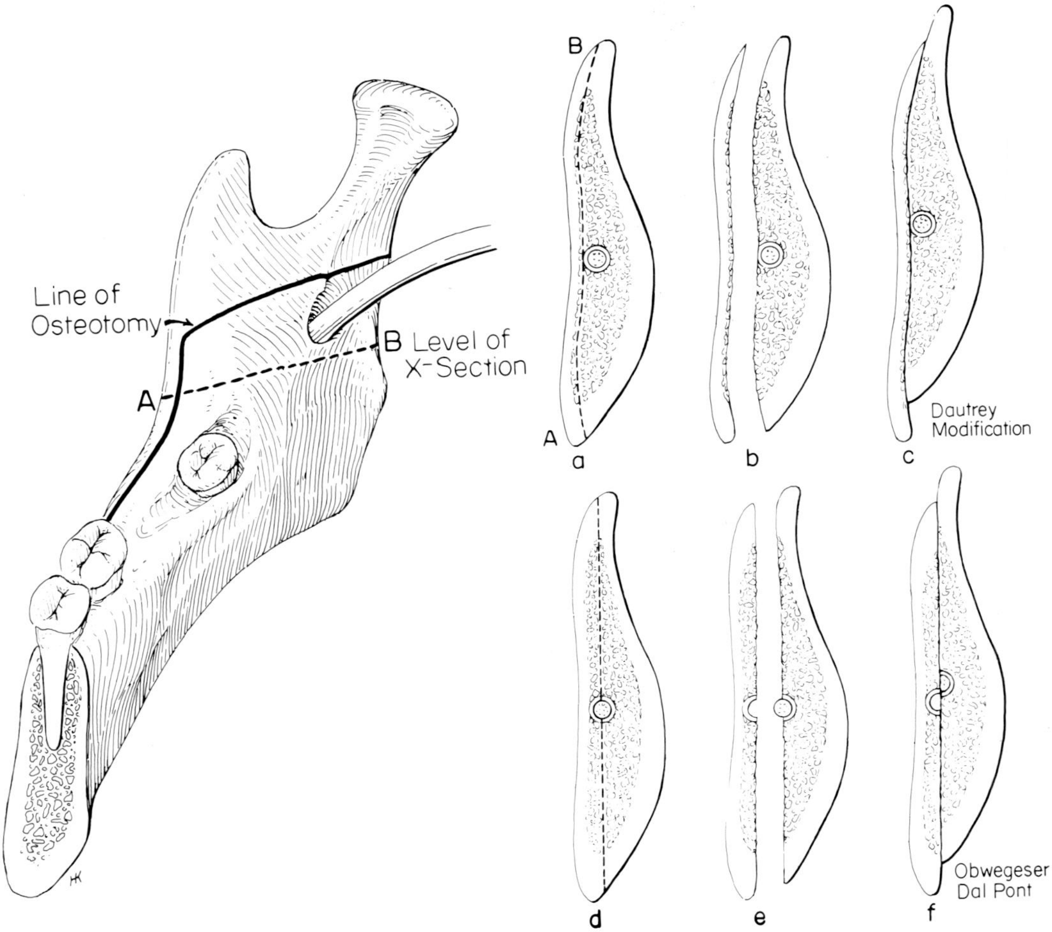

Figure 9.23. Plane of sagittal splitting of ramus. *Dash line A* to *B* represents level of cross section of figures *a* through *f*. Dautrey modification depicted in *a*, *b*, and *c* shows plane of cleavage lateral to mandibular canal. Neurovascular bundle is not exposed. In original Obwegeser-Dal Pont technique shown in *d*, *e*, and *f*, split occurs through canal. Neurovascular bundle can be directly traumatized or compressed when fragments are reapproximated, *f*.

is seen in approximately 50% of the patients.[36, 37] Trauma to the nerve can occur during the splitting action itself or possibly by compression when the two fragments are brought together by the interosseous fixation (Fig. 9.23). By keeping the plane of the split lateral to the canal (Dautrey modification) exposure of the inferior alveolar nerve is avoided and the incidence of hypesthesia is greatly diminished.[35]

MANDIBULAR RETROGNATHIA (MICROGNATHIA)

The word failure best describes the many techniques used in the past to advance the mandible. Technically, it is not difficult to advance the lower jaw. The real problem lies in maintaining the new position and eliminating relapse.

Muscles and soft tissues tolerate stretch in an uncomfortable manner. They retain found memories for old habits. Consequently, advanced mandibles tend to relapse toward their preoperative position.

Again, as with the treatment of mandibular prognathism, an imaginative assortment of osteotomies has been devised to lengthen the lower jaw. In some techniques bone grafts were used to fill any gaps left by the advancement. In others, partial bony contact was maintained and bone grafts were not used. The voids that were created were left to be obliterated by the body's healing process. Unfortunately, all the techniques have fallen into the shadows of disrepute. The sagittal splitting osteotomy has been able to survive though not without criticism.

The steps of the sagittal splitting ramal osteotomy operation are similar to those described in the treatment of prognathism. However, the tooth-bearing segment is now advanced rather than retruded. After intermaxillary fixation is established, interosseous wire fixation is used to coapt the proximal and distal fragments. The proximal fragment must be well seated into the glenoid fossa.

Although the sagittal splitting osteotomy reigns as the most popular technique to advance the mandible, it is far from fool proof. The risk of injuring the inferior alveolar nerve remains. In addition, an unsolved problem of relapse remains. Advancing the mandible places a stretching force on the muscles and the soft tissues. Skeletal relapses of 50–80% have been documented.[38] To minimize the amount of relapse, various maneuvers have been advocated. These measures include preoperative exercises to lengthen the hyoid musculature,[39] suprahyoid myotomies,[40] anterior overcorrection and opening the posterior bite,[38] and postoperative use of a cervical collar.[38, 41] Although the suggested practices may be helpful, the most important factor seems to be the proper seating of the condyle in the glenoid fossa and the use of skeletal mandibular-maxillary fixation for a prolonged period of 10–11 weeks.[39]

Because of the problems associated with the sagittal splitting osteotomy, a "C" shaped osteotomy of the ramus[42] and its modification[43] have been designed (Fig. 9.24). The phenomenon of relapse, however, remains unsolved because of technical difficulties in preventing distraction of the condyle from the fossa.[39] Furthermore, the procedure has the added disadvantage of an external scar.

MICROGENIA AND MACROGENIA

The size and shape of the chin must be analyzed as a separate unit of the lower jaw. Even with a normal mandible with ideal occlusion, the lower facial proportions can be aesthetically unexceptable because of an abnormally shaped chin.

A small chin can be augmented by the insertion of an alloplastic implant or by an osteotomy and advancement of the symphyseal region.

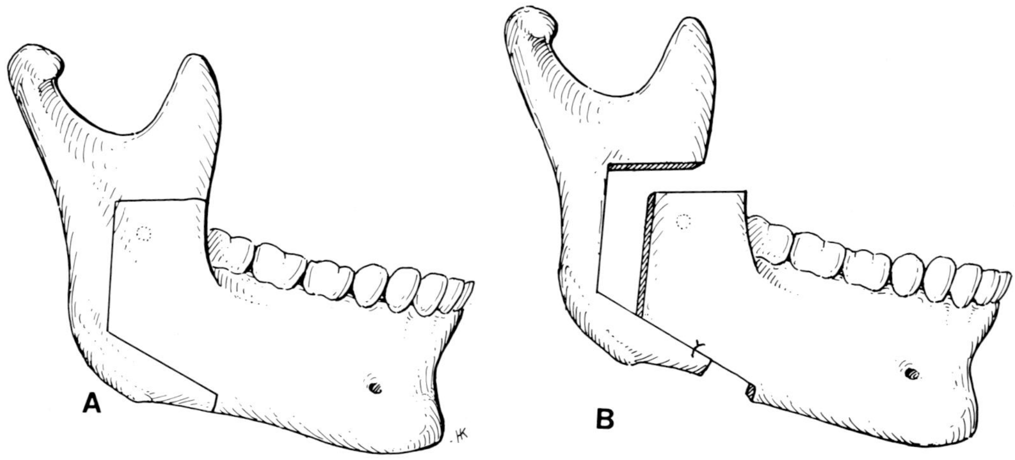

Figure 9.24. "C" osteotomy of mandible. (*A*) Outline of osteotomy avoiding neurovascular bundle. (*B*) Bony contact maintained after advancement and held together with interosseous wire.

Mild to moderate problems with microgenia are commonly corrected by the insertion of an alloplastic implant. Silicone prostheses are the most popular and come ready-made in various sizes. Over the prominence of the chin, a subperiosteal or supraperiosteal pocket is created just large enough to accommodate the implant. An external submental incision or an intraoral approach can be used. Fixation of the prosthesis to the periosteum or to the bone itself is optional.

Augmentation of the chin with an alloplastic implant is a simple procedure which can be performed under local anesthesia. Care must be taken to limit the dissection of the pocket to the size of the implant and to seat the prosthesis over the thick cortical bone of the mental prominence. Awareness of the location of the mental foramen near the apices of the bicuspid root will prevent an annoying paresthesia of the lower lip. Postoperative complication of infection, malposition, and extrusion can also occur. Radiologically, under most of the implants, bony absorption can be detected.[44, 45] This is not necessarily harmful if the implant is properly seated over the thick cortical bone of the mental symphysis. However, should the implant "ride up" onto the thin cortical bone of the alveolar process, the roots of the incisors can be jeopardized by the erosion process (Fig. 9.25).

Microgenia of greater proportion is best treated with a horizontal osteotomy of the mental symphysis region. The chin is exposed through the intraoral degloving technique (Fig. 9.26).[45] An incision is made 2–3 mm below the mucogingival junction from cuspid to cuspid sparing the labial frenulum. The subperiosteal dissection is carried to the inferior border of the chin and extended posteriorly under the mental foramen. A reciprocating power saw is used to make the horizontal osteotomy. The cut is made at least 5 mm below the apices of the cuspid (Fig. 9.27). The fragment is advanced to obtain the desired amount of projection. The insertions of the geniohyoideus and genioglossus usually need not be detached unless the muscles are placed under excessive stretch.[32, 47] Interosseous fixation stabilizes he fragment. The incision is closed in layers and a pressure dressing applied to complete the procedure.

The advancement achieved of the inferior border of the symphysis is stable. Relapse is minimal. Nonunion is indeed rare. The main complications of the procedure are those of infection and paresthesia of the lower lip.

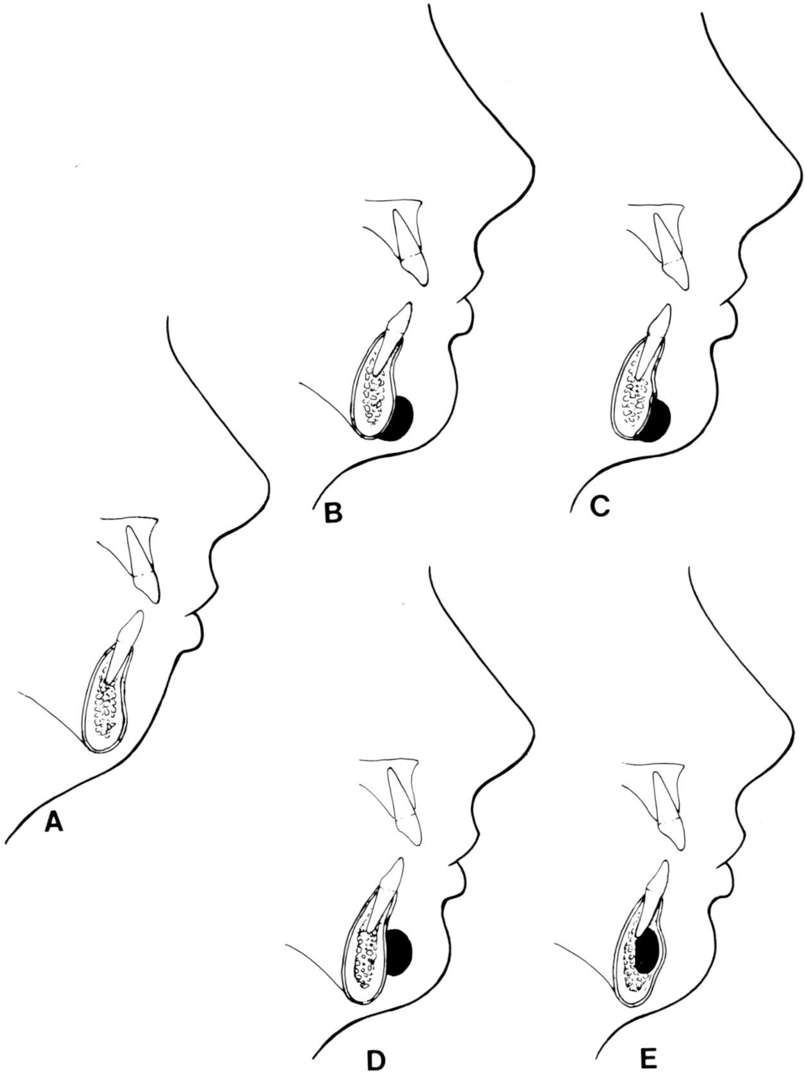

Figure 9.25. Placement of alloplastic implant to correct microgenia. (*A*) Outline of deformity. (*B*, *C*) Correct position of implant over thick cortical bone of symphysis. Mild settling of implant into cortical bone can be expected as shown in *C*. (*D*, *E*) Incorrect placement of implant. Implant has moved up onto thin cortical plate of dentoalveolar complex. Erosion through this thin bone jeopardizes underlying teeth as implant encroaches onto their roots.

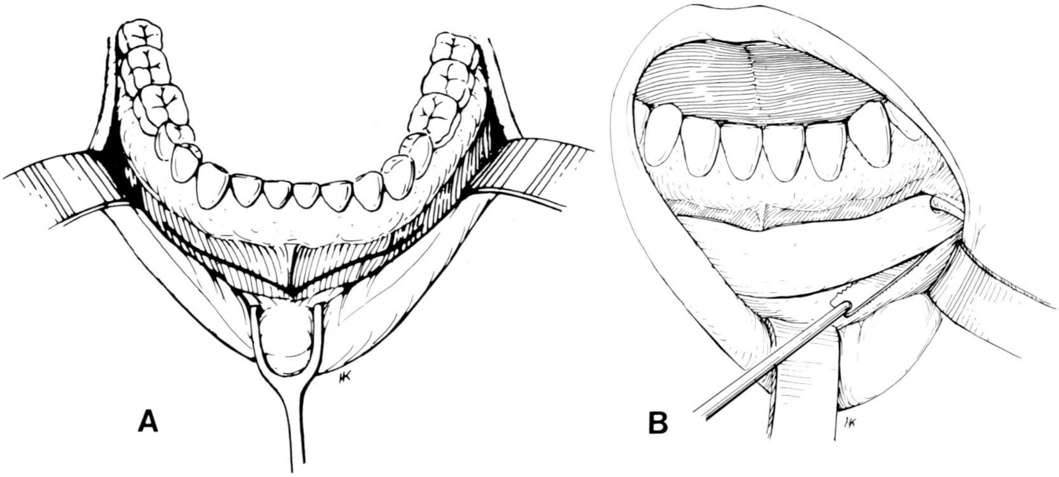

Figure 9.26. Degloving procedure to expose symphysis. (*A*) Mucosal incision below mucogingival junction and extending from first premolar to first premolar region. (*B*) Mucosa has been reflected in subperiosteal plane exposing inferior aspect of mental foramen and nerve. Reciprocating saw slipped under neurovascular bundle to begin the osteotomy.

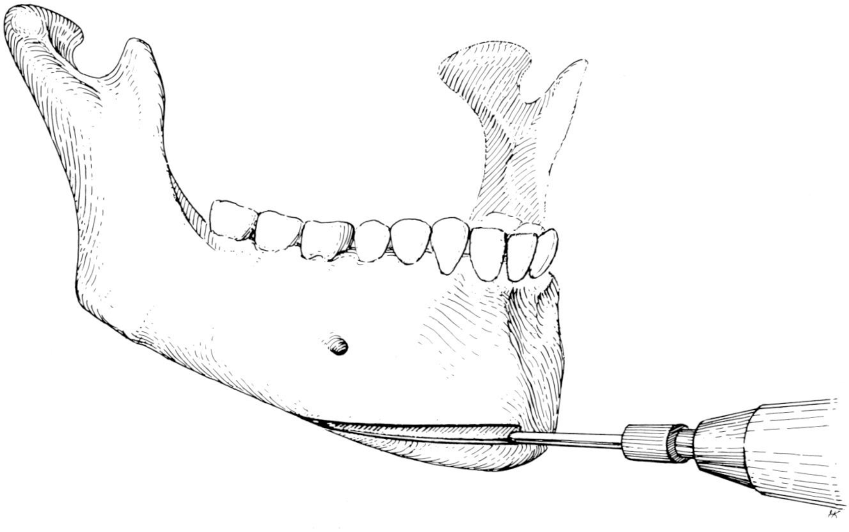

Figure 9.27. Horizontal osteotomy of symphysis. Reciprocating saw beginning its cut through symphysis. Level of cut can be varied to meet needs of deformity but must remain below mental foramen and apices of teeth.

The horizontal osteotomy of the mandible can be used to correct several deformities of the chin (Fig. 9.28). The fragment can be moved laterally to correct problems of a deviated chin. A wedge resection can be performed to reduce the vertical dimension of an enlarged chin. Furthermore, the vertical dimensions can be increased by the interposition of a bone graft.

MAXILLARY DEFORMITIES

Repositioning the entire maxilla is one of the simplest operative procedures of the jaws. The bones are thin, the access is direct, and the strong muscles of mastication are outside the confines of the operative site.

The basic maxillary osteotomies are named after the Le Fort classification of fractures. They generally follow the same lines produced by trauma but depart from the classical pattern in the region of the pterygoid plates. Instead of being carried horizontally across the perpendicular plates, the osteotomy is directed vertically through the pterygopalatine suture line (Fig. 9.29).

The Le Fort I osteotomy can be used to treat a wide range of deformities. It can be applied to correct maxillary retrusion and prognathism, short and long face syndromes, arch width discrepancies, and total anterior open bite deformities.

Basic Technique. The entire procedure is performed through an intraoral route. To minimize blood loss hypotensive anesthesia and the injection of a solution of 1:100,00 epinephrine are helpful measures.

The incision is made 2–3 mm above the mucogingival junction. It begins in the region of the molars and extends around the arch to the opposite side (Fig. 9.30). The labial frenulum is spared. The subperiosteal dissection is carried up to the level of the inferior orbital foramen, around the pyriform aperture, and posteriorly around the zygomatic buttress into the pterygopalatine junction. The nasal mucosa is elevated off the nasal floor and up a short ways along the nasal septum and the lateral nasal wall.

The blade of the reciprocating saw is placed 3–5 mm above the apices of the teeth and a cut is made along the outer wall of the maxilla from the pyriform aperture to the pterygopalatine junction (Fig. 9.31). The saw is then slipped under the nasal mucosa and directed through the lateral nasal wall into the maxillary sinus. The blade should be kept flush with the nasal floor to prevent encroachment onto the opening of the nasolacrimal duct that lies beneath the inferior turbinate. The nasal septum is then divided along the floor with a double guarded osteotome (Fig. 9.32).

Only the pterygopalatine suture line remains as a bony attachment. This suture line is thin and easily sliced with a sharp thin curved osteotome (Fig. 9.33). The vertical dimensions of the suture measure approximately 15 mm.[48] Attention should be paid to keep the osteotomy low and away from the overlying pterygomaxillary fissure. By following this precaution troublesome bleeding from the neighboring internal maxillary artery and the pterygoid venus plexus can be avoided.

With a pair of Rowe disimpaction forceps a downward force is used to separate the maxilla.[49] Blood supply to the maxilla is maintained through the palatal mucosa. In essence, the mobilized maxilla is now a composite flap based on the palatal soft tissues.

Depending on the desired movement, variations on the basic osteotomy can now be made.

Maxillary Hypoplasia and Prognathism. If the maxilla is to be advanced, intermaxillary fixation is established and iliac bone grafts are inserted into the space created in the pterygopalatine region to support the forward movement (Fig. 9.34). Bone grafts are not required if the advancement is less than 5–7 mm. On the other hand, if the maxilla is to be retropositioned, bone must be removed in the tuberosity area. With the maxilla in a downfractured position, the necessary amount of bone can be removed with a curved rongeur.

Long Face and Short Face Syndrome. In case of vertical dysplasia, a horizontal section of

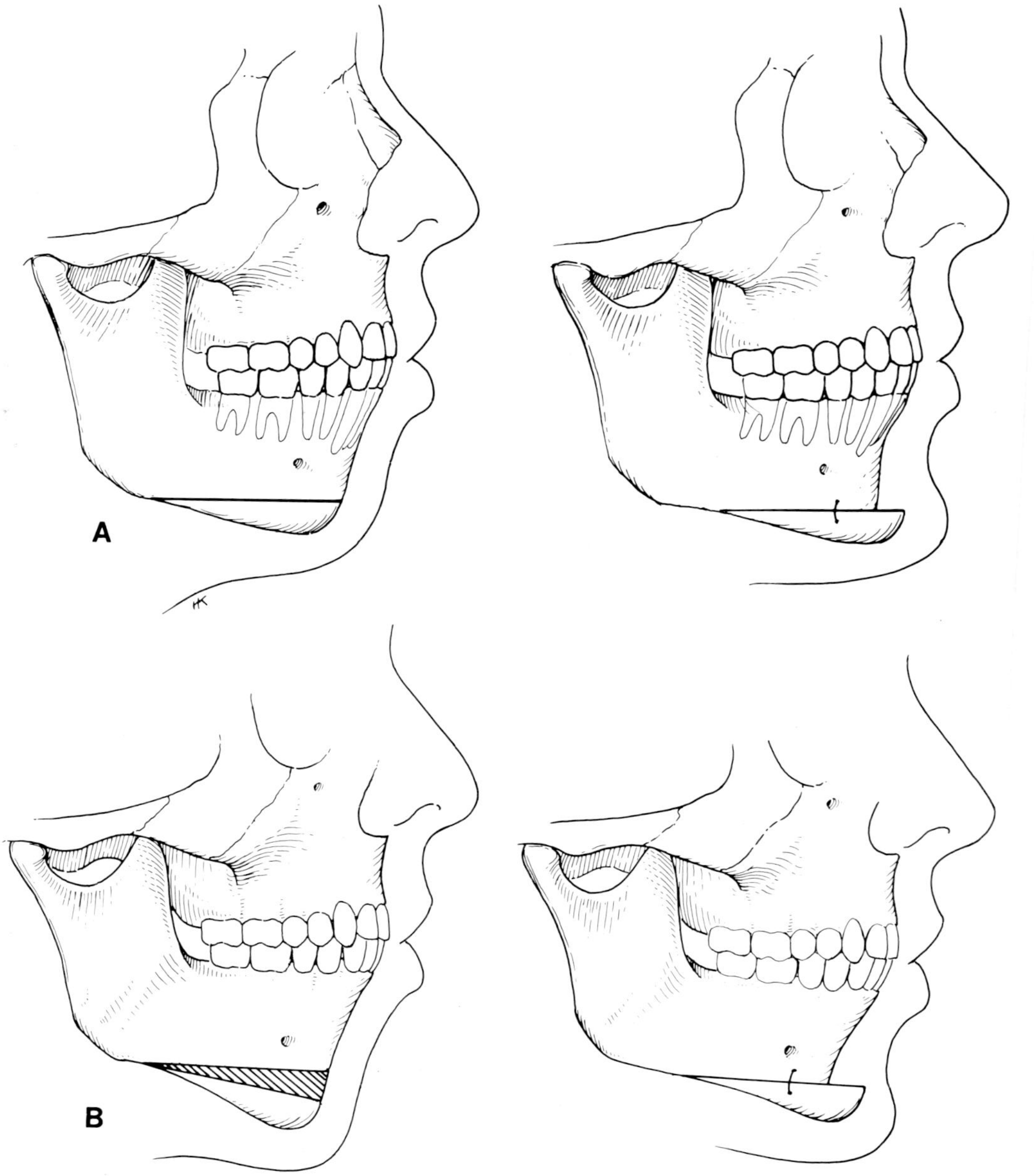

Figure 9.28. Variation of horizontal osteotomy of symphysis. (*A*) Sliding genioplasty to correct microgenia with inadequate anterior projection. (*B*) Wedge resection and advancement to correct vertical excess and inadequate projection. (*C*) Iliac bone graft interpositioned to correct microgenia with in vertical and anteroposterior deficiency. (*D*) Lateral deviation of chin corrected by shift of of symphyseal fragment.

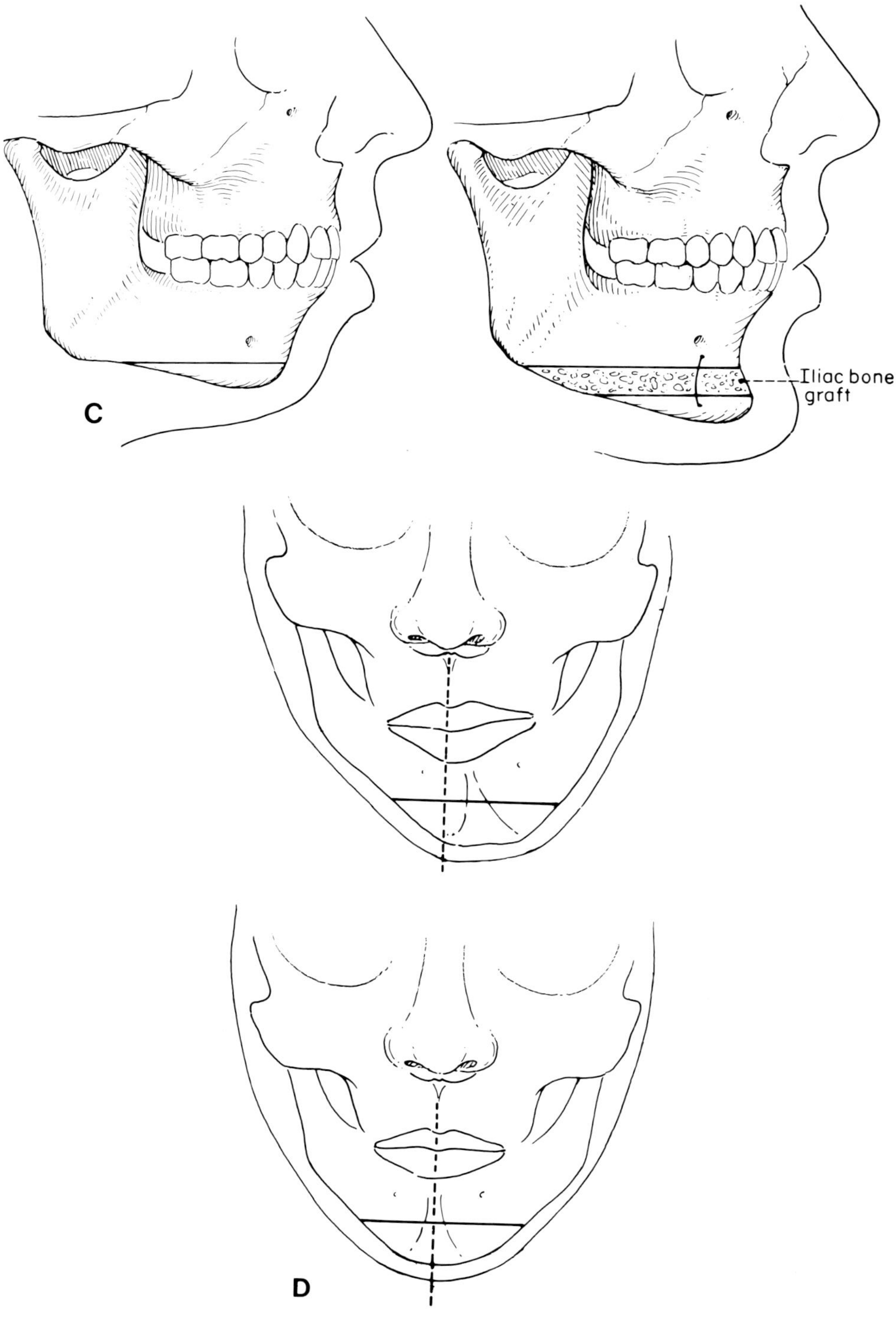

Figure 9.28. (*C and D*)

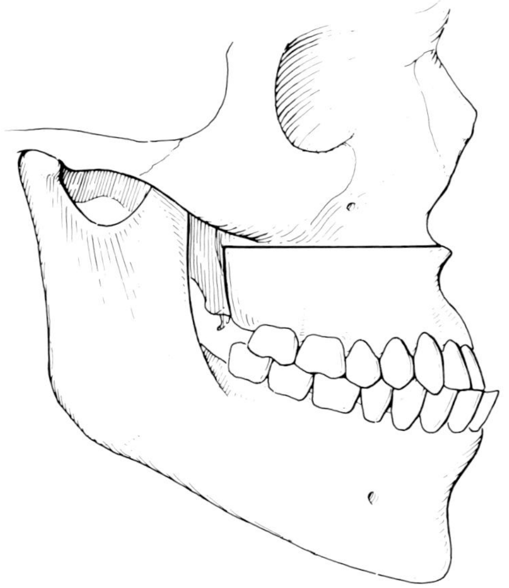

Figure 9.29. Le Fort I osteotomy. Basic outline of osteotomy extending from pyriform aperture, above apices of teeth to pterygopalatine junction.

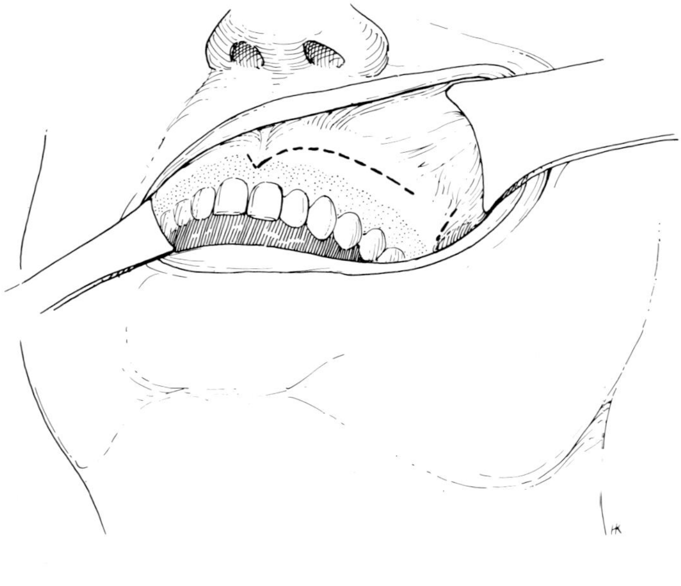

Figure 9.30. Incision to expose maxilla. Incision spares labial frenulum, extends around maxillary arch to molar region, and is placed a few millimeters above mucogingival junction.

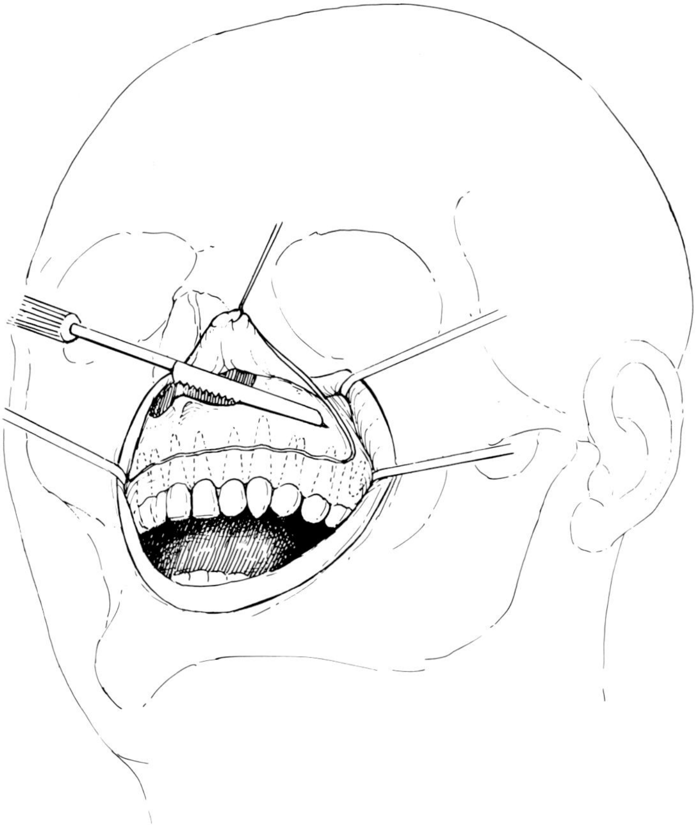

Figure 9.31. Osteotomy of lateral maxillary wall. Power reciprocating saw is placed 3–5 mm above apices of teeth.

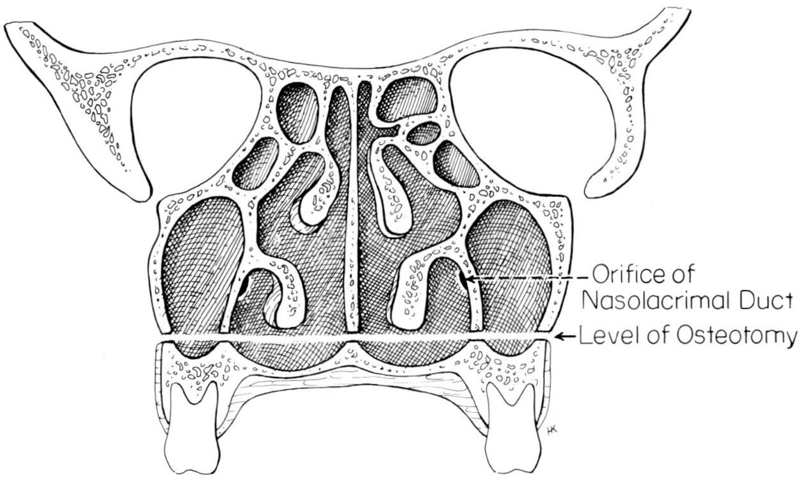

Figure 9.32. Cross section of maxilla. Level of osteotomy through walls of maxilla and across nasal septum. Osteotomy should remain along floor of nose to prevent injury to nasolacrimal duct.

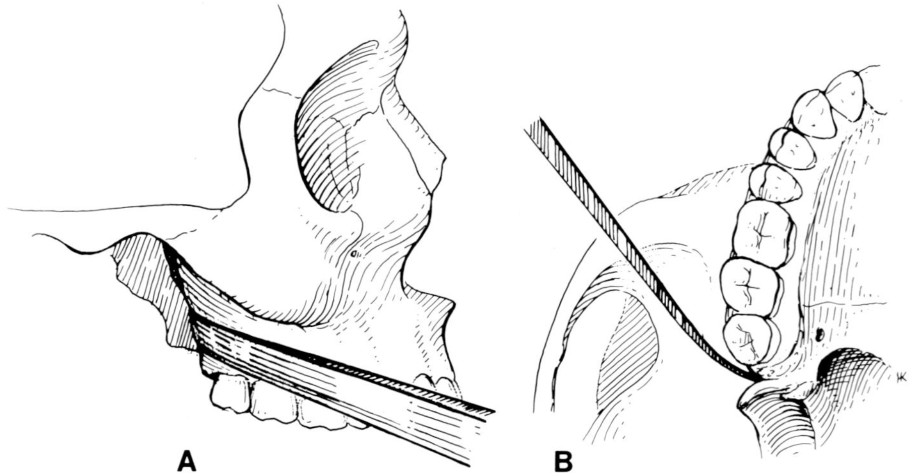

Figure 9.33. Pterygopalatine separation. (*A*) Sharp, thin, curved osteotome is inserted in lower portion of junction. Pterygoid fissure region, located superiorly, must be avoided to prevent injury to internal maxillary artery and pterygoid venous plexus. (*B*) Palatal view showing direction of osteotomy through pterygopalatine junction.

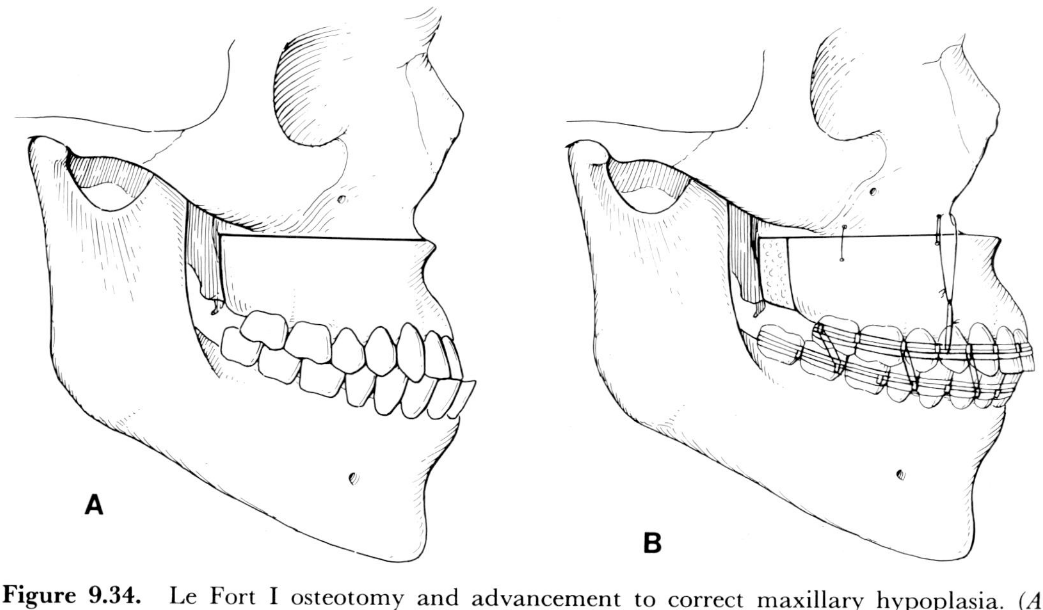

Figure 9.34. Le Fort I osteotomy and advancement to correct maxillary hypoplasia. (*A*) Outline of osteotomy. (*B*) After advancement an iliac bone graft is placed in pterygopalatine junction to support the forward displacement. Note direction of intermaxillary wires which favors advancement of maxilla. Interosseous wires pass through thicker bone of pyriform rim and zygomatic buttress. Suspension wire also passes through pyriform rim.

bone is removed to correct a long face problem. The maxilla can then be impacted to decrease the vertical dimension (Fig. 9.35). If the problem is one of a total open bite, a wedge-shaped section is removed (Fig. 9.36). The posterior portion of the maxilla is again impacted to close the open bite. With a short face problem, iliac bone grafts must be interposed in the osteotomy site to gain the desired amount of lengthening (Fig. 9.37). The amount of vertical change in each instance can be calculated preoperatively in the discussion with the orthodontist.

Multiple Segmental Osteotomies. When problems of width and length of the arch exist, the maxilla can be split into sections to alter its arch configuration. Approaching from the nasal side of the down-fractured maxilla, the maxilla can be subdivided with a burr and fine thin osteotomes to correct the deformity (Fig. 9.38). It is imperative to avoid injury to the palatal mucosa since it provides the sole blood supply to the mobilized maxilla. A prefabricated splint and intermaxillary fixation are used to secure the fragments.

Interosseous wire fixation in the region of the pyriform aperture and the zygomatic-maxillary buttress further immobilizes the fragments. As an added precaution, suspensory circumzygomatic wires or drop wires through the inferior orbital rims can be passed.

The basic Le Fort I osteotomy can, thus, be used to correct a wide range of maxillary deformities. Regardless of the variation on the theme, a period of 6 weeks of intermaxillary fixation is required to launch the consolidation process. At the end of the fixation period, mobility of the maxilla can often be detected since the union is fibrous in nature. If slight in amount, intermaxillary fixation can be discontinued and orthodontic therapy reinstituted. Continuation of fixation is warranted if gross mobility is present.

Infection is a possible complication of every operation. Surprisingly, its occurrence is extremely rare in maxillary osteotomies. The excellent blood supply and prophylactic antibiotic therapy play a contributory role as does the anatomical uniqueness of the maxilla. Surrounded by air spaces and thin walls, the likelihood of a formation of a hematoma or an abscess pocket is small. Such collections are discouraged by the generous drainage routes furnished by the

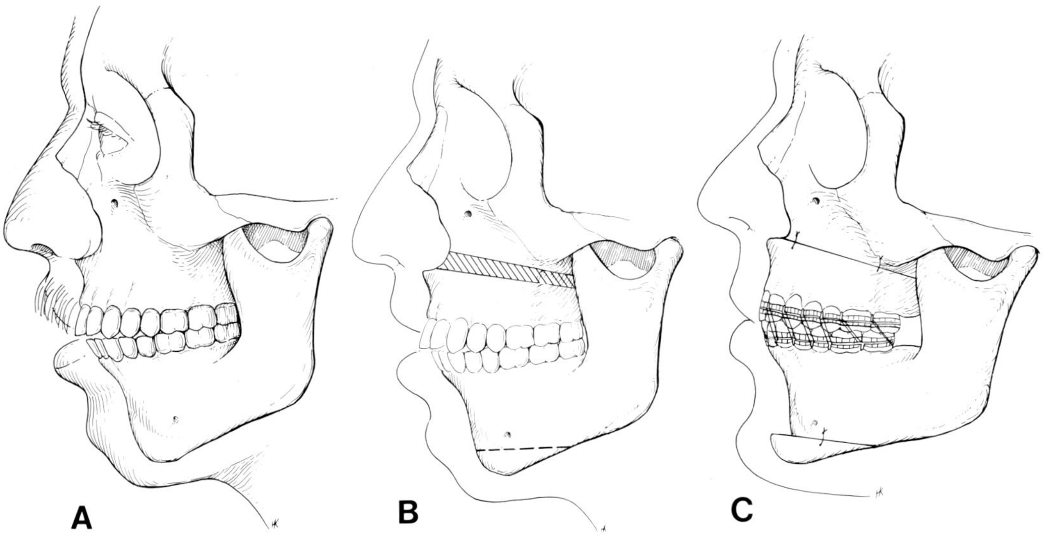

Figure 9.35. Long face syndrome. (*A*) Relationship of soft tissues to underlying skeleton with excess vertical maxillary development. (*B*) Outline of osteotomy. *Shaded area* represents region of resection to shorten midface. Sliding genioplasty is often required to provide additional advancement of chin beyond that achieved by autorotation effect. (*C*) Results following shortening, genioplasty and fixation.

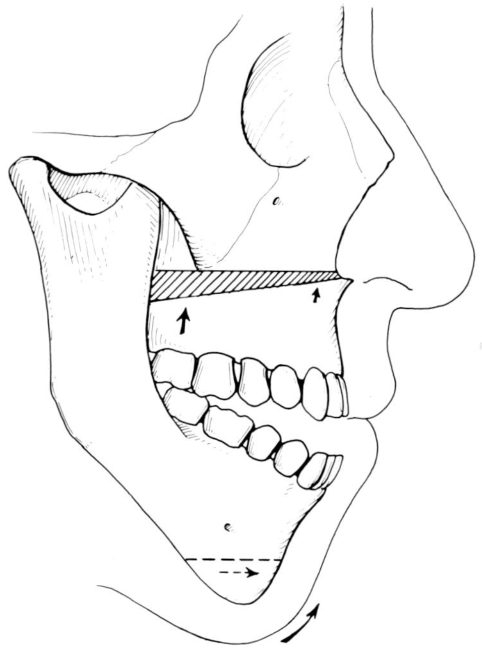

Figure 9.36. Total apertognathia (open bite). *Shaded wedge* indicates area of resection. Greater impaction posteriorly is required to close open bite. Sliding genioplasty may also be needed.

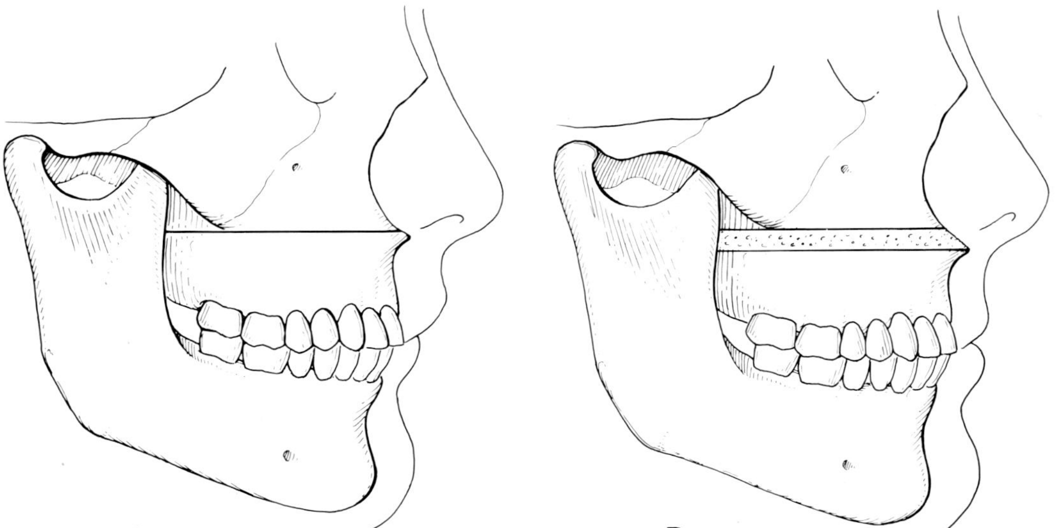

Figure 9.37. Short face syndrome. Vertical deficiency of lower third of face caused by insufficient maxillary growth. (*A*) Line of osteotomy. (*B*) Interposition of iliac bone graft to increase vertical dimension of maxilla and restore facial harmony.

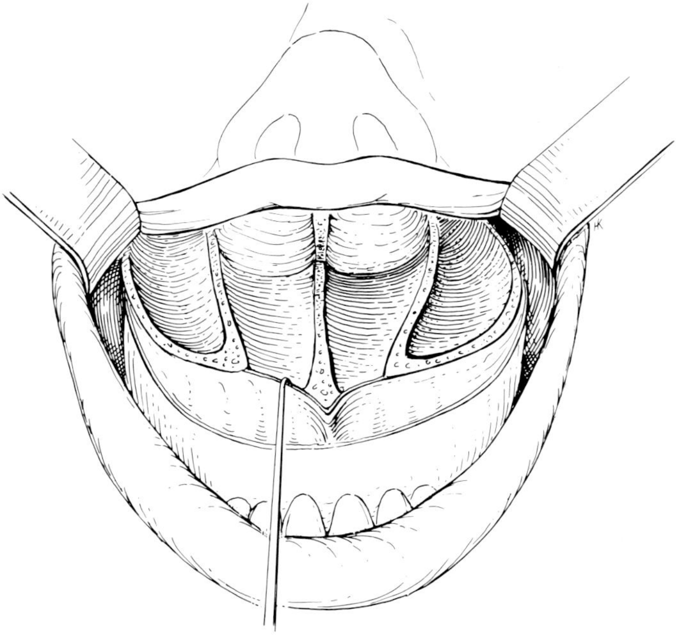

Figure 9.38. Maxilla in down-fractured position after Le Fort I osteotomy. Exposed are floor of maxillary sinus and nasal cavity.

osteotomy. The incidence of maxillary sinusitis, immediately postoperative or long term, is not increased by the operation.

Secondary nasal changes do occur following the Le Fort I osteotomy. When the maxilla is advanced or displaced cephalad, a widening of the alar base is seen. Patients should be informed about this change and the possible need in the future for an alar base resection.

Vertical impaction of the maxilla can also produce impairment of the nasal air exchange. If the caudal edge of the septum is not sufficiently shortened, the cartilagineous septum can be buckled by the cephalad displacement of the maxilla. Furthermore, when the maxilla must be shortened a great amount, impingement on the inferior turbinates can occur. A partial turbinectomy or removing bone from the floor of the nose with a burr should be considered.[50]

Compared with mandibular repositioning, relapse is less of a problem with maxillary movements. Willmar,[51] in an analysis of 106 Le Fort I osteotomies, showed that relapse was negligible in most instances. Greatest relapse tendencies were seen when the vertical dimension was increased in cases of the short face syndrome or when the maxilla was brought forward in patients with clefts of the lip and palate.

Vitality of the teeth is preserved if the roots are not injured. The osteotomy must, therefore, be kept 3–5 mm above the apices of the teeth. Sensibility is temporarily altered since the nerves are severed by the osteotomy. However, with time sensibility is restored.

Though flexible in application, the Le Fort I osteotomy does have its limitations. When the deformity encroaches into the periorbital and nasal complex regions, more extensive mobilization of the craniofacial skeleton is required.

MAXILLARY AND MANDIBULAR ANTERIOR PROTRUSION

The term protrusion denotes a malformation of the dentoalveolar complex in which there is an excessive frontal projection of the anterior teeth. Unlike the previously discussed

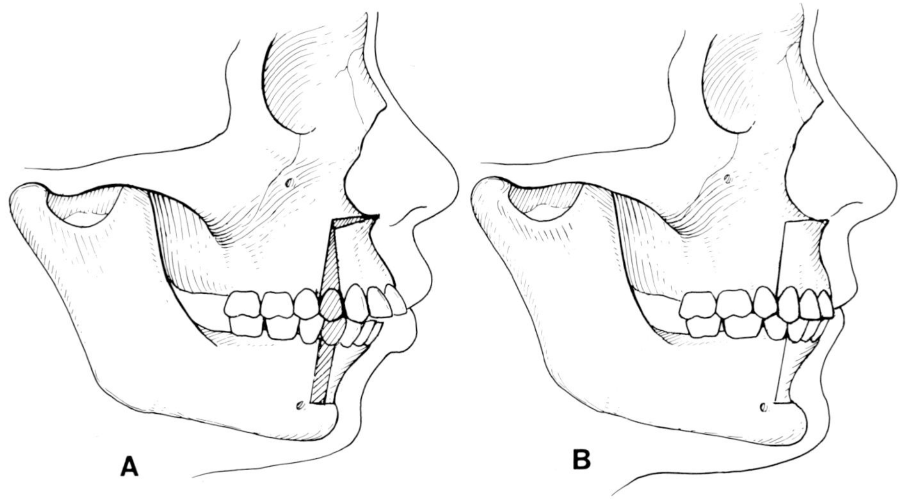

Figure 9.39. Bimaxillary anterior protrusion. (*A*) Fullness of lips caused by excessive protrusion of anterior dentoalveolar complex. *Shaded areas* represent segments to be resected. (*B*) Correction of occlusion and facial profile following repositioning of mandibular and maxillary anterior segments.

deformities, the primary problem is now focused on the dentoalveolar complex and not on the supporting skeletal base. Consequently, massive movements of the jaw is not necessary. To correct these deformities, only the teeth and the immediately surrounding alveolar bone need be relocated.

On a set of dental casts the proposed osteotomies are made. The amount and direction of displacement of the anterior segments are recorded. Once the proper relationships are obtained, an acrylic splint to be used for fixation is fabricated.

Either the labial or lingual (palatal) mucosa must be kept intact to safeguard viability of the mobilized segment. When the setback procedure was originally performed, a two-stage procedure was recommended to prevent necrosis of the segment.[52] However, it has been shown that the operation can be safely performed in one stage if a mucoperiosteal flap is maintained on one side of the composite flap.[53] On the maxilla, either the labial or palatal mucoperiosteum can be preserved. Because of access, on the mandible it is easier to leave the lingual mucosa intact.

The vertical portion of the osteotomy is generally carried through the region of the first premolar (Fig. 9.39). A wedge or a parallel section of bone is removed depending upon the desired change in angulation of the incisors. The pattern is easily determined during the preoperative model surgery on the dental casts. Exposure of the root surfaces adjacent to the resection site must be avoided.

The horizontal component of the osteotomy is made leaving a 3–5 mm clearance of the root of the cuspid which is the longest tooth. On the maxilla, this cut is carried into the pyriform aperture. Division of the anterior part of the nasal septum completes the separation. On the mandible, a degloving approach is used. The osteotomy is made with a power saw leaving the lingual mucoperiosteal flap intact. Intrusion of the mobilized segment is often required. When this is necessary, a horizontal slice of bone is removed to accommodate the change.

During the planning, anteroposterior, vertical, and inclination changes all must be considered. In addition, a potential problem of arch discrepancies exists. The anterior part of the dental arch is narrower than the posterior portion. Therefore, a buccolingual disturbance in arch form can be created as the anterior segment is setback (Fig. 9.40). This stepoff can be

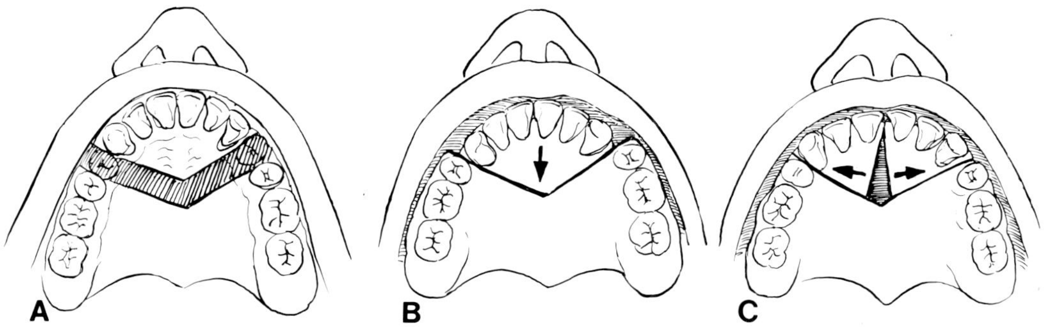

Figure 9.40. Arch realignment following anterior maxillary setback. (*A*) *Shaded areas* represent amount of resection required for posterior displacement of anterior maxillary segment. (*B*) Malalignment of arch due to smaller arc of anterior portion of dental arch. (*C*) Midline split of anterior segment allows for lateral displacement and restoration of arch form. (Reproduced with permission from J. M. Converse, H. K. Kawamoto, D. Wood-Smith, P. J. Cocarro, and J. G. McCarthy: Deformities of the jaws, in *Reconstructive Plastic Surgery*, Ed. 2, edited by J. M. Converse. Philadelphia, W. B. Saunders, Philadelphia, 1977.)

eliminated by splitting the anterior segment in the midline and increasing the width of the arch.

An acrylic splint, fabricated preoperatively from the working dental casts, provides fixation for the mobilized segment. Stainless steel wires are used to ligate the anterior teeth to the splint which is then ligated to the stable posterior teeth (Fig. 9.41). Intermaxillary fixation is not required. Fixation is maintained with the splint for 3 weeks. A continuous labial arch wire is placed by the orthodontist at the end of this time and the splint is removed. Orthodontic therapy can be immediately reinstituted.

Infection, relapse, and nonunion are exceedingly rare. If the apices are not endangered, sensibility returns with the passage of months and is completed by the end of a year.[53] Formation of a periodontal pocket and subsequent periodontal disease is a concern at the osteotomy site. Careful alignment of the segment will minimize this possibility.[55] The main concern is necrotic loss of the entire segment. This can be avoided by guarding the integrity of either the labial or lingual (palatal) mucoperiosteal flap. In addition, the flap must be carefully inspected for any kinking or compression after the setback and the establishment of fixation.

OPEN BITE

Open bite deformities can be seen in the anterior or posterior segments of the dental arch. In severe cases, only isolated contact on the posterior most teeth is seen (total apertognathia). Faulty speech patterns and tongue habits often accompany the deformity and must be controlled if the open bite is to be corrected.

Total Apertognathia. In the past, total open bite was most likely to be treated with a sagittal splitting ramal osteotomy. The mandible was rotated to close the open bite. However, the rotational movement does place a stretching force on the muscles of mastication. Thus, the relapse rate was unexceptably high. This method, therefore, is now reserved for mild cases.

The trend is to correct total open bite deformities with a Le Fort I impaction type of osteotomy. A wedge of bone is resected which will allow a greater impaction of the posterior portion of the maxilla. Correction by this method does not impose a stretching action on the muscles of mastication and the results are stable.

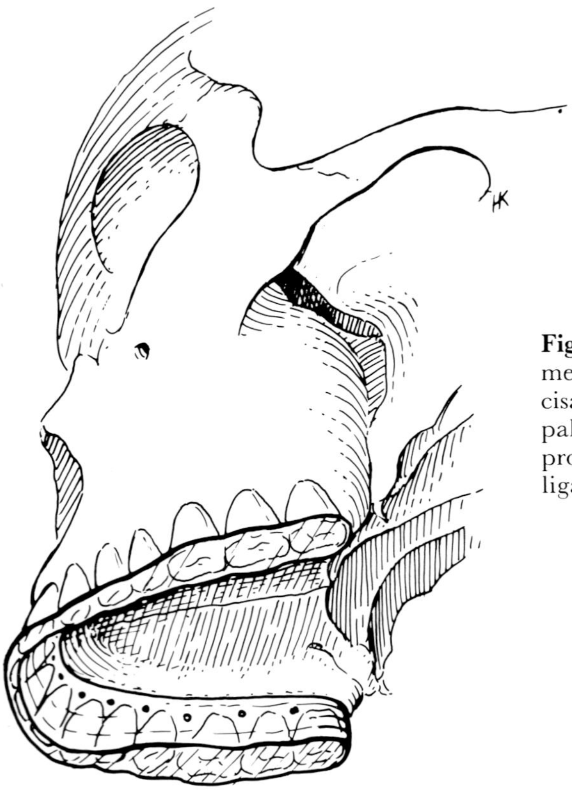

Figure 9.41. Maxillary splint used for segmental osteotomies. Acrylic splint covers incisal and occlusal surfaces and continues on palatal surface for a few millimeters. Interproximal drill holes are used to pass wires to ligate splint to teeth.

Posterior Open Bite. When the open bite is isolated to the posterior region, it is usually unilateral in nature. A common cause is a lateral tongue thrust habit. Control of the faulty lingual activity can correct the deformity. Another cause is the failure of the downward movement of the lesser segment in a unilateral cleft palate patient. Closure is resisted by conventional orthodontic measures and a surgical manipulation is usually required. A hemi-Le Fort I type of osteotomy of the lesser segment can be successfully employed. Iliac bone grafts are placed into the gap caused by the displacement and into the alveolar cleft.

Anterior Open Bite. The anterior open bite is but a sign and the deformity has multiple etiologies. It can be caused by: (1) cephalad placement of the maxillary anterior teeth, (2) caudal location of the mandibular anterior teeth, (3) excessive extrusion of the posterior teeth, or (4) a combination of these problems. The location of the deformity is defined by the clinical examination, dental casts, and cephalograms.

When the only malformation is a cephalad displacement of the maxillary anterior teeth or a caudad displacement of the mandibular anterior teeth, an anterior segmental osteotomy is used to bring the faulty section to the proper incisal level to close the open bite. The technique is similar to that described in the correction of bimaxillary protrusion problems. The gap caused by the displacement is filled with autologous iliac bone grafts (Fig. 9.42). In the maxilla, when the amount of movement is small, the bone graft can be omitted. The mobilized dentoalveolar segments are stabilized in a manner similar to that described in the treatment of maxillary and mandibular protrusion.

Occasionally, a mandibular anterior open bite is found in combination with a chin that is excessively long (Fig. 9.43). Taking advantage of the excess vertical dimension of the chin, Köle[56] described a procedure which simultaneously corrects both deformities. The chin is shortened with a horizontal osteotomy. The redundant bone is removed and transplanted into the defect created by the cephalad displacement of the anterior dentoalveolar complex. In this

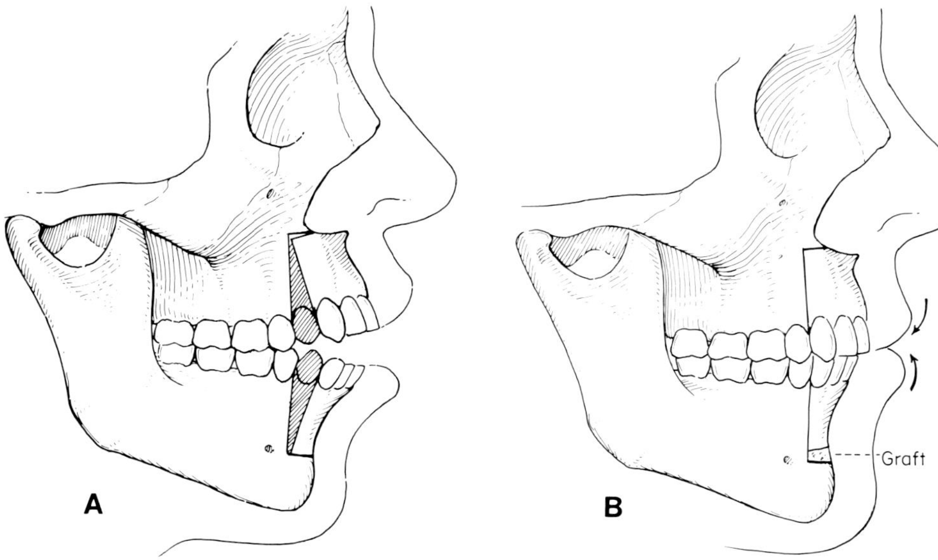

Figure 9.42. Bimaxillary protrusion and open bite. (*A*) Anterior segmental osteotomy and resection required to correct bimaxillary protrusion. (*B*) After repositioning of fragments and insertion of iliac bone grafts to close anterior open bite. *Arrows* indicate direction of migration of lips allowing comfortable lip seal.

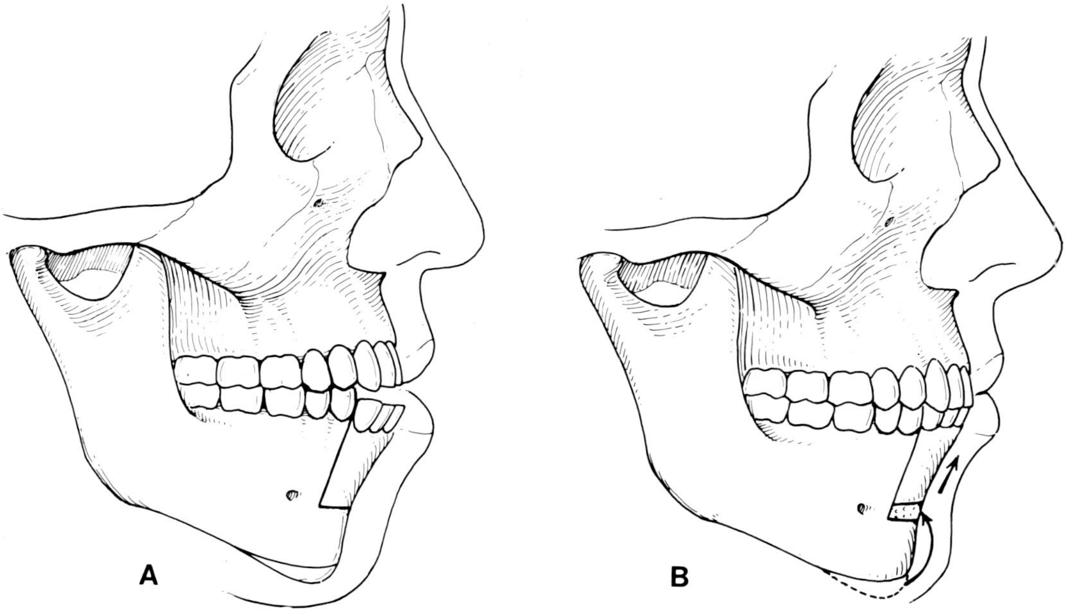

Figure 9.43. Köle procedure. Anterior open bite and vertical excess of chin. (*A*) Outline of anterior segmental osteotomy and sectioning of symphysis. (*B*) Cephalad movement of anterior segment to close open bite. Placement of chin fragments to fill in gap caused by repositioning of anterior segment.

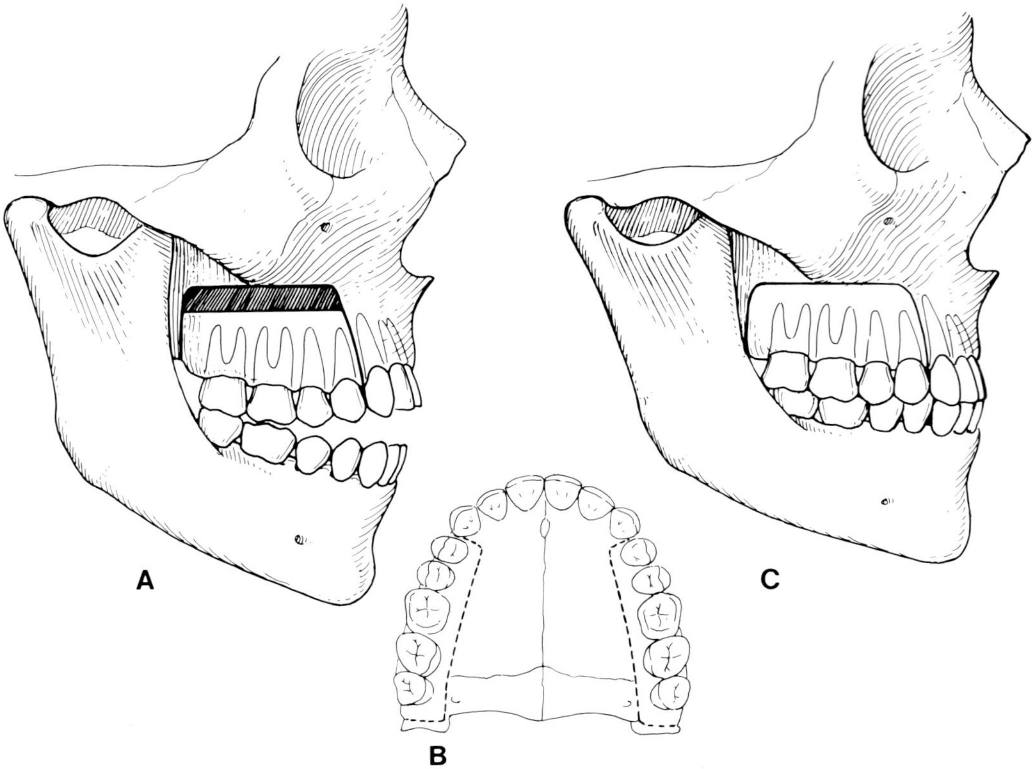

Figure 9.44. Schuchardt procedure to close open bite due to extrusion of posterior maxillary teeth. (*A*) Lateral view of osteotomy with shaded areas indicating portion to be resected. (*B*) Palatal view of line of osteotomy. (*C*) After impaction of posterior segments and closure of anterior open bite deformity.

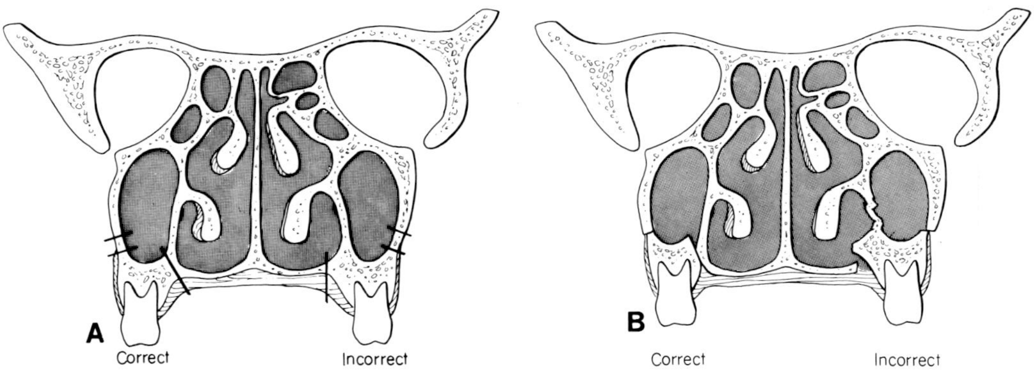

Figure 9.45. Cross section of maxilla in Schuchardt procedure. (*A*) Lines of osteotomy. Palatal cuts should extend into maxillary sinus and not into nasal cavity. (*B*) After impaction of posterior segments into maxillary sinus. Crushed medial wall of maxillary sinus will inhibit superior retropositioning of posterior segments and contribute to relapse.

maneuver, sufficient bone must be preserved between the two horizontal cuts to maintain the integrity and strength of the mandibular arch.

A posterior segmental osteotomy is used to close an anterior open bite which is caused by an overeruption of the premolars and molars. When originally described by Schuchardt[57] in 1955, a two-stage procedure was recommended because of the fear of vascular compromise. This proved to be an overly cautious measure for the osteotomy can be performed in a single stage without danger.[58]

A posterior horizontal incision is made 2–3 mm above the mucogingival junction. The mucosa is reflected off the lateral surface of the maxilla. A horizontal osteotomy is made 3–5 mm above the apices of the teeth with a power saw (Fig. 9.44). A thin osteotome is used to make the vertical cut between the cuspid and the first premolar. The osteotome should be thin to prevent injury to the roots of the teeth. The cut is carried through the palatal bone but leaves the palatal mucosa intact. The pterygopalatine suture is severed with a thin curved osteotome.

Digital pressure applied in a medial direction is sufficient to fracture the remaining palatal bony attachment. Division of the palatal bone by this method has several advantages. The chance of injuring the palatal mucosa, which is the sole blood supply to this composite flap, is minimized. Furthermore, the line of separation will occur through the weakest point. This line extends through the maxillary sinus and not through the thick bone that forms the floor of the nasal cavity (Fig. 9.45). The same steps are performed on the contralateral side. The entire posterior dentoalveolar segment can be impacted into the maxillary sinus to close the anterior open bite. Had the palatal osteotomy been made through the nasal cavity, the medial wall of the maxillary sinus would have to be crushed during the cephalad displacement of the segment. Intermaxillary fixation for 6 weeks is required.

Complications that can be incurred are similar to those mentioned in the treatment of protrusion deformities. In the case of the mandibular anterior segmental osteotomy with the interposition of bone grafts, the return of sensibility can be incomplete.[53] Vitality of the teeth in the mobilized segment is, however, maintained if the roots of the teeth are not violated.

References

1. Angle, E. H.: Classification of malocclusions. *Dent. Cosmos*, *40*:635, 1898.
2. Rowe, N. L.: Fractures of the facial skeleton in children. *J. Oral Surg.*, *27*:497, 1969.
3. Kazanjian, V. H., and Converse, J. M.: *The Surgical Treatment of Facial Injuries*, Ed. 3, Williams & Wilkins, Baltimore, 1974.
4. Panagopoulos, A. P.: Management of fractures of the jaws in children. *J. Int. Coll. Surg.*, *28*:806, 1957.
5. Pheifer, G.: Kieferbruche im Kindersalter und ihre Auswirkungen auf das Wachstum. *Fortschr. Kiefer Gesichtschir.*, *11*:43, 1966.
6. Cornell University Automobile Crash Injury Research: *The Injury-producing Accident: A Primer of Facts and Figures*. Ithaca, N. Y., August 1961.
7. Rowe, N. L., and Killey, H. C.: *Fractures of the Facial Skeleton*. Williams & Wilkins, Baltimore, 1955.
8. McCoy, F. J., Chandler, R. A., Magnan, C. G., Jr., Moore, J. R., and Siemsen, G.: An analysis of facial fractures and their complications. *Plast. Reconstr. Surg.*, *29*:381, 1962.
9. Dingman, R. O., and Natvig, P.: *Surgery of Facial Fractures*. W. B. Saunders, Philadelphia, 1964.
10. Kazanjian, V. H., and Converse, J. M.: *The Surgical Treatment of Facial Injuries*. Williams & Wilkins, Baltimore, 1949.
11. Risdon, F. E.: Ankylosis of the temporomaxillary joint. *J. Am. Dent. Assoc.*, *21*:1933, 1934.
12. Chalmers J. Lyons Club: Fractures involving the mandibular condyle; post-treatment survey of 120 cases. *J. Oral Surg.*, *5*:45, 1947.
13. Gregory, T. G.: As cited in J. M. Converse (ed.): *Reconstructive Plastic Surgery*, Ed. 2, p. 684, W. B. Saunders, Philadelphia, 1977.
14. MacGregor, A. B., and Fordyce, G.: Treatment of fractures of the neck of the mandibular condyle. *Br. Dent. J.*, *102*:351, 1957.
15. Walker, R. V.: Traumatic mandibular condylar fracture dislocations; effect on growth in the *Macaca* rhesus monkey. *Am. J. Surg.* *100*:850, 1960.
16. Leake, D., Doykos, J., Habal, M., and Murray, J.: Long-term follow up of fractures of the mandibular angle in children. *Plast. Reconstr. Surg.*, *47*:127, 1971.
17. Laskin, D. M.: Surgical management of diseases of the temporomandibular joint, in *Oral Surgery*, J. Hayward (Ed.). Charles C Thomas, Springfield, Ill., 1976.
18. Le Fort, R.: Etude experimentale sur les fractures de la machoire supérieure. *Rev. Chir. (Paris)*, *23*:208, 360, 479, 1901.
19. Adams, W. M.: Internal wiring fixation of facial fractures. *Surgery*, *12*:523, 1942.

20. Adams, W. M., and Adams, L. H.: Internal wire fixation of facial fractures. A fifteen-year follow-up report. *Am. J. Surg.*, *92:*12, 1956.
21. Bassett, C. A. L., Hurley, L. A., and Stinchfield, F. E.: The fate of long-term anorganic bone implants. *Transplant. Bull.*, *29:*51, 1962.
22. Markowitz, A.: The use of homogenous bone grafts in mandibular reconstruction. *Am. J. Surg.*, *96:*755, 1958.
23. Mowlen, R.: Cancellous chip bone grafts; report of 75 cases. *Lancet*, *2:*746, 1944.
24. Bromberg, B. E., Walden, R. H., and Rubin, L. R.: Mandibular bone grafts, a technique in fixation. *Plast. Reconstr. Surg.*, *32:*589, 1963.
25. Manchester, W. M.: Immediate reconstruction of the mandible and temporomandibular joint. *Br. J. Plast. Surg.*, *18:*291, 1965.
26. Boyne, P. J.: Autogenous cancellous bone and marrow transplants. *Clin. Orthop.*, *73:*199, 1970.
27. Boyne, P. J., and Zarem, H.: Osseous reconstruction of the resected mandible. *Am. J. Surg.*, *132:*49, 1976.
28. Jaboulay, M.: Les effets de la resection des condyles du maxillaire inférieur sur la situation de la rangée dentaire et la forme du menton. *Lyon Med.*, *75:*519, 1895.
29. Caldwell, J. B., and Letterman, G. S.: Vertical osteotomy in the mandibular rami for correction of prognathism. *J. Oral Surg.*, *12:*185, 1954.
30. Robinson, M.: Prognathism corrected by open vertical condylotomy. *J. South. Calif. Dent. Assoc.*, *24:*22, 1956.
31. Hinds, E. C.: Surgical correction of acquired mandibular deformities. *Am. J. Orthod.*, *43:*161, 1957.
32. Obwegeser, H. L.: In R. Trauner and H. L. Obwegeser: The surgical correction of mandibular prognathism and retrognathia with consideration of genioplasty; I. Surgical procedures to correct mandibular prognathism and reshaping of the chin. *Oral Surg.*, *10:*677, 1957.
33. Dal Pont, G.: Retromolar osteotomy for correction of prognathism. *J. Oral Surg.*, *19:*42, 1961.
34. Hunsuck, E. E.: A modified intraoral sagittal technic for correction of mandibular prognathism. *Oral Surg.*, *26:*249, 1968.
35. Dautrey, J.: Personal communication, Nancy, France, 1974.
36. Pepersack, W. J., and Chausse, J. M.: Long term follow-up of the sagittal splitting technique for correction of mandibular prognathism. *J. Maxillofac. Surg.*, *6:*117, 1978.
37. Willmar, K., Hogeman, K. E., and Thiséus, S.: Sagittal split osteotomy in our experience. *Scand. J. Plast. Reconstr. Surg.*, *13:*445, 1979.
38. Poulton, D. R., and Ware, W. H.: Surgical-orthodontic treatment of severe mandibular retrusion (part II). *Am. J. Orthod.*, *63:*237, 1973.
39. Schendel, S. A., and Epker, B. N.: Results after mandibular advancement surgery; an analysis of 87 cases, *J. Oral Surg.*, *38:*265, 1980.
40. Steinhauser, E. W.: Advancement of the mandible by sagittal ramus split and suprahyoid myotomy. *J. Oral Surg.*, *31:*516, 1978.
41. McNeil, R. W., Hooley, J. R., and Sundberg, R. J.: Skeletal relapse during intermaxillary fixation. *J. Oral Surg.*, *31:*212, 1973.
42. Caldwell, T. B., Hayward, J. R., and Lister, R. L.: Correction of mandibular retrognathia by vertical "L" osteotomy; a new technic. *J. Oral Surg.*, *26:*259, 1968.
43. Hayes, P. A.: Correction of retrognathia by modified "C" osteotomy of the ramus and saggital osteotomy of the mandibular body. *J. Oral Surg.*, *31:*682, 1973.
44. Robinson, M., and Shuken, R.: Bone resorption under plastic chin implants. *J. Oral Surg.*, *27:*116, 1969.
45. Friedland, J. A., Coccaro, P. J., and Converse, J. M.: Retrospective cephalometric analysis of mandibular bone absorption under silicone rubber chin implants. *Plast. Reconstr. Surg.*, *57:*144, 1976.
46. Converse, J. M.: Restoration of facial contours by bone grafts introduced through the oral cavity. *Plast. Reconstr. Surg.*, *6:*295, 1950.
47. Converse, J. M., and Shapiro, H. H.: Treatment of developmental malformations of the jaw. *Plast. Reconstr. Surg.*, *10:*473, 1952.
48. Turvey, T. A., and Fonseca, R. J.: The anatomy of the internal maxillary artery in the pterygopalatine fossa; its relationship to maxillary surgery. *J. Oral Surg.*, *38:*92, 1980.
49. Bell, W. H., Creekmore, T. D., and Alexander, R. J.: Surgical correction of long-face syndrome. *Am. J. Orthod.*, *71:*40, 1977.
50. Verdi, G. D., and Alpert, B.: Correction of the long-face: case report. *Plast. Reconstr. Surg.*, *62:*613, 1978.
51. Willmar, K.: On Le Fort I osteotomy; a follow-up study on 106 operated patients with maxillo-facial deformity. *Scand. J. Plast. Reconstr. Surg., Suppl. 12,* 1974.
52. Wilhelm, W.: The surgical treatment of prognathism of the maxilla. *Bol. Odontol.*, *20:*146, 1954.
53. Wunderer, S.: Die Prognathieoperation mittels frontal gestieltem Maxilla Fragment. *Osterr. Z. Stomatol.*, *39:*98, 1962.
54. Pepersack, W. J.: Tooth vitality after alveolar segmental osteotomy. *J. Maxillofac. Surg.*, *1:*85, 1973.
55. Hinds, E. C., and Kent, J. N.: *Surgical Treatment of Developmental Jaw Deformities.* C. V. Mosby, St. Louis, 1972.
56. Köle, H.: Nouvelles interventions chirurgicales à la hauteur du processus alveolaire en vue de la correction des malformations de l'arcade et des malpositions dentaires. *Rev. Belg. Stomatol.*, *56:*247, 1959.
57. Schuchardt, K.: Formen des offen Bisses und ihre Operativen. Behandlungsmoglichkeiten. *Fortschr. Kiefer Gesichtschir.*, *1:*22, 1955.
58. Kufner, J.: Experiences with a modified procedure for correction of open bite in *Transaction of the Third International Conference of Oral Surgery.* E. & S. Livinstone, London, 1968.

CHAPTER 10

Salivary Glands

John William Little III, M.D.

The salivary glands fall subject to an interesting array of pathologic processes—including inflammatory and neoplastic disease, as well as trauma. The diagnosis and treatment of these conditions is largely the responsibility of the surgeon, and in this pursuit he is confronted by frequent and considerable challenge. Certainly that confident and precise knowledge of anatomy that is necessary to all surgery of the head and neck is nowhere more so than in the successful surgery of salivary gland disease. So too is required a thorough understanding of the biologic potential, growth characteristics, and natural history of these interesting lesions. Too often, the operator of the past has approached these problems in an unenlightened manner, contributing to the high recurrence rate of disease and treatment failure that has become notorious for salivary gland surgery.

ANATOMY

The human salivary glands[36, 52, 57] consist of three paired major glands, the parotid (or greater) glands and the submandibular and sublingual (or lesser) glands, as well as numerous, scattered minor glands. They develop as active, budding epithelial invaginations into subjacent mesoderm.[52]

Parotid Gland

The parotid, the largest of the salivary glands and the only gland with a purely serous output, lies in the preauricular region overlying the masseter muscle, wrapping around the vertical ramus of the mandible. Posteriorly it abuts against the bony and cartilaginous portions of the external auditory meatus, frequently extending to the mastoid process. It may reach as high as the zygomatic arch and inferiorly its "tail" may dip well into the reaches of the upper neck. Anteriorly it extends to the anterior margin of the masseter muscle, around which border its excretory duct (Stensen's) passes, diving deeply through the buccinator muscle and emerging at its ostium in the buccal mucosa opposite the maxillary second molar. The deep relations of the gland include the lateral pharyngeal wall and, posteriorly, the internal carotid artery and jugular vein. Through the substance of the gland (deep to the branches of the facial nerve) pass the superficial temporal artery in company with its vein and the auriculotemporal nerve. The large posterior facial vein passes vertically through the parotid as well, variously deep or superficial to the nerve.

Throughout the substance of the gland occur a discrete number of lymph nodes and these, in association with additional nodes superficial to the gland in the preauricular fat, intervene along the lymphatic drainage of the lateral scalp and facial regions into the superficial and deep lymphatic systems of the neck.

Although there persists disagreement about the presence or absence of a true glandular capsule, a dense fibro-connective layer (commonly called the parotid fascia) encases the gland and is continuous with the temporal fascia above and the deep cervical fascia below. It is this unyielding fibrous envelope that accounts for the severe pain associated with inflammatory swelling of the gland parenchyma, as in infectious viral parotitis (mumps). In any case—there are multiple penetrating septa from this fascia into the parenchyma preventing easy enucleation of the gland.[27]

The most critical of the anatomical relationships of the parotid, however, remains its intimate association with the peripheral facial nerve and its branches (Fig. 10.1). It is this association that removes parotid surgery from the field of straightforward extirpative surgery and places it in a special position of challenge. The facial nerve emerges from its bony conduit at the stylomastoid foramen, posterior to the base of the styloid process. Almost immediately a few small and relatively unimportant branches are given off, including motor branches to the posterior digastric and stylohyoid muscles. The main trunk of the nerve, measuring here some 3 or 4 mm, then penetrates the gland at its posterior aspect, inferior to the auditory meatus. Within the substance of the gland, the nerve customarily divides into two main trunks—the temporal-facial and the cervical-facial divisions. Thereafter the branching occurs in a rapid and highly varied manner as an intercommunicating arborization aptly referred to as the pes anserinus (goose's foot). The fine branches that emerge are generally arranged into five nerves, or groups of nerves. The temporal branch passes lateral to the brow, maintaining

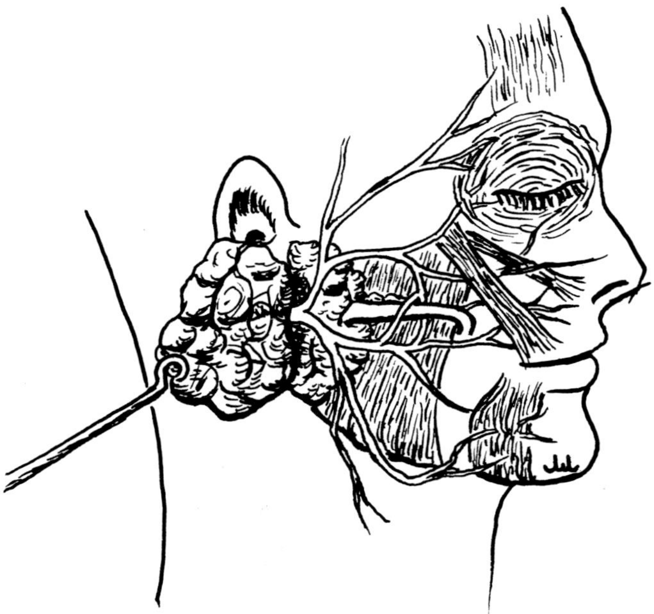

Figure 10.1 Relationship of parotid gland to facial nerve.

elevation of that structure. The all-important zygomatic branch approaches the orbital region for control of the palpebral sphincter. The buccal branch, following the major duct, assures tone in the cheek and upper lip. The mandibular branch passes along the inferior margin of the mandible (frequently dipping below it) under cover of the platysma muscle until reaching the oral commissure, which it maintains in symmetry with its fellow of the opposite side. The expendible cervical branch passes down into the neck to innervate the platysma.

A common misconception concerns the division of the parotid gland into two anatomic lobes by the passage of the facial nerve through the gland, resulting in superficial and deep lobes being joined by a so-called isthmus. A more accurate picture consists of superficial and deep portions of an essentially continuous gland interconnecting widely throughout the interstices of the pes anserinus.[27, 57] Although the anatomic concept of lobes is properly false, the more important surgical concept of "superficial lobectomy" justifies retention of the term. Despite this matter of lobes versus portions, the consideration of practical importance remains the manner of the nerve's passage through the gland. Although the various branches pass through the gland at roughly the same plane, there can be no assurance of this—especially in the presence of pathology. A helpful pattern that can be relied upon, however, is the forward progress of the nerve through the gland—without capricious reversals or doubling-back.[57]

Submandibular Gland

The submandibular gland (or submaxillary gland—as it was once more commonly known) lies tucked beneath the midportion of the horizontal ramus or body of the mandible. It covers the exposed portion of the hyoglossus muscle, overlaping the anterior and posterior bellies of the digastric muscle sling. The submaxillary duct (Warthin's)—along with a consistent deep process of the gland—extends anteromedially, passing beneath the free posterior margin of the mylohyoid muscle and thus into the sublingual space of the floor of the mouth. Here, the glandular process may end in intimate association with the other lesser salivary gland, the sublingual.

The duct itself twice crosses the lingual nerve in the floor of the mouth before terminating in its papilla—or, equally commonly, joined to the major duct (Bartholin's) of the sublingual excretory system to terminate jointly at the prominant sublingual papilla (plica sublingualis). The blood supply of the gland is by way of multiple small branches from the external maxillary or facial vessels (the vein passing superficial to the gland while the artery courses in intimate contact with its deep surface). There is a consistent group of lymph nodes adjacent to the gland within the fascial submandibular space, with a second group appearing along the facial vessels as they emerge over the inferior border of the mandible at the "facial notch." The submandibular gland is also encased in a fibrous capsule, but—unlike the parotid—it remains relatively nonadherent, permitting easier removal. Three important nerve relationships exist around the submandibular gland. The hypoglossal nerve passes deep to the inferior portion of the gland over the floor of the submandibular space or the hyoglossus muscle, where it forms the superior border of Lessor's triangle (the remaining sides composed of the anterior and posterior portions of the digastric sling). Immediately below the floor of this small triangle passes the lingual artery in its course to the tongue. The lingual nerve passes immediately superior to the gland under protection of the horizontal ramus of the mandible. The chorda tympani communications between the nerve and its submandibular ganglion associated with the superior aspect of the gland allow a dangerous displacement of the nerve into the operative field during downward traction on the gland. Finally the mandibular branch, or ramus mandibularae, of the facial nerve passes immediately superficial to the superior aspect of the gland, superficial to the gland capsule and the facial vessels but deep to the platysma muscle, in its course to the angle of the lip.

Sublingual Gland

The sublingual glands are the smallest of the major glands and lie paired to either side of the midline in the floor of the mouth. Unlike the other major glands, drainage is by way of multiple small ducts, although a large single duct often predominates (Bartholin's).

Minor Salivary Glands

The minor glands are numerous aggregates of salivary tissues that occur throughout the oral cavity and much of the embryologic foregut as well. Like the submandibular and sublingual glands, most of the output is mucous or seromucous in nature, as distinguished from the purely serous output of the parotid gland. Some 300–500 glands occur in the oral cavity and oropharynx, where they are most numerous in the palate but are found beneath the buccal, labial and lingual mucosa as well. Extraoral sites include the nasopharynx, the paranasal sinuses and the tracheobronchial tree. The lachrymal glands are histologically indistinguishable.

PATHOLOGY

Neoplastic Disease

Neoplasms of the salivary glands are infrequent, comprising only about 3% of all tumors. Nevertheless, within this small group exists a kaleidoscopic array of tumor types, many of particular fascination. The most common of the benign tumors, for example, is notoriously prone to recurrence—and in recurrent situations may become life-threatening. Three of the more frequent malignancies, on the other hand, tend to progress slowly, coexisting with the host over long periods of time and killing late. Others among the cancers metastasize and kill swiftly. The clinical classification of parotid tumors, then, customarily includes categories for both low grade and high grade malignancies (Table 10.1).

DISTRIBUTION

The parotid gland is by far the most common site of tumor formation, accounting for 80% of all salivary gland tumors. This leaves about 10% each for the submandibular and minor glands, with less than 1% occurring in the sublingual gland.[19] Approximately 80% of parotid neoplasms prove benign. As the size of the salivary gland decreases, however, so does the relative incidence of malignancy; the smaller the gland, the greater the chance for malignant formation. Thus, while the incidence of malignancy in parotid tumors in 20%,[50] that for submandibular tumors nears 40%, and for the rare sublingual gland tumor reaches 80%[7]; the incidence or malignant minor gland tumors is about 50%.[6]

Parotid gland statistics can be approximated in many areas by the figure 80%. Thus 80% of all salivary tumors occur in the parotid. Of these, 80% are in the superficial portion, occurring lateral to the facial nerve. Also, 80% of all parotid tumors are benign, and 80% of these are pleomorphic adenomas (benign mixed tumors). Three salivary gland tumors can be considered essentially limited to the parotid: Warthin's tumor, oncocytoma, and acinic cell carcinoma.[52]

Table 10.1
Classification of Salivary Gland Neoplasms

BENIGN
Pleomorphic adenoma (benign mixed tumor)
Adenolymphoma (Warthin's tumor)
Benign epithelial lesion
Oncocytoma
Others
LOW GRADE MALIGNANT
Low grade mucoepidermoid carcinoma
Acinic cell carcinoma
Adenoid cystic carcinoma (cylindroma)[a]
HIGH GRADE MALIGNANT
Carcinoma expleomorphic adenoma (malignant mixed tumor)
High grade mucoepidermoid carcinoma
Adenocarcinoma
Epidermoid carcinoma (squamous cell carcinoma)
Anaplastic carcinoma

[a] High grade?

A benign parotid mass is apt to represent—in decreasing likelihood—pleomorphic adenoma (80%), Warthin's tumor (10%), benign epithelial lesion, or oncocytoma. Among malignant lesions no one type predominates, carcinoma expleomorphic adenoma (malignant mixed tumor) and mucoepidermoid carcinoma occurring with equal frequency, at twice the rate of adenoid cystic carcinoma and acinic cell carcinoma.[7]

Submandibular gland malignant disease occurs at twice the rate as that of the parotid (40% vs. 20%). Perhaps more significant is an equally higher incidence of aggressive malignant behavior as evidence by metastatic rates of 75% vs. 43%.[19] Benign tumors are virtually confined to pleomorphic adenoma, as Warthin's tumor involves this gland rarely, if at all.[7] Thus a benign submandibular gland mass is apt to represent either benign mixed tumor or an inflammatory lesion, the tumor occurring 4 times more frequently than a discrete inflammatory mass.[21] Among malignant tumors, adenoid cystic carcinoma, adenocarcinoma and anaplastic carcinoma predominate at similar frequencies.[7]

Sublingual gland tumors, while infrequent, remain important becuase of a striking predominance of malignant types (as high as 90%),[51] with adenoid cystic and mucoepidermoid carcinomas accounting for about 40% each.

Minor salivary glands occur over a wide field (including the mucosa of lips and cheek, hard and soft palates, floor of mouth, posterior tongue, as well as nasopharynx, larynx, trachea, lachrymal glands, paranasal sinuses), with their distribution of tumor formation equally wide. The majority of such tumors however, occur in the intraoral sites, with the palate accounting for over one-half of these. Here, the distribution of malignant tumors favors the hard palate, while benign tumors are more common in the soft. Interestingly, minor salivary gland tumors rarely occur in the midline (as opposed to the common, benign bony excrescence known as torus palatinus), but rather lie to either side.[7] While the palate is the most common site for both malignant and benign forms, it is followed by the upper lip and the buccal mucosa for benign lesions, and by the tongue for malignant ones.[25] Pleomorphic adenoma is again the most common of all tumors, and accounts for most of the benign variety (here, intraorally, it is felt to have a lower-than-usual recurrence rate as compared with major glands).[52] The most frequent malignant tumor is adenoid cystic carcinoma occurring diffusely through both intra- and extraoral sites, followed by mucoepidermoid carcinoma (most common in the palate, then the jaws and floor of the mouth), and the adenocarcinomas, which are especially lethal in the mouth.[7]

BENIGN NEOPLASMS

Pleomorphic adenoma (benign mixed tumor) is a slowly growing, benign tumor with a pronounced tendency to local recurrence if inadequately treated (enucleated without a margin of normal gland). It is the most common tumor of the major salivary glands (65%) and involves the lessor and minor glands as well. In the parotid it occurs largely in the superficial portion of the gland (lateral to the facial nerve) and often is limited to that portion behind the mandibular branch, the so-called tail.[7] The tumor has a modest predilection for females and appears most commonly in the 5th decade (those of the minor glands 1 decade later). It presents as an asymptomatic, painless mass which remains moveable, lobulated and smooth. These are solitary tumors, multiple nodularity being a sign of recurrent tumor or malignancy. Histologically the "mixed" epithelial and mesenchymal elements are present in patterns of considerable diversity, with an inner row of epithelial cells and an outer layer of myoepithelial cells associated with a variable stroma which may appear mucoid, chondroid, myxoid, or in combinations of these.[52] The prognosis of primary pleomorphic adenoma is very good, providing adequate surgical treatment (superficial lobectomy) is undertaken. Recurrence rates in the past literature, on the other hand, have approached 50%,[52] reflecting the inadequacy of simple enucleation alone. Careful examination of the gross specimen shows multiple pseudopod extensions beyond the gross "capsule" of the tumor. Malignant change occurs in up to 15% of pleomorphic adenomas,[24] most commonly after multiple benign recurrences. Signs of such transformation include rapid growth, nodularity, ulceration, and nerve weakness.

Warthin's tumor (adenolymphoma or papillary cystadenoma lymphomatosum) is an interesting benign tumor that is essentially limited to the parotid gland (although it has occasionally involved other sites, including the submandibular gland and the minor glands of the lips and antrum).[7] The tumors appear over a wide age range, peaking during the 6th decade, and show a striking 5 to 1 male predilection. Its 10% incidence of bilaterality, as well as multifocal occurrence within a single gland, remains unique among salivary gland tumors. Clinically, Warthin's tumors are asymptomatic and grow slowly, often associated with a long interval before diagnosis is sought. They are well defined, and may impart a feeling of softness or fluctuation on palpation. The most interesting histological aspect is the invariable presence of lymphoid tissue, usually surrounding an epithelium that describes a typical tubulopapillary-cystic pattern.[52] Numerous histogenic theories have been put forward to explain this unusual association of lymphoid and epithelial elements, the most commonly accepted implicating neoplasia of heteroptopic salivary gland tissue within lymph nodes themselves, these occurring either external to or within the parotid.[63] The prognosis for the adequately excised lesion is excellent, and reports of recurrence probably reflect inadequate surgery or unrecognized multifocality.[7]

Benign epithelial lesion is the name associated with a single mass of reactive or inflammatory disease masquerading as a neoplastic process. It probably represents a focal presentation of more diffuse autoimmune conditions, including Sjogren's syndrome.[52] Certainly its incidence is higher in the presence of such conditions, and histologically it is indistinguishable. So, too, does it follow the same female predilection. In any case, the prognosis in the absence of systemic signs and symptoms of autoimmune disease appears good; recurrences are infrequent and malignant forms of the disease, if they do occur at all, are rare.

Oncocytoma is an uncommon salivary gland tumor that is confined almost exclusively to older age groups. It appears most frequently in the parotid, occurring as a solid tumor. When involving the minor glands, however, it does so more frequently in papillary or cystic forms.[52] Microscopically, the lesion is composed of sheets of oncocytes, the large polygonal cells that often occur as areas of hyperplasia in otherwise normal, aging salivary glands.[7] The behavior of the tumor is that of a slow growing, benign lesion with little tendency to recur. Rare malignant forms, have been reported.

Other benign tumors of a monomorphic pattern account for less than 2% of salivary gland tumors. These include sebaceous adenoma, basal cell adenoma, and the rare clear cell adenoma.[52] Among nonepithelial tumors that affect the salivary glands, hemangioma is by far the most frequent—parotid hemangioma comprising the most common salivary gland tumor of infancy and childhood.[22] Spontaneous resolution is the rule for this lesion, unlike the less common lymphangioma.

MALIGNANT NEOPLASMS

Mucoepidermoid carcinoma represents a spectrum of malignant disease. It is among the most common of salivary gland malignancies and shows a slight female predominance. The lesion most commonly presents in the 5th and 6th decades, but is not uncommon before the age of 15 and, in fact, represents the most common salivary gland malignancy of childhood.[52] The presentation of this lesion reflects the diversity of its clinical behavior, the low grade lesions often remaining as painless lumps for long periods before diagnosis, the high grade lesions presenting after a much shorter course of time associated with pain, trismus, bloody saliva, and facial nerve weakness. Histologically the tumor—as its name implies—contains both squamous cells and glandular mucin-secreting cells, and latter often is responsible for mucinous cyst formation. There is in this lesion a significant correlation between the histologic appearance and the clinical behavior and—hence—prognosis.[7] Thus, low grade lesions show well differentiated components of both elements with frequent papillary epithelium and cyst formation. High grade lesions, on the other hand, show predominantly squamous cell types, with few acinar or mucinous elements. The prognosis for mucoepidermoid carcinoma depends in large, but by no means total, measure upon its histologic presentation.[7] Low grade lesions carry a good prognosis, many behaving more like pleomorphic adenoma than carcinoma. Nonetheless, even for these well differentiated lesions the recurrence rate remains significant (approaching 30% in some series) and metastases, though rare, do occur.[7, 52] High grade lesions, by contrast, display a marked tendency to local invasion and recurrence, with a third of these metastasizing to regional lymph nodes and more distant sites. Five- and 10-year survival figures for the low grade tumor generally range between 90 and 100%, while those for their high range counterparts range from 40% down to a dismal zero.[22]

Acinic cell tumor, by contrast, is a neoplasm capable of benign or malignant behavior quite apart from its histological appearance. It is an uncommon tumor—accounting for only 1% of all salivary gland tumors—and is, with few exceptions, confined to the parotid gland.[7] The tumor shows a 2 to 1 female predominance and is found in all age groups, including children.[24, 52] Typically this lesion presents as a slow growing, painless mass, but one with indistinct margins. Fixation to skin or deeper structures may occur. Microscopically the tumor appears benign and unimpressive, displaying collections of granular cells in near-normal acinar form.[52] The prognosis of this lesion has been the source of some argument, but high recurrence rates, significant metastatic rates, and low but definite tumor-related death rates all demand that it be treated with respect.[7] Five-year survival statistics are in the range of 90%, but these fall off by significant degrees with the passage of years,[20] as in other carcinomas of the salivary gland that exhibit a benign, protracted course.

Adenoid cystic carcinoma (cylindroma) is a slow growing, but highly stubborn malignancy that occurs throughout the distribution and range of salivary gland tissue. It is relatively uncommon in the parotid, occurring here at less than half the frequency of mucoepidermoid carcinoma.[7]

It has, on the other hand, a far greater relative frequency among the lesser and minor glands and is the most common malignancy of both the submandibular gland and the intraoral minor salivary glands[41]—where it has a predilection (along with mucoepidermoid carcinoma) for the hard palate.[7] Other sites of involvement include the minor glands of the nasopharynx, paranasal sinuses, larynx and tracheobronchial tree, as well as the ceruminous glands of the ears and the lachrymal glands. The lesion is most frequently diagnosed in the late 5th decade; it is distinctly uncommon in childhood. Most present as an asymptomatic mass, although signs of nerve involvement occur relatively early, given the predilection of this tumor for neural and perineural invasion. Thus pain and muscle weakness are not uncommon symptoms. Microscopically, small cells within a fibrous-hyaline stroma assume varying patterns that are sheetlike trabecular, or glandular (cylindromatous).[52] Most show early invasion along perineural spaces. The prognosis for this lesion must remain guarded. Recurrence is the rule (over two-thirds) but, while it nearly always spells eventual demise, it frequently permits extended survival. Similarly, one-third demonstrate metastasis to regional lymph nodes and distant sites. Five-year surgical statistics are thus notoriously inaccurate in assessing the ultimate prognosis.[52] Such 5-year figures as 65% survival are reduced to less than half in 5–10 years.[8, 24] In general, the minor gland lesions carry a poorer prognosis than those of the major glands.[16] The most favorable prognostic indicator is the absence of tumor involvement at the microscopic margin of the surgical specimen,[52] a status requiring wide and aggressive resection of this incidious, infiltrating lesion with its early invasion of nerve and bone. Thus, while slow growth allows extended survival in the presence of recurrent disease and has prompted some to consider this a low grade malignancy, its stubborn persistence with ultimate unhappy survival rates has recommended its placement among the high grade lesions. Certainly its inclusion here tends to emphasize the need for aggressive initial surgery, with adjuvant therapy where indicated (see fig. 10.6). This emphasis certainly is appropriate in view of a general history of past undertreatment with staggering recurrence rates.

Carcinoma expleomorphic adenoma (malignant mixed tumor) is an aggressive, lethal cancer that almost invariably arises within a pre-existing benign pleomorphic adenoma.[7] Its distribution, then, is similar to that of the benign lesion and the parotid is easily the most common site, where this tumor accounts for approximately 10% of malignant forms. The tumor appears approximately 10 years later than its benign precursor (the 6th rather than the 5th decade).[23] Typically a benign pleomorphic adenoma has existed for many years—with or without recurrence—when a sudden acceleration of growth prompts presentation. Pain and facial nerve involvement often coexist, but the mass may as often remain asymptomatic. Histologically the critera for a diagnosis of malignancy may be difficult to fulfill for a given lesion, and this is especially true on frozen section examination. In general the infiltrative index is the most reliable,[18] but the lesion remains frequently misdiagnosed—or rather, overdiagnosed—toward an interpretation of malignancy.[28] The prognosis is poor.

Adenocarcinoma of the salivary gland refers to that group of glandular malignancies that cannot be classified within one of the more distinctive preceding categories. Histologically these lesions tend to resemble the better known adenocarcinomas of the gastrointestinal tract. There has been some support for the notion that, similar to mucoepidermoid carcinomas, they may be divided into low grade and high grade types.[8] In any case, among malignancies of the intraoral glands, adenocarcinoma—which accounts for as many as one-quarter of these—carries the worst prognosis,[7] with recurrence rates exceeding even those of adenoid cystic carcinoma.

Squamous cell carcinoma (epidermoid carcinoma), indistinguishable from that occurring elsewhere in the body, does occur in the salivary glands. Its frequency is uncommon, with its distribution limited to the major glands, accounting for no more than 3% of parotid tumors, perhaps 12% of submandibular ones.[7] It affects males more often, with the peak incidence in the 6th and 7th decades. These lesions are indurated when first seen, often with fixation to skin or deep structures, and half are ulcerated.[52] The clinical course is often rapid profusion to death from distant metastasis or, more commonly, uncontrollable local disease. Difficulties in differential diagnosis occur both with mucoepidermoid carcinoma in which the epidermoid component predominates and with metastatic squamous cell carcinoma to intra- and periparotid lymph nodes.[7] In advanced lesions replacing much of the gland, differentiation from the latter condition may not be possible. Five-year survivors number around 25%.[24]

Undifferentiated carcinomas are rare and highly malignant tumors that do not lend themselves to inclusion within the foregoing categories. Although they occur most commonly in the 7th and 8th decades without sex preference, they can occur at any age. More than one-third appear to arise in the presence of a mixed tumor, one usually of a long duration.[23] These tumors infiltrate aggressively and metastasize widely. Five-year survival figures are similar to those for epidermoid disease, that is—approximately 25%.[61]

Other malignant neoplasms involving the salivary glands include metastatic carcinoma, which can, of course, involve any of the intra- or periparotid lymph nodes. The source of metastasis is most often malignant melanoma or epidermoid carcinoma arising in the scalp, temple or ear regions. Other areas of the face may occasionally contribute, as well as the palate and nasopharynx. Malignant lymphomas arising in salivary glands also occur, albeit rarely.

Inflammatory Disease

While many systemic inflammatory disorders[7, 52] may affect the salivary glands incidentally, certain conditions are quite specific for these organs.

ACUTE SUPPURATIVE PAROTITIS

Also called postoperative parotitis, this condition occurs as a painful, rapidly developing parotid swelling—most common after the stress of a major surgical procedure or prolonged febrile illness in an elderly, chronically debilitated patient.[52] In such typical circumstances of advanced age and reduced resistance, this complication carries a grave prognosis with mortality rates approaching 20%.[40] The suppuration occurs as an ascending infection (via Stensen's duct) by gram-positive organisms (especially penicillinase-resistant staphylococcus), and is favored by a state of poor oral hygiene and diminished salivary flow—this latter condition often the result of dehydration or certain medications (anticholinergics, diuretics).[39] The severe pain is typical of acute inflammations of the gland within its tough, unyielding capsule. Multiloculated abscesses may partially decompress themselves via the parotid duct. Generally the untreated condition progresses through pain, fever, malaise, trismus and generalized sepsis.

SIALOLITHIASIS

Acute and chronic inflammation of the salivary glands may be associated with calculus formation and the submandibular gland is especially prone to such development—10 times more so than the parotid.[52] There is evidence to suggest that sialith precipitation occurs as the primary event in the submandibular gland with inflammatory changes secondary to it—while in the parotid the converse situation is likely to prevail, with primary inflammatory changes leading to calculus formation.[7, 52] The disease is characterized by intermittent, painful swelling of the gland occurring after meals. However, calculi may remain asymptomatic, or, on the other hand—they may precipitate acute exacerbations of severe degree, proceeding to frank suppuration and systemic sepsis.

UVEOPAROTID FEVER

A local form of sarcoidosis may involve the salivary glands and the uveal tract of the eye. Such uveoparotid fever, or Heerfordt's syndrome, may occur independently or in association with systemic disease.[52] Typically a prodromal fever and malaise is followed by painless parotid swelling that resolves spontaneously after many months. The other major salivary glands may become involved, as well. Uveitis is frequent—occasionally progressing to blindness—and cranial nerve paresis—especially of the seventh nerve—also occurs.[52] The frequent past confusion with Sjogren's syndrome, in which salivary and ocular symptoms also predominate, is readily appreciated.[7]

AUTOIMMUNE DISEASES

Benign lymphoepithelial lesion refers to the histopathologic description of a related group of autoimmune diseases, that include significant salivary gland dysfunction. Mikulicz's disease, recurrent parotitis of childhood—and that of adulthood—and Sjogren's syndrome all represent various aspects of these poorly understood disorders and may constitute a progressive spectrum with—for example—Mikulicz's disease constituting but a mild or incomplete form of Sjogren's syndrome.[52] In any case, the coexistence of a systemic collagen disease with any of these disorders essentially justifies the designation of full blown Sjogren's syndrome.

Sjogren's syndrome[52] is a symptom triad of keratoconjunctivitis sicca, xerostomia, and a systemic collagen disease—most frequently rheumoid arthritis.[9] It afflicts predominantly women in their later years and characteristically presents with arthritis as the earliest complaint. Ocular symptoms typically follow, including redness, itching, burning and foreign body sensation. The oral symptoms appear last and consist of dryness and burning, difficulty with denture wear and dental decay. The parotid glands become subject to intermittent ductal obstruction and resultant inflammation and infection. The histologic picture is one of progressive lymphocytic infiltration at the expense of glandular parenchyma.[7] As a sobering prognostic note, it has lately become apparent that the full blown syndrome predisposes to the late development of carcinoma and especially malignant lymphoma.[60]

OTHER INFLAMMATORY DISEASES

Acute viral parotitis, or mumps, is a common, often epidemic malady of childhood that bestows upon its victims a lifelong immunity.

Ranula refers to cystic degeneration of an obstructed sublingual gland. The resulting cyst of the floor of the mouth may displace the tongue considerably and even, upon occasion, interfere with respiration.

Necrotizing sialometaplasia[1] is a rare, benign inflammatory condition affecting the minor salivary glands of the palate. The typical presentation is one of focal ulceration of the palate mimicking malignancy. Histologically, a picture of lobular necrosis with squamous metaplasia often shows a marked similarity to mucoepidermoid carcinoma. Unwarranted maxillectomy has been performed for this sheep in wolf's clothing. Untreated, this lesion of unknown etiology resolves spontaneously.

DIAGNOSIS

The mainstay in diagnosis of diseases of the salivary glands remains a careful history and physical examination, with confirmation by tissue examination performed only while treatment, usually surgery, is underway.

History

Symptoms are carefully investigated as to their onset and duration and their possible association with previous disease and trauma. The presence of pain or numbness is especially important in the evaluation of a discrete tumor as it usually heralds nerve involvement and hence malignancy. A history of intermittent pain and swelling, on the other hand—especially when related to mastication—is more suggestive of calculus disease. Autoimmune disease, of course, may be associated with systemic symptomatology, which should be sought.

Physical Examination[52]

Inspection and palpation, including intraoral and bimanual palpation, offer much information in the diagnosis of salivary gland disease. Tenderness is often a component of inflammatory disease, and calculi themselves can often be detected, especially in the floor of the mouth. Inspection and gentle probing of the various ductal orifices may yield additional information about inflammatory states. Localization of mass lesions is important, remembering the predilection of pleomorphic adenoma and Warthin's tumor for the tail portion of the parotid gland. The consistency of the mass is helpful, most benign masses presenting a firm, smooth feeling, while malignant ones are more likely to be irregular and hard. Warthin's tumor, on the other hand, is frequently softer than other types, and hemangioma frankly compressible. Motor nerve weakness must be specifically sought by facial muscle and tongue testing, as it may remain subtle in early lesions. Its presence, of course, is tantamount to a diagnosis of malignancy, although rare exceptions occur. When a diagnosis of malignancy is likely—as in the presence of fixation, nerve involvement, or ulceration—a careful search for systemic symptoms and signs of metastatic disease is mandatory and enlarged regional lymph nodes are always sought.

Following penetrating trauma of the cheek region, physical examination becomes especially important in ruling out injury to the facial nerve or parotid duct. Careful testing of the facial musculature is mandatory, and a doubtful response requires exploration of the wound under optimal conditions (under magnification in the operating room). If the course of the parotid duct—which parallels the middle third of a line connecting the tragus of the ear to the philtrum of the lip—is at risk, then retrograde cannulation or instillation of fluid is indicated via the ductal orifice; the appearance of cannula or fluid in the wound confirms ductal breech.

Special Diagnostic Procedures

Although helpful to a degree, special studies have not proven as valuable in the investigation of diseases of the salivary glands as they have in those of other parenchymatous organs.

LABORATORY TESTS

In suspected autoimmune disease, standard rheumatoid workup is indicated, including serum protein electrophoresis and latex fixation testing. Bacteriologic workup and skin testing becomes important in infectious and granulomatous conditions.

ROENTGENOGRAPHIC STUDIES

A standard chest plate is taken of any patient with a salivary gland mass to examine for the pulmonary metastasis of malignant disease, as well as evidence of other unsuspected systemic conditions. Plain films of the jaw region in various projections may also reveal salivary calculi, of which 80% are radiopaque.[52]

Sialography[52] is the study of the salivary ductal system by the introduction of radiopaque media via the appropriate ductal ostium. Although it enjoyed a considerable vogue at one time, most surgeons rarely utilize the technique in the diagnosis of surgical disease of the salivary glands. This is largely so because the technique yields only general and nonspecific information for salivary gland neoplasm, adding little useful information in the management of this condition. In the presence of chronic inflammatory disease (its use is contraindicated during acute episodes), calculus, and autoimmune disease—on the other hand—it is often of particular value, helping to confirm the diagnosis and grade the severity of involvement, and to localize focal pathology such as calculus obstruction. Its use today is, for the most part, reserved for these conditions.

Other radiologic studies include radioisotope scintillation scanning, ultrasound, and arteriography, and these specific procedures may have limited application in the diagnosis of salivary gland disease.[52] In general, like sialography, the information they yield is nonspecific and adds little to the management of most surgical disease. An interesting exception occurs with the first of these, as technetium-scanning of the parotid gland consistently gives a "hot nodule" pattern for Warthin's tumor, whole other types appear variously as "warm" or "cold."[60]

ELECTRODIAGNOSTIC STUDIES

Electromyography and related tests play a significant, albeit limited, role in the management of extracranial facial nerve lesions. Nerve division, for example, can usually be confirmed by the appearance of fibrillation potentials within about 2 weeks after injury.[52] So too can early reinnervation be demonstrated by a decrease in such hyperirritability and by the appearance of polyphasic, multiunit action potentials.

Biopsy

The final diagnosis for all surgical disease rests, of course, with tissue diagnosis. Here salivary gland tumor present a special problem. Aspiration, or needle biopsy, as well as incisional biopsy, are contraindicated as preoperative maneuvers in most circumstances. The notoriously high recurrence rates for these tumors (adenoid cystic carcinoma and pleomorphic adenoma, for example) speak to the great risk of tumor dissemination during such biopsy procedures. With respect to the major glands, most neoplasms are contained within the narrow tissue space between the facial nerve and the superficial subcutaneous tissues of the cheek. Biopsy procedures make contamination of the deep and superficial limits of this space likely, negating the otherwise highly effective, yet conservative procedure of superficial parotidectomy. Also the seventh nerve itself is placed at risk by these procedures. With respect to the lesser glands, it must be remembered that tumors here are more likely to be malignant and, when malignant, more aggressive. There is, therefore, no place for incisional biopsy of these small glands.

The general guideline has therefore developed that the minimal surgical procedure—biopsy or otherwise—to be performed upon the major salivary glands should be formal, superficial parotidectomy, and upon the lesser glands total extirpation. As with all guidelines—and these are good ones—there may be exceptions. Specifically, early discrete tumors of the parotid when fortuitously located may be removed within a block of normal parotid tissue, dissecting out the appropriate facial nerve branches in the immediate vacinity, but avoiding complete lobectomy with its concominant flattening of contour and otherwise unjustified total nerve dissection. With respect to the lesser glands, there can be no such advantage to partial sparing of the gland and, therefore, total extirpation remains indicated.

To confirm a diagnosis of Sjogren's syndrome, the simple expedient of labial gland biopsy from the inner lower lip is highly effective, as the histologic picture in these minute glands accurately reflects those of the greater glands in this condition.[42]

TREATMENT

The treatment[52, 53] of most disease of the salivary glands remains surgical, although such adjuvant modes as radiotherapy and chemotherapy are playing an increasingly important role in overall management.

Neoplasms

The initial treatment of virtually all undiagnosed salivary gland tumors remains surgical, as surgery alone yields the intact specimen for tissue diagnosis and, hence, proper management. In many cases, this initial biopsy procedure (superficial parotid lobectomy or total removal of the submandibular gland) is therapeutic as well, and no further treatment is necessary.

SURGICAL THERAPY

Major gland (parotid) surgery for both diagnosis and treatment most frequently comprises lateral, or superficial, lobectomy. The greater majority of primary lesions presenting early for treatment are contained within the block of tissue encompassed by this procedure. To invoke this practice for all parotid lesions, however, is to overtreat those certain early lesions that present in favorable locations, but to do so is always preferable to enucleation or excision without dissection of the facial nerve. Thus small, benign lesions residing in the superior, preauricular portion or in the tail portion behind and below the main nerve trunk and its cervicofacial division may be removed within a block of engulfing normal gland, requiring dissection of only a portion of the nerve. To subject the entire nerve to dissection in such cases is to present it undo risk of injury. In the case of lesions overlying the pes anserinus and those of greater dimensions, lateral superficial parotidectomy remains indicated. Individualization of treatment in the surgical approach, then, is encouraged as long as principles are not violated. In the case of the initial biopsy procedure, these principles remain the removal of the lesion within a bloc of normal tissue and the protection of the facial nerve through formal dissection of all branches that are at risk during the procedure.

A proposed approach to the management of the undiagnosed mass lesion of the parotid gland follows. The entire hemi-face and neck are prepared and left exposed with the patient under general anesthesia without nerve blocking agents. The incision should follow aesthetic lines to the greatest degree possible, while permitting the necessary exposure for safe surgery. Many patterns have been described, most on a Y pattern, incorporating the ear lobule within the arms of the Y (Fig. 10.2*A*). Such patterns yield an undesirable vertical scar that runs against the line of relaxed skin tension in that portion of the neck below the lobule. In favorable cases with a low likelihood of malignancy, an alternative approach combines the standard rhytidectomy, or facelift, incision with a high transverse, or skin-crease, incision of the neck, running some 2 cm below the mandibular border (Fig. 10.2*B*). This incision begins behind the tragus and passes into the skin crease along the anterior lobule, which structure it follows into the postauricular sulcus. Here the incision reaches to the height of the auditory meatus and passes sharply backward across the postauricular skin to follow the hairline to the

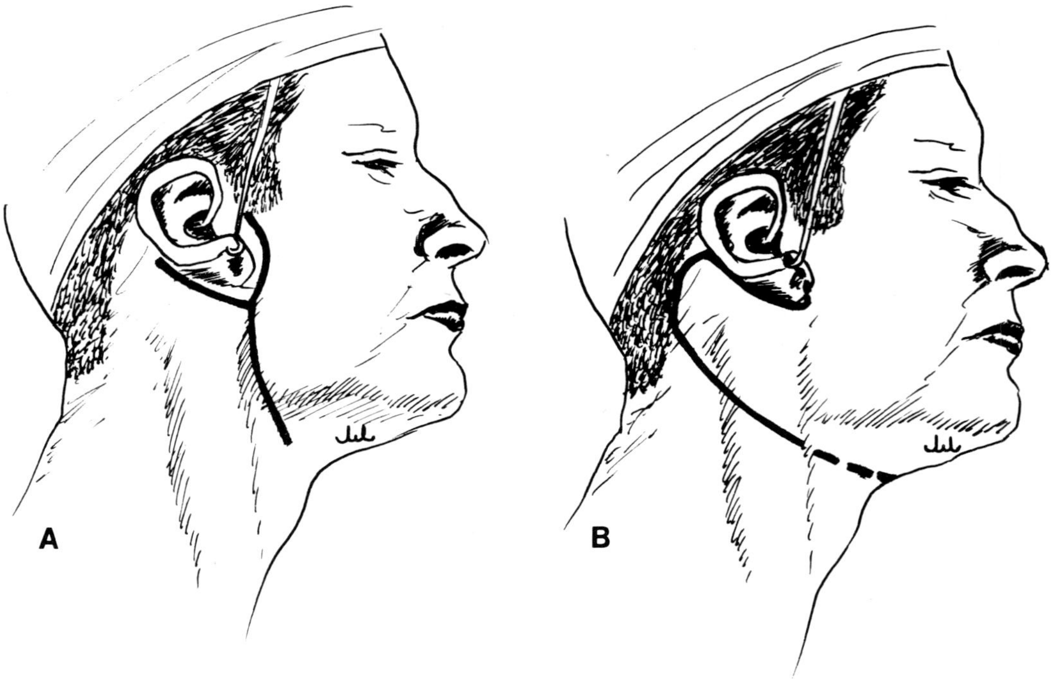

Figure 10.2 Incisions for parotidectomy. (*A*) Traditional "Y" incision. (*B*) Aesthetic alternative for favorable cases (due care is required in handling of postauricular flap).

point where it joins the high cervical incision. Only that portion of the incision is made that is necessary for exposure of the given tumor according to the considerations of size and location. Thus a small preauricular lesion may be approached without need for the cervical extension and, where necessary, the cervical portion is limited in terms of its anterior extent to what is strictly required. When combined neck dissection is indicated the anterior incision can be extended to the submental region as the upper arm of the favored parallel incisions of McFee. This scheme avoids a vertical incision in any portion of the neck. The posterior skin flap overlying the sternocleidomastoid muscle is sharply dissected from investing fascia of the muscle, thereby protecting those branches of the greater auricular nerve that will not be sacrificed with the tissue bloc; the flap over the cheek is sharply elevated with the knife at the deep rhytidectomy plane, leaving adequate layers of subcutaneous tissue both on the flap and over the underlying bloc. Now the facial nerve is sought and identified before the dissection of the gland is commenced. Loupe magnification (2½X to 6½X) now becomes a great aid to the further surgery. In the standard situation the main trunk of the nerve is sought immediately distal to its exit from the skull where it is surrounded by a group of palpable skeletal landmarks, including the cartilaginous external auditory meatus, the transverse process of the second cervical vertebrae, and the mastoid process.[52] In exposing the nerve in this region one proceeds superior and deep to the exposed posterior belly of the digastric muscle with particular care. Here the main trunk is identified by blunt dissection and this fact confirmed with the nerve stimulator as a one-time test. Further use of the stimulator is unnecessary as the nerve dissection is continued under visualtization and in continuity at all times. The dissection then rapidly proceeds along the course of the major trunk to its two divisions. The technique used is one of blunt development of a tunnel above the course of the nerve, followed by sharp division of the sides of that tunnel with the exposed nerve ahead under constant view. Bipolar electrocoagulation maintains hemostasis, while great care is taken to avoid unnecessary handling of the nerve itself.[57] As dissection along any branch advances the intact gland behind the advance may be divided safely with confidence in the fact that the nerve does not turn back upon itself. This process is continued branch by branch until the entire specimen has been cleared and thus delivered en bloc. In certain cases, as mentioned before, it may be possible to subject only a portion of the gland to dissection and in such case it is often to advantage to locate first a peripheral branch of the nerve (Fig. 10.3). One such retrograde approach[12] locates the posterior facial vein along the anterior border of the sternocleidomastoid muscle and follows this structure superiorly into the gland. Shortly after entering the gland substance, the cervical-facial division can be consistently located some few millimeters anterior to the vein. This major divison can then be followed back to the main bifurcation. Another site for retrograde dissection[59] is the parotid duct, which is isolated at the anterior border of the masseter muscle. The accompanying buccal branch of the nerve can then be traced backward.

An additional maneuver that has been described is the retrograde instillation of methylene blue via the ductal orifice immediately prior to surgery.[54] The parenchyma of the gland is thereby stained a deep blue, while the facial nerve remains, by contrast, a glistening white. Neoplasms remain unstained, as well.

Whatever the manner of dissection, the entire superficial specimen is submitted intact for frozen section diagnosis when possible. If it becomes clear during the dissection, however, that the neoplastic process involves branches of the nerve, then a decision must be made whether to sacrifice the nerve or to dissect the tumor from it. In this single instance is incisional biopsy

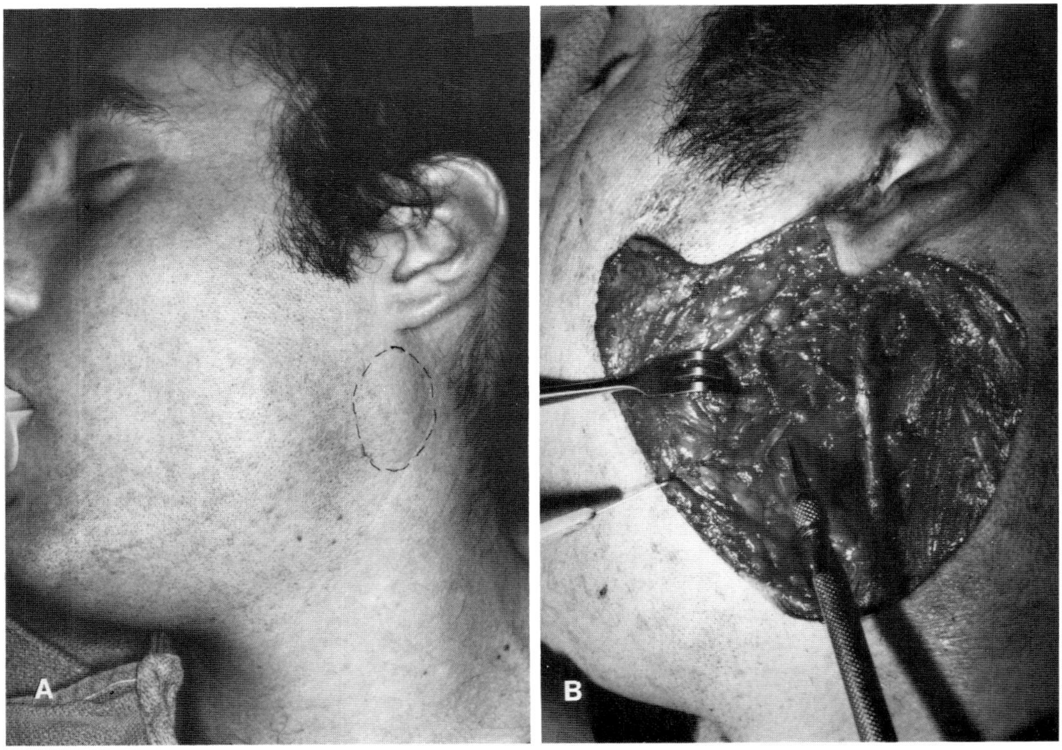

Figure 10.3 (*A*) Small mass in tail region of parotid (*dotted line*). (*B*) Retrograde dissection allows partial lobectomy, exposing only cervical-facial trunk.

advisable during the course of the procedure. Even so, great effort is made to minimize the possibility of tumor spillage and contamination, and here needle aspiration into the bloc may be the best approach. If the incisional biopsy confirms the presence of malignant disease, the appropriate branches or the entire nerve are then sacrificed, whereas in the presence of primary benign disease the dissection is continued closely along the nerve while sparing it.

If the pathology report of the intact superficial specimen indicates the presence of a benign tumor, the procedure is terminated as adequate treatment has also been accomplished. If malignant disease is present an estimation must be made of the grade of malignancy. In the case of a typically low grade malignant lesion, such as acinic cell carcinoma or low grade mucoepidermoid carcinoma, the remaining portions of parotid gland are removed, including the deep lobe, while the branches of the facial nerve are left intact—so-called total parotidectomy with preservation of the facial nerve.[52] While some argue that superficial lobectomy constitutes adequate treatment in such circumstances, personal experience with intraparotid metastasis from miniscule primaries of such low grade cancers dictates complete removal of the gland. With respect to preservation of the nerve, adenoid cystic carcinoma remains a borderline consideration and decisions must be individualized. In the case of clearly high grade malignancy, a radical parotidectomy is completed with sacrifice of the nerve. Immediate nerve grafting may then be performed. In those instances primarily involving the deep lobe, the same approach is followed; it is necessary to remove the superficial lobe to ensure the safety of the nerve before a diagnosis can be established by separate dissection of the deep lobe with the nerve thus visualized. This scenario need not be followed in recurrent cases nor in those of obvious malignancy. In the case of stubborn recurrence of pleomorphic adenoma, it is frequently necessary to sacrifice specific branches of the facial nerve to ensure likelihood of control in these difficult circumstances. Immediate nerve grafting is then indicated. So too should the entire previous scar be included with the specimen. In the case of almost certain malignancy, preliminary biopsy may well be justified as a prelude to formal radical parotidectomy with sacrifice of the nerve. Any specimen that reveals malignancy and is associated with palpable nodes in the ipsilateral neck indicates in continuity neck dissection. In the case of such highly malignant lesions as squamous cell carcinoma and anaplastic carcinoma, neck dissection is often indicated in the absence of clinical nodes. When lower grade malignancies are encountered, node sampling from the upper neck may be done, but in the absence of confirmed metastasis, neck dissection is not justified. In larger lesions the extent of surgery is enlarged to encompass the lesion, as with any malignancy. Involvement of the masseter muscle, for example, dictates mandibulectomy.

Lesser gland (submandibular and sublingual) surgery requires a minimal operative procedure of total extirpation with preservation of the lingual, hypoglossal and mandibular nerves. Only then is diagnosis made by frozen section means. If malignancy is found, there is greater justification for elective neck dissection with these lesions because of their more aggressive nature as compared with those of the parotid. Certainly in high grade malignancy, such should be considered. Primary extirpation in the case of likely malignancy should include complete dissection of the submandibular triangle, as well as portions of the mandible and oral lining, if indicated.

Minor salivary gland diagnosis is most often by incisional biopsy, and it is thus important to incorporate the entire previous biopsy site in the extirpation of proven tumor. The tendancy of the past has been to undertreat malignant lesions, and to avoid this firm adherence to all principles of tumor surgery remains critical here. Cases of malignancy involving the hard palate for example, must include full removal of subjacent bone with the specimen. The special tendency of adenoid cystic carcinoma for nerve invasion must be born in mind, and in the region of major nerves (i.e., greater palatine) such invasion must be sought out and eradicated. Thus relatively small and innocuous lesions may require considerable sacrifice of lining and underlying bone and nerve [see Fig. 10.6]. Doubtful cases must be pursued until surgical margins are clear of tumor by frozen section examination.

ADJUVANT THERAPY

Radiation therapy has traditionally played a small role in the treatment of salivary gland malignancy—at least in this country.[52] A general impression of radioresistance, however, has recently given way to concepts of enhanced control through the postoperative, adjunctive use of this modality.[13, 33, 56] Thus the postoperative application of radiation therapy may allow the surgery to conserve a facial nerve that otherwise would be lost to surgical control alone. Emerging and ever clearer indications for postoperative treatment include known tumor residual following surgery, microscopic tumor at the margin of resection, and unresectable tumor.[52] Lymphoma and metastatic carcinoma remain conditions for radiation treatment, as well. Neck specimens showing greater than three tumor-positive nodes also represent indications for this postoperative therapy.

Chemotherapy remains of limited value for most salivary gland malignancies except the epidermoid variety, which here responds, as elsewhere, to such agents as methotrexate and bleomycin.[52]

Inflammatory Disease

Inflammatory conditions are best managed by a combination of medical and surgical therapies.[52]

SIALADENITIS

Acute bacterial infections are treated by rest, liquid diet without salivary stimulants, oral rinses, and appropriate antibiotics. Gentle probing of major duct orifices may promote gland drainage and decompression. When abscess formation complicates the picture, external incision and drainage is required—taking special care to avoid injury to the facial nerve branches. While such intervention usually spares function in the parotid gland, subsequent excision is frequently required of the lesser glands. With respect to the chronic cystic degeneration of the sublingual gland known as ranula, total excision is preferred over marsupialization. Viral parotitis is treated by supportive measures similar to those used in bacterial disease, with the exception of antibiotics.

SIALOLITHIASIS

First-time major ductal obstructions can frequently be relieved by transoral incision of the duct and removal of the calculus. Recurrent or chronic disease usually indicates total excision of the lesser glands or segmental excision of the parotid, such as superficial parotidectomy. Again, supportive measures, as well as antibiotics, play a role.

AUTOIMMUNE DISEASE

No curative treatment exists for Sjogren's syndrome, although symptomatic therapies are offered, including artificial tears and salivary substitutes—to ameliorate the sicca complaints. Inpeccable oral hygiene becomes mandatory in preventing dental complications. Corticosteroids may temporarily limit troublesome parotid swelling, but otherwise are ineffective. Superficial parotidectomy may improve intractable symptoms, but otherwise does not alter the disease course. In view of the clear risk of malignant degeneration that has become apparent, immunosuppressive agents such as cyclophosphamide are recommended by some.[4]

RECONSTRUCTION[52, 53]

Post-Traumatic

Although injury may occur to any area bearing salivary tissue, the problem of salivary gland trauma is essentially confined to penetrating injury of the parotid gland and division of either or both of its associated structures, the parotid duct and the facial nerve. Laceration of the parotid gland parenchyma without division of the major ductal system requires only soft tissue repair of overlying tissues.[17, 47] Occasional collections of saliva may be treated by needle aspiration and, in any case, disappear within a few weeks. Persistent parotid fistula is no more likely after such injury than after routine amputation of the tail of the gland during radical neck dissection. Persistent drainage, on the other hand, indicates ductal injury and requires repair. When the diagnosis of ductal injury is made, early repair should be undertaken before local tissue inflammation complicates the picture.[17, 47] Direct periductal anastomosis should be performed under magnification utilizing fine sutures. Approximation of neighboring parenchyma should relieve all tension from the repair, which should be completed over a Silastic tube splint brought out through the ductal orifice and sutured in place to the buccal mucosa for 2 weeks.[52] When an established external fistula (internal fistula into the mouth is uncommon and does not require treatment) is seen, successful treatment is more difficult to achieve. Solutions include dissection of the fistulous tract including its cutaneous stoma and translocation into the mouth[46] or construction and delivery of a buccal mucosal flap (with or without tubing) into a cystic portion of the fistula or to the proximal ductal end.[17]

Division of a major branch of the facial nerve results in considerable functional as well as cosmetic deformity and such division and its resulting deficit should be repaired and restored whenever possible. This is not the case for smaller, peripheral branches, where spontaneous return of function following division is the rule. A vertical line dropped from the lateral canthus is a helpful guide in determining which injuries require repair as those lateral to this line require treatment, while those medial to it, in general, do not.[17] When the diagnosis of disruption has been made, confirmation should be carried out by wound exploration under magnification in the operating room. Immediate repair should follow, whenever possible. Exceptions include unusual contamination with a likelihood of infection and massive soft tissue injury with uncertain viability of covering tissues. In these instances nerve ends should be identified and tagged for later repair, which should follow soon after a closed healed wound is achieved—within 4–6 weeks. If complex injury renders anatomy and nerve identification confusing, a proximal dissection of the nerve as in superficial parotidectomy should be undertaken, following the branches out to the level of division.[52]

Immediate repair offers the best chance for nerve restoration while tissues remain soft and supple without changes of inflammation, proximal nerve ends have not yet begun neuroma formation, and distal nerve ends remain excitable to nerve stimulation—a condition persisting some 72 hours and one that greatly simplifies nerve-end location. It must be remembered that motor unit atrophy progresses with the interval of denervation, rendering late nerve repair less and less effective. Nevertheless, attempts at late repair may be indicated as long as 18 months following injury especially where electromyographical studies confirm muscle response.[3]

Repair may be accomplished by either conventional epineural alignment or by perineural or fascicular repair, as long as universally accepted principles of nerve repair are adhered to, including the use of fine (8-0 to 10-0) suture materials placed under magnification (operating microscope) without tension.[55] The breakage of these fine suture materials during attempted repair is evidence of unacceptable tension and a clear indication for interpositional nerve graft. The intraparotid seventh nerve is a pure motor nerve with multiple interconnections among its branches. Cases of spontaneous recovery without repair of major branches occur from time to time, and recovery following proper repair is to be expected. Function should reappear by 6 months and such function can be anticipated by a matter of weeks through electromyography.[52]

Post-Surgical

Unintentional injury to the facial nerve during parotid surgery should occur rarely, and such injury should never go unnoticed. In such an event, repair is immediately performed as in traumatic division. The far more common source of nerve injury during surgery is, of course, the intentional sacrifice of all or part of the nerve during tumor extirpation. Here repair is by nerve graft,[15] utilizing the greater auricular or lesser occipital nerves for replacement of partial loss and the more proximal cervical plexis for total loss. During surgery for carcinoma, when the neck is positive for metastatic disease or when the tumor type suggests this eventuality (as with epidermoid and anaplastic carcinomas), the contralateral neck should serve as the donor site. A distant, less favorable source, remains the sural nerve. Repair of the zygomatic branch for lid control assumes special importance, but the remaining temporal, buccal, and mandibular nerves should all be restored, as well. Again, immediate restoration offers the best chance for recovery and should be carried out whenever tumor control appears a reasonable expectation. This decision should not depend upon considerations of pre- or postoperative adjuvant therapy, such as radiation. The outcome of such grafting procedures can be predicted by the rule of fourths.[10] One-fourth of cases achieve excellent results with both active animation and display of emotion; a second quarter achieve good results with active motion alone; a third 25% are benefited only to a fair degree showing symmetry in repose; finally a quarter so treated have poor results with little or no improvement. Once again, some evidence of function should be seen within 6–8 months and this can be anticipated by electromyography.[11] Certain facial muscle deficits cannot be safely tolerated for such a period, chief among these the lid weakness and lagophthalmos that accompanies division of the zygomatic branch. The resulting corneal exposure threatens desiccation of that structure and potential perforation of the globe. Therefore, a prudent adjunct to repair of this branch is temporary lateral tarsorrhaphy,[52] fusing the denuded margins of the lids together laterally, thus limiting palpebral aperture and corneal exposure. When temporary interruption of function is predicted, as after a difficult dissection of tumor from the intact branch, a simple suture tarsorrhaphy may be helpful for several weeks, while lid tone recovers. Temporary weakness may also go untreated, except for education of the patient to the avoidance of exposure. Eye drops may be helpful during the day and Bell's phenomenon (the rolling of the globe upward beneath the upper lid during attempted closure) is often protective of the cornea during the critical hours of sleep.

Additional reconstructive measures may be helpful simultaneous with or subsequent to nerve repair, including both static and dynamic support procedures. An example of the former is one- or two-stage support to the angle of the mouth through fascia lata grafts that extend to the zygomatic arch, where they are fixed to produce slight overcorrection of the drooping oral commissure.[26] Synthetic slings[5] may also be buried within the lid margins and tightened to narrow the palpebral fissure, and weights[37] may be imbedded in the upper lid to exploit gravity in aiding lid closure. Dynamic supports include partial masseter muscle transfer[2] to the angle of the mouth, retaining both the zygomatic orgin of the muscle and its intact nerve supply through the motor branches of the mandibular division of the fifth nerve. The temporalis muscle[29, 43] and its fascia can be similarly used to encircle the eyelids with a dynamic effect.

Additional late ancillary procedures include skin excisions on the flaccid side (brow lift, nasolabial excision, hemirhytidectomy or facelift)[26] and selective myomectomy[48] (usually of muscles acting at the modiolus or angle of the mouth region) on the active, now exaggerated side. Nerve transfers are also available, anastomosing the 11th or accesory[14] and the 12th or hypoglossal[38] nerves to the interrupted facial. As one might predict, however, the resulting activity is crude and "mass-action" in nature. Furthermore, added additional deformities are incurred from interruption of the donor nerves (shoulder drop and dysarthria). The recent description of nerve transfer from isolated motor branches of the masseter muscle[58] offers theoretical advantages over previous transfers. Nonetheless, results from such heterogeneous transfers are clearly inferior to facial-to-facial grafting. Thus these procedure are largely reserved for situations in which the facial nerve lesion exists proximal to the extracranial course of the nerve, as in Bell's palsy. Even so, transfacial nerve grafting from selected peripheral branches of the contralateral facial nerve is superceding nonfacial transfers in unilateral disease.[3] Here an added benefit results from division of the donor nerves and, hence, less exaggerated facial posture on the unaffected side. In any case, such nerve transfers are effective only until irreversible denervation atrophy occurs in the muscle units of the injured side.

In the presence of such atrophy, free muscle grafting[64] has lately been described, with free innervation of the transplanted units occuring presumably from local intervated muscles in the vicinity, including the muscles of mastication on the affected side and the facial musculature of the normal side. Although there can be no doubt about clinical successes following such free muscle grafting, the consistency and magnitude of such success appears limited and unpredictable to the point that clinical application is questionable. The more recent transfer of muscle as revascularized free grafts utilizing microvascular anastomosis,[34] on the other hand, offers real promise. Reinnervation is by way of transfacial nerve grafts implanted during a preliminary first stage. This arrangement, although technically demanding and far from clinically established, offers perhaps the greatest promise for late reanimation of the paralyzed face.

The remaining reconstructive considerations following parotid gland surgery are, for the most part, straightforward. Following most surgery for benign and low grade malignancy, repair is simply by return and suture of the overlying facial flap. The most common resulting deficit relates to the sunken contour behind the angle of the mandible—a moderate depression after lateral lobectomy that becomes more significant following total gland removal. Although dermal fat grafts are an obvious solution to these contour problems, they have proved less effective and lasting than the transfer of local dermal fat flaps denuded of covering epithelium.[52] This relatively simple adjunctive measure may be performed primarily or secondarily, but carries with it the disadvantage of additional scarring in the neck. An alternative that we have used is the transfer of muscle flaps to fill this depression (Fig. 10.4). At the completion of a total parotidectomy the tendon of origin of the sternocleidomastoid muscle is detached over its anterior two-thirds from the mastoid process, this under full view of the exposed nerve trunk. The tendon is then opened up or unfurled and the muscle brought across the retromandibular depression to be sutured to the masseter muscle between the branches of the nerve. This maneuver is similar to the transfer of the expanded sartorius muscle from the anterior superior iliac spine to the inguinal ligament as protection for the exposed neurovascular bundle following groin dissection. Portions of the temporalis muscle, with or without attached outertable bone[44] (Fig. 10.5*F*), can also be brought down beneath the zygomatic arch to fill out surrounding areas of soft tissue deficit.

A remaining problem following surgical treatment of the parotid gland is gustatory sweating which occurs in roughly 25% of patients some 6 months following parotidectomy. First described by Fry and known variously as Fry's syndrome and auriculotemporal syndrome, this complication is characterized by flushing and sweating of the parotid region of the face following eating. Although the phenomenon has prompted a number of complex theories, the most likely explanation is a simple one. The auriculotemporal sensory nerve carries the postganglionic parasympathetic fibers from the otic ganglion of the glossopharyngeal nerve to the excretory apparatus of the parotid. Following the routine division of this nerve during

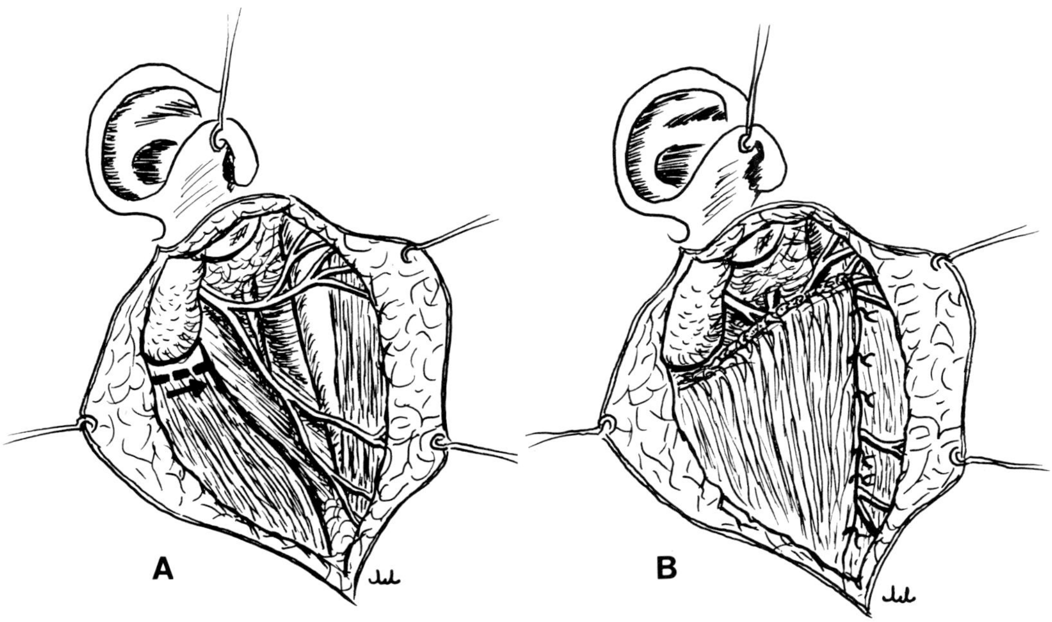

Figure 10.4 Sternocleidomastoid expansion. (*A*) Retromandibular defect following total parotidectomy with preservation of the facial nerve. *Dotted line* shows line of division of sternocleidomastoid muscle. (*B*) Muscle brought across depression and sutured to masseter between nerve branches.

parotidectomy, regenerating fibers are felt to realign themselves in part with divided sympathetic fibers destined for the sweat glands of the overlying skin. The visceral efferent impulse from a gustatory stimulus then activates not only the proper target cells of the parotid excretory mechanism but also the inappropriate and mistargeted sweat glands of the overlying skin.[35] Most cases are mild and all that is required is an explanation to the patient. Some, however, are quite distressing and account for significant morbidity. Surgical therapies have included tympanic neurectomy dividing Jacobson's branch of the glossopharyngeal nerve in the middle ear,[65] but such interruption has frequently proven ineffective. Efforts to interpose multiple autogenous tissues, such as dermis or fat, between the surgical bed and the overlying skin have also failed. Medical treatment in the form of systemic anticholingerics has been effective, but at the price of considerable systemic side effects. One of the best medical treatments has been topical scopolamine cream applied directly to the involved area. Most recently, interposition of fascia lata grafts has been described as highly effective and this may supplant previous surgical corrections.[66]

In the case of advanced malignancies, of course, the scope of the operation must expand to include the extent of the disease and the resulting defects may be considerable. Here, all of the principles of major head and neck reconstruction apply. When the loss has been limited to a moderate deficit in the covering tissues of the cheek, the most expeditous replacement is by local flaps from the neck and retroauricular areas (see Chapter 3). When larger defects are present or previous radiation prevents the use of local tissues, more distant sites, such as the deltopectoral area and beyond, may be used. Portions of maxilla and mandible as well as oral lining may require replacement as with intraoral malignancies (see Chapter 8). In complex circumstances reconstruction may prompt the transfer of distant tissues to the area by microvascular anastomoses (see Fig. 10.5 and Chapter 16).

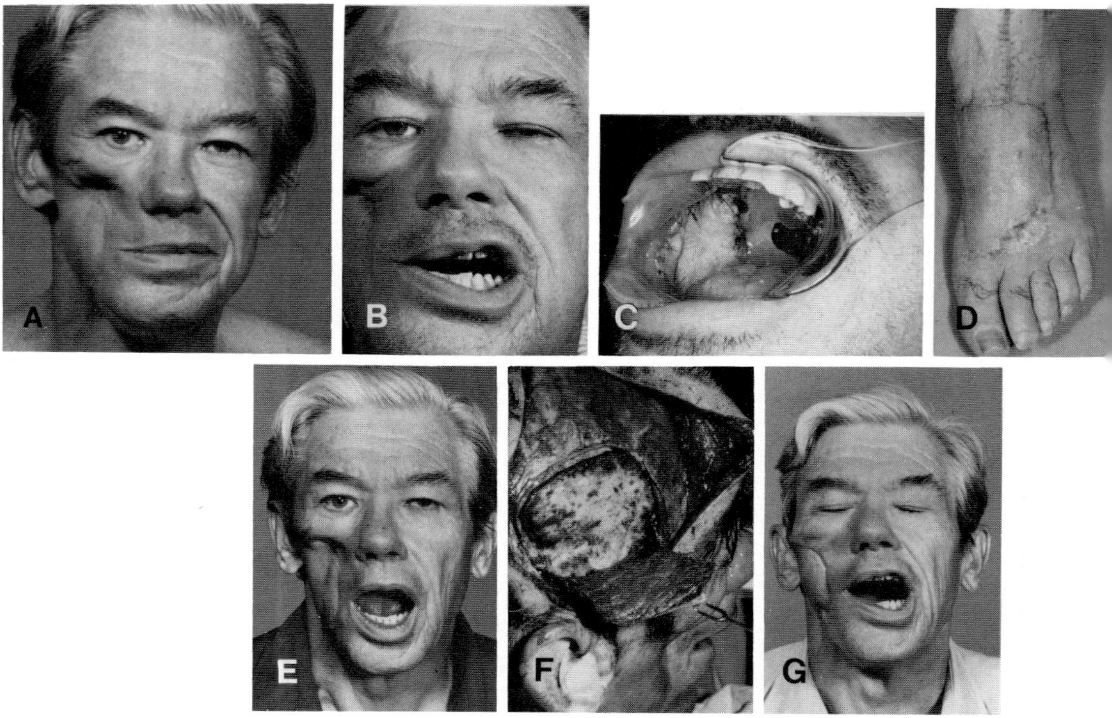

Figure 10.5 (*A*) Patient 3 months after radical excision by a different service for recurrent parotid adenoid cystic carcinoma followed by radiotherapy. Full thickness defect repaired by skin-graft-lined deltopectoral flap, with (predictable) subsequent loss of lining during radiation. (*B*) Maximal opening demonstrates cicatricial ankylosis now causing weight loss, further deterioration in speech (partial seventh nerve loss) and inadequate oral hygiene. (*C*) Scar lining replaced with dorsalis pedis flap from foot. Long vascular pedicle allows microvascular anastamoses to transverse cervical artery and external jugular vein—well outside radiation field. (*D*) Grafted donor site. (*E*) Result at 6 months shows excellent opening, but maxillectomy defect evident. (*F*) Second-stage turn-down of partial temporalis muscle flap with attached outer-table bone, brought beneath zygomatic arch to fill out contour defect from maxillectomy. (*G*) Result at 2 years shows good opening, improved contour, and no evidence of malignancy.

The reconstructive considerations after submandibular gland surgery are similarly those of general reconstruction of the head and neck area. Tumor extirpation may require mandibulectomy with or without inclusion of the sublingual gland and portions of the floor of the mouth. Intensional sacrifice of a portion of the hypoglossal nerve may be replaced with interpositional nerve graft. The functional deficit from interruption of the lingual nerve, however, is not so great as imagined and is considerably less than with loss of the glossopharyngeal branches to the posterior tongue. In any case, nerve graft has proved disappointing for lingual deficits and probably is not warranted.

Reconstruction following extirpation of minor gland tumors is again essentially that following all intraoral malignancy, particularly when these lesions affect the tongue, lips, floor of mouth and buccal surfaces. The palate, aside from being the most common site of malignant involvement, is a site of particular challenge in reconstruction. Here the goal must be full restoration of hard and soft palatal integrity such that velopharyngeal closure is possible for the normal functioning of speech and deglutation. Such competence can be rendered by skillful prosthodontics, but this solution is, in general, inferior to reconstruction by autogenous tissues. Here three favored sources of local tissues are available, including the posterior pharyngeal mucosa, the buccal mucosa, and the mucoperiosteum of the hard palate (Fig. 10.6). The pharyngeal mucosa is most often brought into place as a superiorly based posterior pharyngeal flap, usually supplying nasal lining to the palate. The buccal tissue is added as a

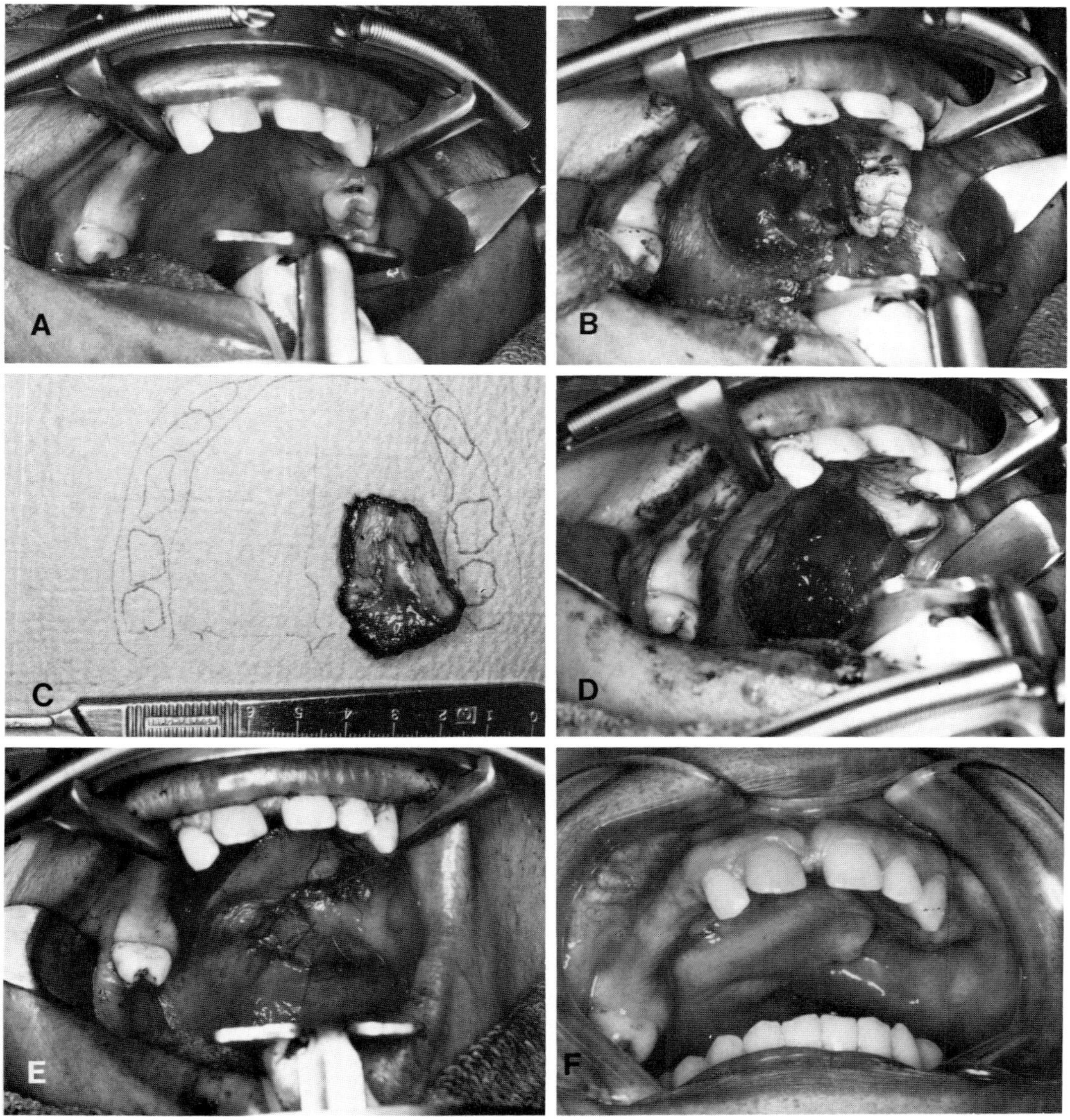

Figure 10.6 (*A*) Subtle mass over greater palatine foramen diagnosed is adenoid cystic carcinoma by dental biopsy. (*B*) Wide, local excision includes portions of maxilla, palatine bone, and pterygoid plates as well as greater palatine nerve. (*C*) Initial specimen. Frozen sections reveal tumor, nests at proximal cut end of nerve. (*D*) Excision extended to include maxillary alveolus and tuberosity, antral floor, and pterygoid plates to base of skull. Repeat frozen section examination negative for tumor. (*E*) Reconstruction by remaining palatal mucoperiosteum rotated on contralateral greater palatine vessels and large buccal mucosal transposition flap. Adjuvant radiotherapy followed. (*F*) Result at 1 year with excellent speech, no antral fistula, no evidence of malignancy.

simple transposition. The most effective way to utilize the hard palatal mucoperiosteum is with palatal island flaps based on the greater palatine vessels.[45] Thus an entire velum can be reconstructed using a single superiorly based posterior pharyngeal flap and double island flaps of hard palatal mucosa. An additional source of local tissue remains the tongue, but usually its use requires two stages.[32]

A final reconstructive consideration remains the surgical management of uncontrolled drooling from such diverse causes as cerebral palsy in children and postsurgical deformity following head and neck cancer ablation in adults. Parotid salivary flow is diverted by ductal lengthening and transposition into the tonsillar fossa by way of buried, untubed flaps of buccal mucosa. When combined with submandibular gland excision, such diversion has been worthwhile.[67] Recently, the more complicated transposition procedure has been replaced by simple duct ligation, which appears equally effective.[30]

References

1. Abrams, A. M., Melrose, R., and Howell, F.: Necrotizing sialometaplasia. *Cancer, 32:*130, 1973.
2. Adams, W.: The use of masseter, temporalis and frontalis muscles in the correction of facial paralysis. *Plast. Reconstr. Surg., 1:*216, 1947.
3. Anderl, H.: Reconstruction of the face through cross-face nerve transplantation in facial paralysis. *Chir. Plast. (Berl.), 2:*17, 1973.
4. Anderson, L., Cummings, N., et al.: Salivary gland immunoglobulin and rheumatoid factor synthesis in Sjogren's syndrome. *Am. J. Med., 53:*456, 1972.
5. Arion, H. G.: Dynamic closure of the lids in paralysis of the orbicularis muscle. *Intern. Surg., 57:*48, 1972.
6. Batsakis, J. G.: Neoplasms of the minor and lesser major salivary glands. *Surg. Gynecol. Obstet., 135:*289–298, 1972.
7. Batsakis, J. G.: *Tumors of the Head and Neck, Clinical and Pathological Considerations*, Williams & Wilkins, Baltimore, 1974.
8. Blanch, C., Eneroth, C. M., and Jakobson, P. A.: Mucus-producing adenopapillary (nonepidermoid) carcinoma of the parotid gland. *Cancer, 28:*676, 1971.
9. Bloch, K. J., Buchanan, W., Wohl, M., and Buhnn, J.: Sjogren's syndrome. *Medicine, 44:*187, 1965.
10. Boles, R: Management and rehabilitation of the facial nerve in parotid surgery. *Otolaryngol. Clin. North Am., 10:*443, 1977.
11. Buchthal, F.: Electromyography in paralysis of the facial nerve. *Arch. Otolaryngol., 81:*463, 1965.
12. Byars, L. T.: Preservation of the facial nerve in operations for benign conditions of the parotid area. *Ann. Surg., 136:*412, 1952.
13. Catterall, M.: The treatment of patients with fast neutrons from the Medical Research Council's cyclotron at Hammersmith Hospital, London, in *Particle Accelerators in Radiation Therapy, Conference Proceedings*, pp. 135–139. U.S. Atomic Energy Commission, March 1973.
14. Colman, C. C., and Walker, J. C.: Technique of anastomosis of the branches of the facial nerve with the spinal accessory for facial paralysis. *Ann. Surg., 131:*960, 1950.
15. Conley, J. J.: Facial nerve grafting. *Arch. Otolaryngol., 73:*322, 1961.
16. Conley, J., and Dingman, D. L.: Adenoid cystic carcinoma in the head and neck (cylindroma). *Arch. Otolaryngol., 100:*81, 1974.
17. Converse, J. M.: Early treatment of facial injuries, in *Kazanjian and Converse's Surgical Treatment of Facial Injuries, Vol. 1*, Ed. 3, Williams & Wilkins, Baltimore, 1974.
18. Eneroth, C. M.: Histological and clinical aspects of parotid tumours. *Acta Otolaryngol. (Suppl.), 191:*1, 1964.
19. Eneroth, C. M.: Salivary gland tumors in the parotid gland, submandibular gland, and the palate region. *Cancer, 27:*1415, 1971.
20. Eneroth, C. M., Hamberger, C. A., and Jakobson, P. A.: Malignancy of acinic cell carcinoma. *Ann. Otol. Rhinol. Laryngol., 75:*780, 1966.
21. Eneroth, C. M., and Hjertman, L.: Benign tumors of the submandibular gland. *Pract. Otorhinolaryngol., 29:* 166, 1967.
22. Eneroth, C. M., Hjertman, L., and Moberger, G.: Mucoepidermoid carcinoma of the palate. *Acta Otolaryngol., 70:*408, 1970.
23. Evans, R. W., and Cruickshank, A. H.: *Epithelial Tumors of the Salivary Glands.* W. B. Saunders, Philadelphia, 1970.
24. Foote, F. W., Jr., and Frazell, E. L.: Tumors of the major salivary glands. *Cancer, 6:*1065, 1953.
25. Frable, W. J., and Elzay, R. P.: Tumors of minor salivary glands: a report of 73 cases. *Cancer, 25:*932, 1970.
26. Freeman, B. S.: Facial palsy, in *Reconstructive Plastic Surgery*, edited by J. M. Converse, W. B. Saunders, Philadelphia, 1964.
27. Gaughran, G. R. L.: The parotid compartment. *Ann. Otol., 70:*31, 1961.
28. Gerughty, R. M., Scofield, H. H., Brown, F. M., and Hemmigar, G. R.: Malignant mixed tumors and salivary gland origin. *Cancer, 24:*471, 1969.
29. Gillies, H. D.: Experience with fascia lata grafts in the operative treatment of facial paralysis. *Proc. Roy. Soc. Med., 27:*98, 1934.
30. Glass, L. W., Nobel, G. L., and Vecchione, T. R.: Treatment of uncontrolled drooling by bilateral ex-

cision of submandibular glands and parotid duct ligations. *Plast. Reconstr. Surg.*, *62*:523, 1978.
31. Grove, A. S. and DiChiro, G.: Salivary gland scanning with technetium-99m pertechnetate. *A.J.R.*, *102*:109, 1968.
32. Guerro-Santos, J.: Tongue flaps, in *Skin Flaps*, edited by W. C. Grabb and M. B. Myers, Little Brown, Boston, 1975.
33. Guillamondegui, O., Byers, R. M., and Tapley, N.: Malignant tumors of salivary glands, in *Textbook of Radiotherapy*, edited by G. H. Fletch, Lea & Febiger, Philadelphia, 1973.
34. Harii, K., Ohmori, K., and Torii, S.: Free gracilis muscle transplantation, with microneurovascular anastomoses for the treatment of facial paralysis. *Plast. Reconstr. Surg.*, *57*:133, 1976.
35. Hemenway, W. G.: Gustatory sweating and flushing. *Laryngoscope*, *70*:84, 1960.
36. Hollinshead, W. H.: *Anatomy for Surgeons*; *Vol. I*: *The Head and Neck*, Ed. 2, Harper & Row, New York, 1968.
37. Jobe, R. P.: A technique for lid loading in the management of the lagopthalmus of facial palsy. *Plast. Reconstr. Surg.*, *53*:29, 1974.
38. Kessler, L. A., Moldaver, J., and Pool, J. L.: Hypoglossal facial anastomosis for treatment of facial paralysis. *Neurology*, *9*:118, 1959.
39. Kripparhne, W., Hunt, T., and Dunphy, J.: Acute suppurative parotits. *Ann. Surg.*, *156*:251, 1962.
40. Lary, B.: Postoperative suppurative parotits. *Arch. Surg.*, *89*:653, 1964.
41. Leafstedt, S. W., Gaeta, J. F., Sako, K., Marchetta, F. C., and Shedd, D. P.: Adenoid cystic carcinoma of major and minor salivary glands. *Am. J. Surg.*, *122*: 756, 1971.
42. Mandel, L.: The labial accessory salivary glands in the diagnosis of systemic disease. Third Trans. International Conference on Oral Surgery, New York, September 1968.
43. Masters, F. W., Robinson, D. W., and Simons, J. N.: Temporalis transfer for lagophthalmos due to seventh nerve palsy. *Am. J. Surg.*, *110*:607, 1965.
44. Millard, D. R.: Personal communication, 1975.
45. Millard, D. R., and Seider, H. A.: The versatile palatal island flap: its use in soft palate reconstruction and nasopharyngeal and choanal atresia. *Br. J. Plast. Surg.*, *30*:300, 1977.
46. Morel, A. S., and Firestein, A.: Repair of traumatic fistulas of the parotid duct. *Arch. Surg.*, *87*:623–626, 1963.
47. Musgrave, R. H.: Special problems of soft tissue repair of the eyelids, nose, lips, parotid gland, facial nerve, and ears, in *Plastic and Maxillofacial Trauma Symposium*, edited by N. G. Georgiade, *Vol. 1*, pp. 161–172, C. V. Mosby, St. Louis, 1969.
48. Niklison, J.: Facial paralysis: moderation of non-paralyzed muscles. *Br. J. Plast. Surg.*, *18*:379, 1965.
49. Paff, G. H.: *Anatomy of the Head and Neck*, W. B. Saunders, Philadelphia, 1973.
50. Rankow, R. M.: Surgical decisions in the treatment of major salivary gland tumors. *Plast. Reconstr. Surg.*, *51*:514, 1973.
51. Rankow, R. M., and Mignogna, F.: Cancer of the sublingual salivary gland. *Am. J. Surg.*, *118*:790, 1969.
52. Rankow, R. M., and Polayes, I. M.: *Disease of the Salivary Glands*, W. B. Saunders, Philadelphia, 1976.
53. Robinson, D. W., and Masters, F. W.: Surgical treatment of diseases of the salivary glands, in *Reconstructive Plastic Surgery*, edited by J. M. Converse, Ed. 2, Vol. 5, W. B. Saunders, Philadelphia, 1977.
54. Robinson, D. W., Master, F. W., and Forest, H. J.: Clinical experience with supravital staining in surgery of the parotid gland. *Surg. Gynecol. Obstet.*, *110*: 121, 1960.
55. Rubin, L. R.: *Reanimation of the Paralyzed Face; New Approaches*, C. V. Mosby, St. Louis, 1977.
56. Smith, L. C., Lane, N., and Rankow, R. M.: Cylindroma (adenoid cystic carcinoma): a report of fifty-eight cases. *Am. J. Surg.*, *110*:519, 1965.
57. Southwick, H. W.: Salivary glands, in *Operative Surgery*, edited by P. F. Nova, Lea & Febiger, Philadelphia, 1972.
58. Spira, M.: Anastamosis of masseteric nerve to lower division of facial nerve for correction of lower facial paralysis. *Plast. Reconstr. Surg.*, *61*:330, 1978.
59. State, D.: Superficial lobectomy and total parotidectomy with preservation of the facial nerve in the treatment of parotid tumors. *Surg. Gynecol. Obstet.*, *89*: 237, 1949.
60. Talal, N., and Bumin, J.: The development of malignant lymphoma in the course of Sjogren's syndrome. *Am. J. Med.*, *36*:529, 1964.
61. Thackray, A. C., and Lucas, R. B.: Tumors of the major salivary glands, in *Atlas of Tumor Pathology, Second series, Fascicle 10*, Armed Forces Institute of Pathology, Washington, D.C., 1974.
62. Thackray, A. C., and Sobin, L. H.: International Histological Classification of Tumours, No. 7; "Histological Typing of Salivary Gland Tumours," World Health Organization, Geneva, 1972.
63. Thompson, A. S., and Bryant, H. C., Jr.: Histogenesis of papillary cystadenoma lymphomatosum (Warthin's tumor) of the parotid salivary gland. *Am. J. Pathol.*, *26*:807, 1950.
64. Thompson, M.: Treatment of facial paralysis by free skeletal muscle grafts, in *Fifth International Congress on Plastic and Reconstructive Surgeons*: *Transactions*, *Melbourne, Australia*, p. 66, Butterworth, London, 1971.
65. Wallenborn, W.: Parotid gland atrophy produced by transtympanic destruction of tympanic plexus. *Laryngoscope*, *78*:132, 1968.
66. Wallis, K. A., and Gibson, T.: Gustatory sweating following parotidectomy: correction by a fascia lata graft. *Br. J. Plast. Surg.*, *31*:68, 1978.
67. Wilke, T. E.: The surgical treatment of drooling. *Plast. Reconstr. Surg.*, *45*:549, 1970.
68. Wolfe, J. J.: Congenital hemangioma of the parotid gland. *Plast. Reconstr. Surg.*, *29*:692, 1962.

CHAPTER 11

Surgery of the Paranasal Sinuses

Thomas C. Calcaterra, M.D., F.A.C.S.

Although surgery of the paranasal sinuses is usually performed to treat chronic sinusitis, the emphasis of this chapter will be on reconstructive surgery related to the paranasal sinuses and methods or orofacial rehabilitation following extensive extirpative surgery for cancer. The paranasal sinuses comprise a series of pneumatic cavities occupying approximately one-quarter of the skull volume, and thus they are closely associated with various important anatomic structures such as the orbit, anterior cranial fossa, nose and oral cavity. Reconstructive surgery of the sinuses, therefore, must necessarily consider the structural and functional needs of these other adjacent structures.

The sinuses begin their pneumatic expansion from the nasal cavity in fetal life and this continues until early adulthood; the frontal sinus is the last to develop completely. The degree of pneumatization of the sinuses varies considerably among individuals and for this reason each patient is unique with respect to the type of injuries sustained and the method of surgical repair required.

The paranasal sinuses perform several functions. Each is lined by a respiratory epithelium over an inner layer of thin periosteum, and the respiratory cells largely consist of ciliary mucus cells that produce a continual blanket of mucus sweeping toward the natural ostium of each sinus. This mucus serves to moisten inspired air for respiration while lubricating the pharynx and larynx to enable swallowing and phonation. The sinus cavities lighten the weight of the skull and provide resonators for the voice.

The paranasal sinuses are susceptible to a variety of disease processes. Infection constitutes the most common disease affecting the sinuses. Trauma and neoplasm are less frequent but may cause infection of the involved sinus by blocking its natural ostia and thereby complicating therapy.

TRAUMA

Inasmuch as trauma of the face often involves the underlying paranasal sinuses, this subject will be covered in other chapters. This chapter deals with the frontal sinus and nasofrontal complex, both of which are subject to numerous complications that may stem from injuries in this area.

Acute Frontal Sinus Injuries

The air-filled frontal sinuses are capable of absorbing a blunt traumatic force, thereby protecting the contents of the cranial vault. Nevertheless, numerous sinus injuries may be incurred by such trauma. The most common injury results from the head striking the dashboard during an automobile collision, particularly when the injured person is wearing only a lap seat belt. Frontal sinus fractures represent 5–10% of all facial fractures.[1]

Clinical Findings and Diagnosis

The external manifestations of frontal sinus injuries may be deceptive. If there is no facial laceration (closed injury), the patient may simply present with generalized forehead swelling which makes palpation of the frontal bone and supraorbital rims difficult. Other findings may include anesthesia of the forehead, indicating injury of the supraorbital and/or supratrochlear nerves, and diplopia which can result from hematoma formation within the orbit or mechanical restriction of upward rotation of the globe due to infringement of the superior rectus and superior oblique muscles. The latter two findings are generally associated with fractures of the sinus floor and supraorbital rim.

Because the acute physical findings are unreliable when assessing the degree of the injury, x-rays are mandated for all patients with a suspected frontal sinus fracture. Anteroposterior (A-P), lateral and Waters' views are satisfactory to rule out significant fracture, but laminagrams are often necessary to delineate the precise extent of the fracture. Lateral laminagrams best assess the integrity of the anterior and posterior tables, and especially the status of the nasofrontal duct. The presence of intracranial air invariably indicates a dural tear with leakage of cerebrospinal fluid. A fluid level in the sinus may represent blood, retained mucus or cerebrospinal fluid, and it usually indicates damage to the nasofrontal duct.

Treatment

The treatment plan is predicted on the extent of the injury, which can be classified into three general categories: anterior table, nasofrontal duct, and posterior table fractures.[2] Combinations of these fractures obviously also occur.

Anterior Table Fractures

This is the most common type of fracture sustained, usually occurring as a linear or depressed fracture of the glabella. When there is an overlying facial laceration, the anterior table of the sinus is routinely examined after any debris or devitalized soft tissue is removed. Nondisplaced fractures require no treatment and the soft tissue laceration is closed appropriately. Antibiotics are employed whenever there is a compound fracture. If a displaced fracture is encountered, the fragment or fragments are elevated and wired back into normal position whenever possible. In addition to interosseous wiring, the periosteum may also be sutured to secure the bony fragments inasmuch as bone usually heals rapidly in this area and there are no muscular forces tending to displace the fragments. When there is no associated laceration and laminagrams show a depressed fracture, it is often better to wait 48–72 hours for partial resolution of the swelling to ensure that the patient has suffered no intracranial injury. The anterior table fracture can then be approached and elevated through a brow incision or a transverse forehead crease. A follow-up sinus x-ray should be obtained to determine whether the sinus is draining properly.

Nasofrontal Duct Fractures

These injuries can be the most difficult to assess.[3, 4] The duct is a funnel-shaped channel that passes between the cancellous bony anterior wall underlying the glabella and the anterior ethmoidal air cells. Blunt trauma to the forehead is capable of driving the anterior wall posteriorly, collapsing the nasofrontal duct. Occasionally this may cause only minimal visible deformity, manifested simply by edema of the duct orifice.

The application of endonasal vasoconstricting agents in the middle meatus is of little value in restoring patency of the injured nasofrontal duct. All patients with radiographic evidence of fracture adjacent to the nasofrontal duct should be surgically explored. If the duct orifice appears patent, the sinus may be closed although it is often advisable to leave a small plastic tube through the fracture site. The patency of the nasofrontal duct can be tested by irrigating sterile saline through the tube. When the saline passes readily to the nose, the plastic tube is removed. If the nasofrontal duct appears completely disrupted, the surgeon must decide whether to attempt reconstruction of the duct or obliterate the frontal sinus. Although many reports have been published describing successful long term obturation of the duct or repair with mucosal flaps, a large percentage of patients will eventually develop chronic frontal sinusitis and osteomyelitis of the frontal bone secondary to delayed stenosis of the nasofrontal duct. If the surgeon prefers reconstruction of the nasofrontal duct, the intersinus septum should be removed so that the opposite nasofrontal duct will serve as a reserve drainage route.

The current favored method of managing a disrupted nasofrontal duct is sinus obliteration.[4] The sinus mucosa is completely removed and the nasofrontal mucosa rolled back into the nose. The bony nasofrontal orifice is sealed with a pericranium graft and the sinus cavity packed gently with adipose tissue usually obtained from the left lower quadrant of the abdomen. This method is advantageous because it prevents late mucocele formation and provides temporary support for the bone fragments when there is comminution of the anterior table.

Posterior Table Fractures

Posterior table fractures represent the most serious type of frontal sinus injury because of the relatively frequent association with intracranial complications such as subdural or extradural hematoma, laceration of the dura and frontal lobe with spinal fluid leakage, and late epidural abscess formation (Fig. 11.1). Such fractures are often managed in cooperation with a neurosurgeon; indeed, if a significant dural laceration is anticipated, a frontal craniotomy will provide the best access for dural repair.[5] All suspected posterior table fractures warrant exploration as soon as the patient's condition permits. This injury is likely to be associated with extensive fractures of the anterior table.

A coronal scalp incision is preferred unless there is extensive forehead laceration. Any depressed posterior table fragments are elevated and usually removed. The dura is inspected and, if lacerated, it is widely exposed by removing adjacent posterior wall bone and then repaired by direct suture or with autogenous fascial or pericranial grafts. If the anterior wall is shattered beyond reasonable possibility of reapproximation, then the sinus must be ablated by removing the remnants of the anterior wall and medial orbital rims (Fig. 11.2). All mucosa

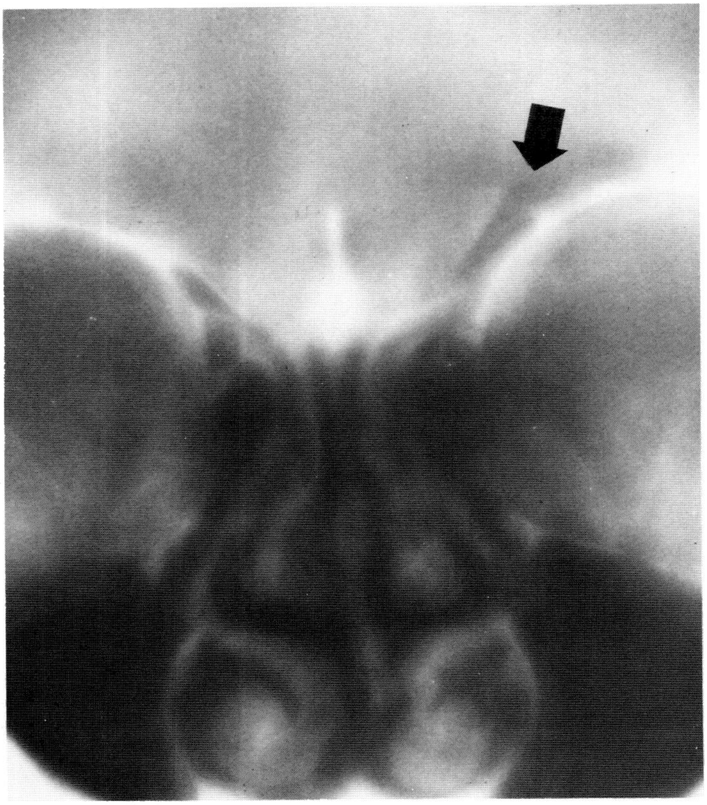

Figure 11.1 Coronal laminagram demonstrating a fracture of posterior table of the left frontal sinus.

is removed from the posterior wall and floor of the sinus, and the forehead skin and frontalis muscle are allowed to collapse into the former sinus cavity. Although this undeniably causes a considerable cosmetic deformity, particularly when unilateral, it is the safest method of management. Another but less safe alternative would be to obliterate the cavity with autogenous adipose tissue. This involves the risk that in the immediate postoperative period the devascularized fat might be subject to infection which, when adjacent to recently exposed or damaged dura, could cause meningitis, cerebritis, or brain abscess. One other possibility is that of packing this cavity with autogenous iliac cancellous bone chips. This obviates the contour defect that would result if no immediate reconstruction were done.

SECONDARY RECONSTRUCTION OF FRONTAL BONE DEFECTS

Improved acute head injury care now enables far more patients to survive extensive frontal cranial trauma. However, in many instances the frontal bone fragments are so comminuted, particularly when there is frontal lobe injury, that primary reconstruction is impossible. In such cases the patient is often left with a severe disfigurement of the forehead. A similar type of deformity also results when it is necessary to remove bone for osteomyelitis secondary to chronic frontal sinusitis. Over half of these patients will have developed frontal osteomyelitis following frontal sinus trauma which impaired the drainage of the nasofrontal duct. Although antibiotic therapy should be attempted when frontal osteomyetlitis is diagnosed, generally it

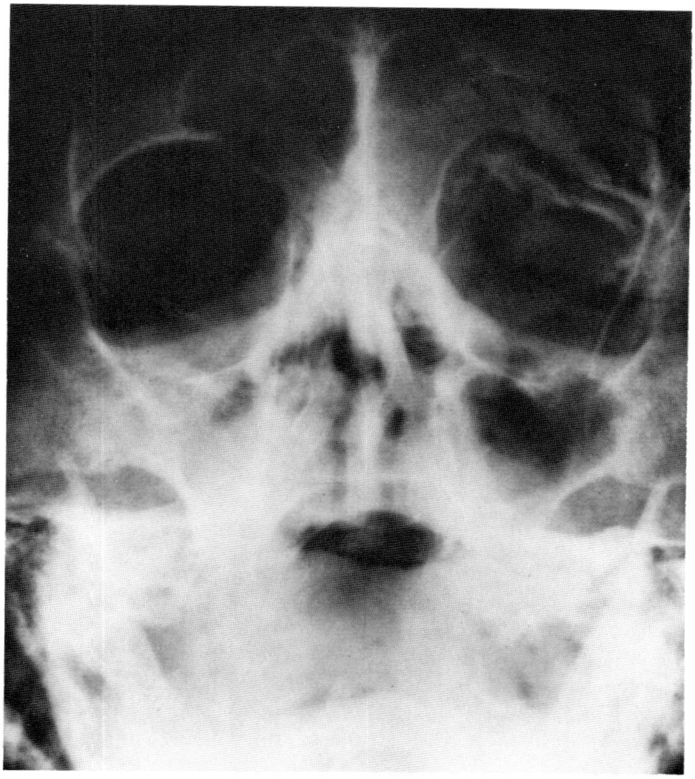

Figure 11.2 Caldwell view of sinuses showing a severely fragmented fracture of the left frontal sinus with displacement of bone fragments into the orbit.

is necessary to surgically excise all of the diseased bone and ablate the sinus. Correction of the forehead deformity should be delayed until complete healing and resolution of any inflammatory reaction in the bone have occurred, often as long as 6 months.

Several methods of secondary frontoplasty (cranioplasty) have been reported and the subject has recently been reviewed.[6, 7] The primary indications for reconstruction are to correct an unsightly defect and provide mechanical protection for cranial contents not covered by bone. The ideal implant material should be easy to contour, durable, and resistant to rejection or infection.

Various types of metals were used for the earliest implants, including gold, silver, lead, aluminum, stainless steel, tantalum and Vitallium. However, metals are disadvantageous because they are difficult to mold, thermally conductive (which can lead to headache), and subject to pressure or dislodgment (which can lead to skin erosion and perforation).

Bone Graft Frontoplasty

Various types of autogenous tissue have also been employed to restore contour of the forehead, chiefly split rib grafts[8] (see Chapter 2, Fig. 2.17) and iliac crest bone chips.[7] Both of these methods expose the cancellous trabeculae, thereby improving the survival of the osteocytes. This technique is particularly helpful when dealing with young patients, in whom the skull is still growing, because there is evidence of dynamic growth of the bone grafts and fusion with the skull.[6] In adults, however, free bone grafts tend to undergo some resorption, giving the forehead an irregular or "cobblestone" appearance. The acquisition of bone requires a secondary operative procedure and the hospitalization period may be prolonged because of the discomfort at the donor site, particularly the iliac crest.

Methyl Methacrylate Frontoplasy

Use of alloplastic implants constructed of acrylic has become prominent during the past decade. Methyl methacrylate is an acrylic resin known by the trade name of Cranioplast, probably the most widely used material for frontal bone reconstruction owing to its availability, radiolucency, inertness, and precise sculpturing quality.[9] The polymer is prepared by adding a liquid catalyst to the resin powder and this liquid mixture is poured into the defect and allowed to harden. During this hardening process, considerable heat is released by the chemical reaction, and therefore continuous cool saline irrigation is recommended. When the acrylic is firm, a mastoid burr is employed to obtain the desired contour. Because methyl methacrylate is somewhat brittle and subject to fracture, an aluminum or stainless steel wire mesh has been advocated to prevent fragmentation and reduce the danger of brain damage.[10]

Silicone Elastomer Frontoplasty

The author prefers silicone elastomer sponge for use in restoring the contour to the forehead.[11] Whenever possible, a coronal scalp incision is employed to avoid proximity of the implant to the skin incision and ensure an ample blood supply of the skin over the implant. The anterior scalp flap is elevated to the level of the remaining supraorbital rim, completely exposing the frontal defect.

The silicone sponge is not used in a preformed block; rather, the vulcanizing process is carried out just prior to implantation. A catalyst (stannous octoate) is added to the liquid silicone polymer and the solidifying mixture is poured immediately into the frontal bone defect. A firm sponge forms in about 5 minutes, precisely fitting the irregularities of the frontal bone defect. The outer surface of the newly formed sponge is trimmed with a wide knife blade or with scissors to restore the previous forehead contour. The implant is secured by anchoring sutures to the adjacent periosteum, although there is little tendency to shift since the implant exactly fits the recesses of the defect.

There are several advantages afforded by silicone sponge. The implant has a consistency similar to soft tissue, and will retain it for a long time (Fig. 11.3, *A* and *B*). Histologic studies made after silicone sponge implantation reveal minimal, if any, tissue reaction. Moreover, connective tissue grows into the open cells of the implanted sponge, promoting its stability. The one major disadvantage of any alloplastic material (including silicone) is the possibility of tissue necrosis or infection in the region of the implant which invariably leads to its extrusion. This complication has not occurred in the author's use of silicone elastomer in eight patients who have been followed for periods as long as 9 years.

EXTRACRANIAL REPAIR OF CEREBROSPINAL RHINORRHEA

Skull trauma with dural tearing is unequivocally the most common cause of cerebrospinal rhinorrhea.[12] Usually the fracture involves some portion of the anterior cranial fossa floor. The leaks occur through the cribriform plate or ethmoid sinus roof into the nose, inasmuch as this is the most delicate bone in the area, and the dura is highly adherent. As mentioned earlier, another common anterior fossa fracture site is the posterior wall of the frontal sinus through

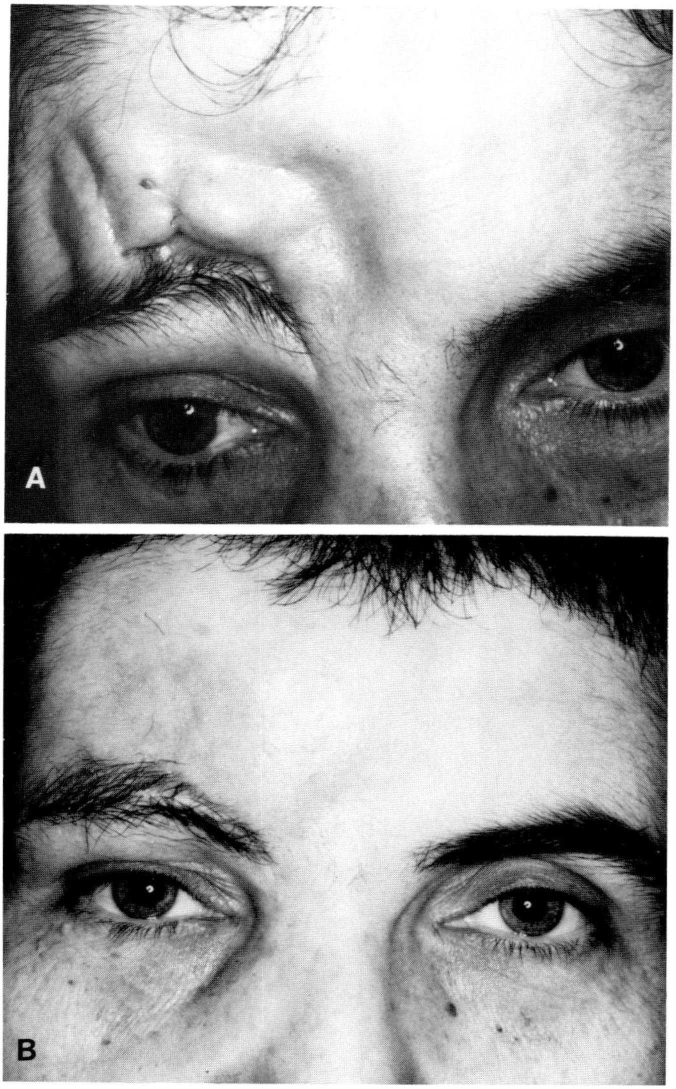

Figure 11.3 (*A*) Retraction of frontal skin over previously placed free cortical bone grafts which have partially absorbed. (*B*) Postoperative appearance following removal of the cortical bone grafts and reconstruction of the forehead defect with silicone elastomer sponge.

which cerebrospinal fluid can escape into the nose via the nasofrontal duct. Less common are middle cranial fossa fractures that can cause leakage to the nose via the sphenoid sinus or eustachian tube. For reasons that are not well understood, cerebrospinal rhinorrhea may develop as late as several months after skull fracture. It is probable that the fractured area allows herniation of dura which, with continued pulsations of the brain, cause separation of the dural fibers and eventual leak.

Diagnosis

Diagnosing the presence of cerebospinal rhinorrhea is not likely to be difficult, particularly when there are antecedent factors such as head trauma. Shortly after the injury, the fluid may be sanguineous but later a clear watery discharge persists, almost always from one nostril. It is increased by having the patient assume a prone position with the head hanging or by compression of the jugular veins. The patient may complain of a salty taste when lying supine.

Confirming that the rhinorrhea is in fact spinal fluid is best accomplished by chemical determination of the glucose content of a fluid sample. Any concentration of glucose exceeding 30 mg/100 ml is considered diagnostic. However, glucose determination by glucose oxidase test papers is unreliable because of the reducing substances present in the lacrimal gland secretions and nasal mucus.

Precise localization of the leak is a more challenging task. There may be factors in the patient's history that may be helpful in identifying the site of the leak. A gush of fluid that occurs when the head changes position suggests a collection of fluid in one of the sinuses, particularly the sphenoid. A deficient sense of smell indicates injury near the olfactory area. Numbness in the forehead suggests fracture of the frontal bone adjacent to the supraorbital or supratrochlear nerves.

Tomography of the anterior skull base and paranasal sinuses is often extremely helpful because it enables visualization of a fracutre site or bone dehiscence (Figs. 11.4 and 11.5). An air-fluid level may be seen in one of the sinuses.

Intrathecal Dye Localization Test

Injection of various types of marking substances into the intrathecal space have been utilized to localize the dural defect. Although radioisotopes are helpful in determining whether a leak

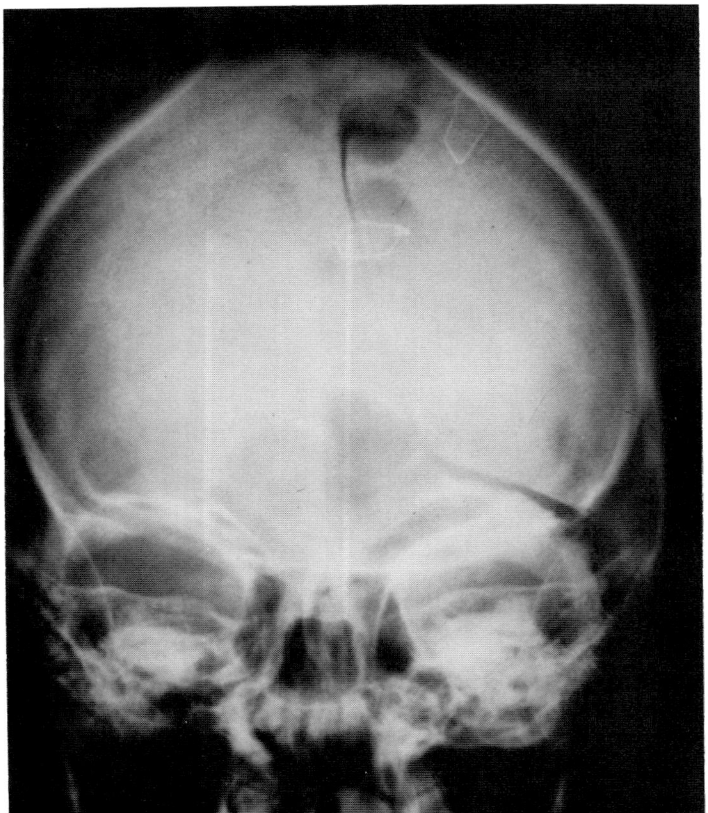

Figure 11.4 Skull view showing a craniotomy bone cut which inadvertently entered the left frontal sinus, causing persistent postoperative cerebrospinal fluid rhinorrhea.

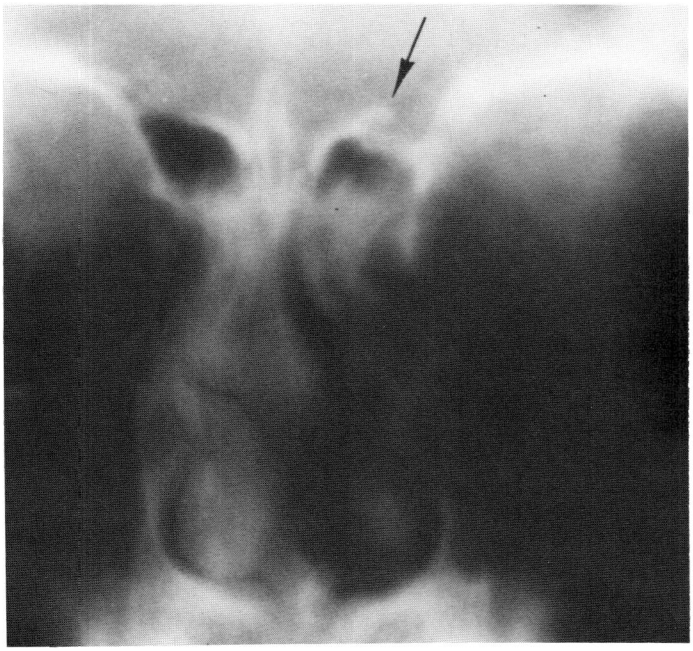

Figure 11.5 Coronal tomogram through the ethmoid sinuses revealing a displaced fracture fragment of the left ethmoid roof into the anterior cranial fossa.

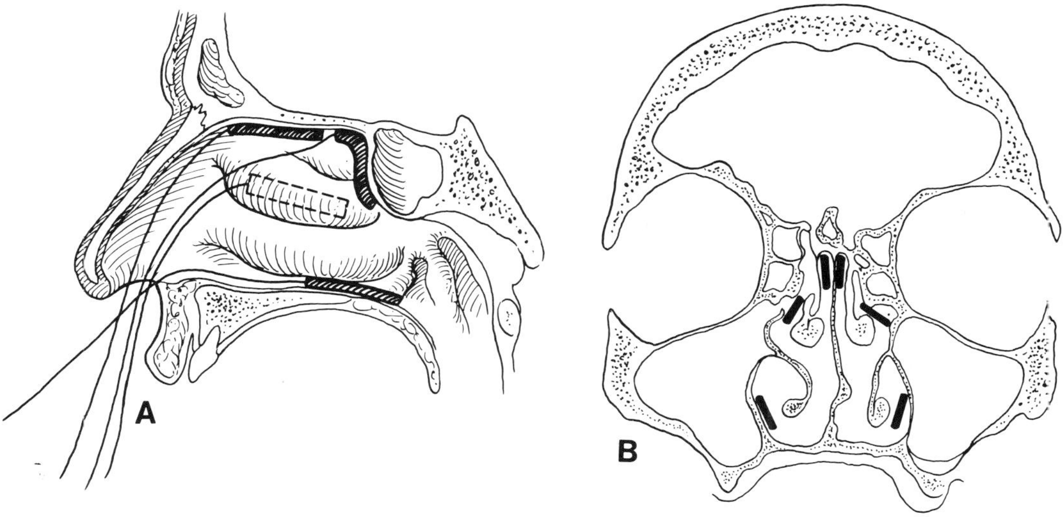

Figure 11.6 Lateral (*A*) and frontal (*B*) topographical locations of cottonoid pledgets.

is present, they usually cannot reveal the fine detail required to localize the site of the leak. In the author's experience, vital dyes such as fluorescein or indigo carmine used in conjunction with cottonoid pledgets placed strategically in the nose have provided the best information (Fig. 11.6, *A* and *B*). At least 10 ml of spinal fluid is withdrawn from a lumbar puncture and mixed with a small amount of dye (0.5 ml 5% fluorescein), and then slowly injected into the intrathecal space. After the patient has been recumbent for about 30 min, his nose is examined and the cottonoid pledgets are removed. The area of cottonoid staining identifies the site of the leak. If the pledget removed from the middle meatus is stained, the leak is located in the frontal sinus. If the cottonoid retrieved from the anterior fossa is stained, a leak exists at the cribriform plate or anterior ethmoid roof. When the pledgets placed in the posterior nasal roof and sphenoethmoid recess are discolored, either the posterior ethmoid region or sphenoid sinus is involved. It is important to recognize whether cerebrospinal fluid is emanating from the eustachian tube orifice and this can be detected by staining of a cottonoid pledget placed below the posterior end of the inferior turbinate, by staining of the posterior pharyngeal wall, or by the appearance of dye behind the tympanic membrane.

General Treatment Considerations

Acute leaks from head trauma or various types of cranial surgical procedures are managed conservatively whenever possible. This treatment generally consists of a 2-week trial of bedrest in a semisitting position, daily lumbar taps, and the administration of prophylactic antibiotics (although the latter measure remains controversial).

On the other hand, a trial of conservative management is generally not advisable if the injury is severe enough to warrant surgical intervention for other reasons, or whenever meningitis occurs. In these instances the surgical repair of the dura is accomplished as soon as the patient's general condition permits or when the meningitis is cleared with antibiotics. Because delayed leaks developing subsequent to head trauma or nontraumatizing leaks rarely heal spontaneously, surgical repair is usually carried out without awaiting preliminary observation.

Since 1926 when Dandy[13] documented the first successful intracranial repair of a cerebrospinal fluid leak, management of this condition has almost exclusively been by craniotomy. With the advent of the operating microscope and more refined methods of localizing the dural defect, extracranial methods of dural repair have come to the forefront because of their inherent lower morbidity.

Operative Treatment

In order to pinpoint the dural defect intraoperatively, intrathecal dye is injected during the operation just after the induction of general anesthesia. An indwelling spinal catheter is placed in the lumbar subarachnoid space, and about 30 min before the anticipated exposure of the dural leakage site, spinal fluid mixed with dye is slowly injected. A discrete flow of spinal fluid can be seen trickling from the dural defect. The spinal catheter can also be used to maintain a low spinal fluid pressure by intermittent drainage 3–5 days after operation, thereby ensuring better healing of the dural repair.

Frontal sinus leaks are generally approached by an osteoplastic frontal bone flap through a coronal or eyebrow incision.[14] This operation enables visualization of the posterior wall of the frontal sinus where the dural defect will usually be found. The area of the dural tear is exposed by removing adjacent bone with a drill burr or forceps, and the dura is closed by direct suture approximation or by mattress suture of a connective tissue graft such as frontalis fascia. To further ensure the seal, the frontal sinus may be packed with fat after all mucous membrane has been removed.

Leaks in the region of the cribriform plate and ethmoid roof are exposed through a curved naso-orbital incision. Access to this area requires a complete ethmoidectomy during which the dural defects are sealed with mucoperiosteal flaps rotated either from the lateral nasal wall or the nasal septum. On occasion a fascia graft obtained from the thigh may be glued to the undersurface of the dura with tissue adhesives. Further stabilization of the flaps or grafts are obtained with absorbable packing such as oxidized cellulose.

Leaks in the region of the sphenoid sinus may be approached between the nasal septal membranes or through the ethmoid sinuses.[15] The transeptal approach has the advantage of avoiding a facial incision and allowing sphenoid sinus packing without an open communication with the nasal cavity. In either case the intersinus septum is removed and the sphenoid sinus denuded of its mucosa under visualization with the operating microscope. The sinus is then packed with thigh muscle fragments buttressed by septal bone.

TUMORS OF THE PARANASAL SINUSES: CLASSIFICATION AND PATHOLOGY

Tumors of the paranasal sinuses constitute about 5% of all tumors arising from the respiratory tract. The peak incidence occurs in the 6th and 7th decades, with a slight male predominance, as in cases of head and neck cancer, but the association with tobacco smoking is not as strong as with carcinomas in other parts of the respiratory tract.

No widely accepted classification of sinus malignancies exists inasmuch as such tumors are rarely confined to one anatomic area when first diagnosed. Localized tumors of the maxillary sinus have been arbitrarily divided into two groups by Ohngren's line (a theoretic plane passing between the medial canthus of the eye and the angle of the mandible). Tumors occurring below the plane have a more favorable prognosis whereas those developing above this plane, called suprastructure tumors, have a less favorable outlook owing to their proximity to the orbit and cranium.

The type of tumor generally found in the paranasal sinuses is the squamous cell carcinoma, representing about 80% of the total. Squamous cancers are typically intermediate in differentiation, tending to metastasize late to the cervical lymph node network. Moreover, distant metastases are quite rare until late in the course of the disease.

Clinical Features

Among paranasal sinus tumors, those occurring in the maxillary sinus predominate and, unfortunately, they tend to grow large before becoming symptomatic. If the drainage of the sinus is impaired by the tumor, concomitant sinusitis is likely to develop. With progressive tumor growth the patient may experience cheek pain, nasal airway obstruction and blood-streaked nasal mucus. Dental symptoms such as tooth pain or looseness of the molar teeth followed by later actual displacement of the palate may occur. Fullness over the cheek, particularly accompanied by numbness over the distribution of the infraorbital nerve, strongly suggests a maxillary sinus cancer. Since the orbit is surrounded on three sides by paranasal sinuses (maxillary, ethmoid, and frontal), orbital symptoms are frequently associated with paranasal sinus cancer. The earliest symptom is simple displacement of the orbital contents away from the involved sinus. If the cancer invades the orbital contents, diplopia and ultimate blindness will develop. Posterior extension of maxillary sinus tumors is often manifested by trismus as the pterygoid muscles are invaded. Ethmoid sinus cancers are prone to invade the anterior cranial fossa, cavernous sinus and orbit. However, frontal sinus cancers are quite uncommon, typically invading the anterior cranial fossa before diagnosis. The rarest kind, primary sphenoid sinus cancers, become apparent by affecting the neurovascular structures that surround the sinus.

The radiographic signs of cancer may be difficult to differentiate from inflammation, but suspicion is raised by bony erosion, patchy bony sclerosis, a discrete soft tissue mass, and enlargement of the osseous foramina. The anatomic extent of the suspected tumor can be better detailed by tomography. Diagnosis requires histologic confirmation by biopsy. If transnasal biopsy is not feasible or productive, then it will be necessary to obtain representative tissue by direct sinusotomy of the involved sinus, employing various approaches such as the Caldwell-Luc operation, external ethmoidectomy or frontal sinusotomy.

Treatment

No uniform consensus exists regarding the optimal treatment method for these cancers; nevertheless, during the past decade a combination of radiation and surgery has been emphasized to maximize the cure rate. Some clinicians favor preoperative irradiation followed by immediate surgery.[16] Although this planned combined therapy does maximize the cure rate, it needlessly sacrifices the sinus or possibly the eye in instances where irradiation has been successful. Sometimes a modification of planned combined therapy is used, consisting of surgical removal of the alveolar ridge and hard palate beneath the involved maxillary sinus 6–8 weeks after full-dose irradiation. Multiple biopsies of the maxillary and ethmoid sinuses are then examined by frozen section. If viable tumor is encountered, a total or extended maxillectomy is immediately performed. On the other hand, if no tumor is found, the defect is obturated with a prepared prosthesis that is later incorporated as part of a denture. This palatal opening can then be used for future inspection of the sinus cavity to determine any sign of recurrence.

The type of surgery chosen for nasal and sinus tumors is predicted on the anatomic extent of the tumor. For tumors occupying the nasal fossa, a lateral rhinotomy and medial maxillectomy allowing an en bloc resection of the septum and lateral nasal wall are often employed.[17] Tumors confined to the maxillary sinus are treated by total maxillectomy which may or may not involve removal of the sinus roof (orbital floor).[18] This surgery is performed by elevating the cheek skin off the maxilla by splitting the lower lip and carrying the incision alongside the nose and just below the palpebral border to the lateral orbital rim (Webber-Fergusson incision). The maxillary sinus is then removed en bloc by cutting the hard palate medially, the zygoma laterally, the ethmoid sinus superiorly and the pterygoid plates posteriorly. The undersurface of the cheek flap is dressed with a split-thickness skin graft and the resultant surgical cavity obturated with a prepared prosthesis which is attached to the remaining maxillary teeth. If the maxillary sinus roof is removed, the orbital contents can be suspended on a flap of temporalis muscle attached to the medial portion of the orbital rim. If the cancer invades the orbit, orbital extenteration is recommended at the time of maxillectomy. Tumors arising in the ethmoid sinus usually require removal of the orbital contents because of the thin partition between the sinus and orbit (lamina papyracea). The ethmoid roof and cribriform plate can be resected if tumor closely approximates this area, occasionally necessitating craniotomy.[19, 20]

Tumors are usually considered inoperable if there is significant erosion of the pterygoid plate indicating deep invasion of the pterygoid muscles, as well as computerized tomography (CT) scan evidencing involvement of the anterior cranial fossa or sphenoid sinus and cavernous sinus. In the latter instances, polytomography will typically demonstrate that the cribriform plate is absent, the crista galli is tilted or the lateral wall of the sphenoid sinus and foramen rotundem is eroded.

Close cooperation with a maxillofacial prosthedontist is mandatory for optimal rehabilitation of these patients. Indeed, all of the surgically treated patients will require some type of obturator to seal the sinus and nasal fossa from the oral cavity. While it will sometimes be necessary to resect the nose or cheek, a prosthesis can be worn to fill the defect and achieve an acceptable facial appearance.[21]

Management of patients with advanced nasal and paranasal sinus cancer is clearly the greatest challenge. In many instances, palliation alone becomes the therapeutic goal. Chemotherapy has assumed an increasingly effective role for patients who suffer recurrent disease, and it is also being evaluated as an adjunctive modality immediately following initial therapy. Recurrent disease can also be palliated with cryotherapy or local endocavity radiation.

Prognosis

Five-year survival rates for patients with tumors of the nasal fossa and paranasal sinuses are difficult to summarize because staging is obscure and tumor types vary widely. Tumors arising close to the cranial fossa, e.g., frontal and sphenoid sinus cancers, have an unfavorable prognosis; in fact, prolonged survival is rare. Tumors involving or extending to the ethmoid sinus and orbit have an intermediate prognosis; with aggressive combined therapy, the 5-year survival rate ranges between 30 and 40%. Tumors confined to the nasal fossa and maxillary sinus cavity have the best prognosis, ranging between 45 and 55%.

ORBITAL DECOMPRESSION FOR GRAVES' DISEASE

Graves' disease remains a perplexing and unpredictable disorder which is related in some unknown way to thyroid dysfunction. Among the various symptoms of the disease, the eye component usually becomes the paramount concern to the patient and his physician. The ophthalmic manifestations stem from the extreme hypertrophy of the orbital fat and muscles, with interstitial edema and lymphatic infiltration producing increased intraorbital pressure and forward displacement of the globus. The intraorbital pressure may be sufficient to cause optic nerve damage and the proptosis severe enough to lose the eyelid protection of the cornea, thus allowing exposure keratitis to develop. Other symptoms include orbital pressure, pain, diplopia, excessive lacrimation and photophobia.

General Management Considerations

The management of the ophthalmic component of Graves' disease depends on its severity. Mild proptosis without any impairment of vision can readily be managed conservatively by prescribing eye drops and eyelid-taping at night. Unfortunately, many patients with this condition develop relentless proptosis and increasing intraocular pressure which threaten the vision. Currently, three different methods are employed in the treatment of this advanced disease: steroids, irradiation, and orbital decompressive surgery. Systemic steroids tend to provide only a temporary remission. Supervoltage orbital radiotherapy has been unpredictable and runs the risk of late irradiation damage to the orbital structures. While surgery has the longest therapeutic record, many different surgical approaches have evolved because of limitations of each technique (Fig. 11.7).

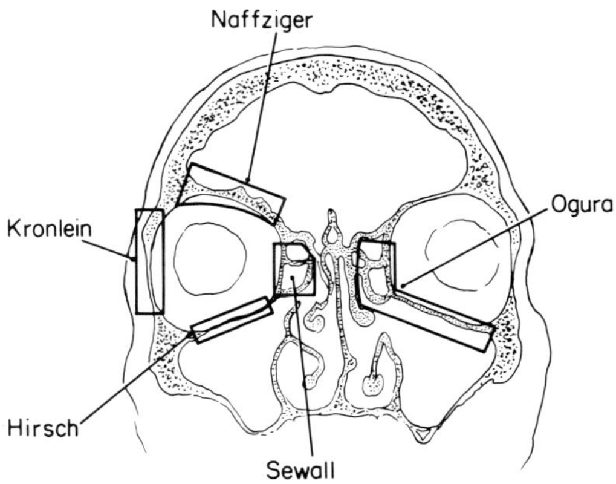

Figure 11.7 Schematic illustration showing various techniques for removing a portion of the orbit.

In 1911 Dollinger first reported orbital decompression by removing the lateral wall of the bony orbit (Krönlein's operation) to allow the orbital contents to herniate into the temporal fossa. Two decades later, Naffziger published the first report of decompression of the orbital contents into the anterior cranial fossa via a transcranial approach. Use of the paranasal sinus cavities to decompress the orbit was first described by Sewall, who removed the common wall between the ethmoid sinuses and the orbit to provide a medial decompression. Hirsh later reported inferior decompression into the maxillary sinus by removal of the orbital floor. Walsh and Ogura combined the operations of Hirsh and Sewall, removing both the medial and inferior walls of the orbit. This antral-ethmoid method of orbital decompression has been the author's preference.[22]

Patients have a variety of signs and symptoms related to the increased intracranial pressure, but the predominant complaints are the excessive tearing and photophobia. Any patient with ocular pain and/or decreasing vision who has evidence of optic neuropathy or exposure keratitis refractory to medical management is considered a candidate for surgery. Other indications for surgery include disfiguring proptosis which may be asymmetrical. Decompressive surgery is also performed preliminary to extraocular muscle surgery for diplopia.

Operative Technique

Clinical hyperthyroidism is corrected medically whenever possible before operation. Documentation of adequate sinus pneumatization and freedom from inflammatory disease is ascertained by sinus x-ray films. Patients currently or recently receiving systemic steroids are prepared by parenteral corticosteroids given on the evening and morning before the operation.

Decompression is carried out with the patient under general endotracheal anesthesia in a semisitting position. The eyes remain uncovered so that they can be observed during the operative procedure. A sublabial incision is made to approach the maxillary and ethmoid sinuses. The ethmoid cells are exenterated posterior to the lacrimal crest and superior to the cribriform plate. The orbital floor and lamina papyracea are fractured in an eggshell fashion and removed, while preserving the orbital periosteum, infraorbital nerve and orbital rim. Orbital periosteum tends to sag considerably after removal of bone. Additional recession may be achieved by radial incisions of the orbital periosteum to allow the fat to herniate through the incisions. The degree of orbital recession is monitored by a gas-sterilized exophthalmometer while increasing the number and extent of the periosteal incisions until the desired position of the eye is accomplished. The more proptotic eye is approached first, preserving some periosteal support; the other eye is then decompressed until both eyes are approximately equal. In no instance is periorbital fat dissected from around the muscles. It is important to anticipate and allow for an additional 1–2 mm of recession that invariably develops within the first postoperative month. A conventional nasal antrostomy is created through the inferior meatus of the nose. The entire procedure may be performed on both orbits in approximately 1 hour, and the patient is usually discharged on the 2nd postoperative day.

Decompression of the swollen orbital contents into the ethmoid and maxillary sinuses has the advantage of utilizing an air-containing space. This technique is more effective than a lateral or a superior (cranial) decompression inasmuch as the soft tissue compromises the space available for orbital recession, and rarely more than 3 mm of recession can be accomplished in either of the latter two approaches. The antral-ethmoid approach permits greater recession and the degree of recession can be controlled (Figs. 11.8, *A* and *B*, and 11.9 *A* and *B*). On the other hand, the cranial approach involves an extensive procedure with risk of intracranial complications, and the lateral approach requires facial incisions that extend posteriorly from the lateral canthus.

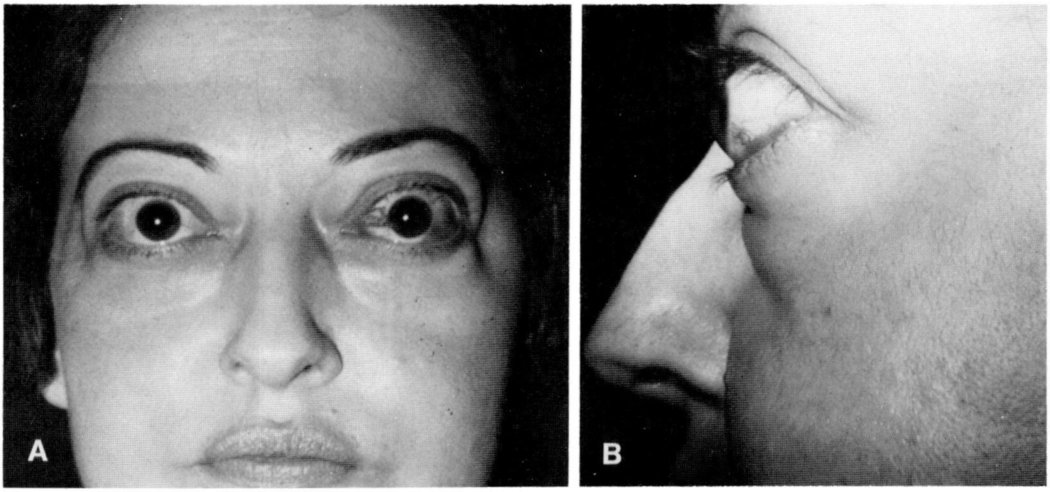

Figure 11.8 Preoperative anterior (*A*) and lateral (*B*) views of a patient with severe proptosis secondary to Graves' disease.

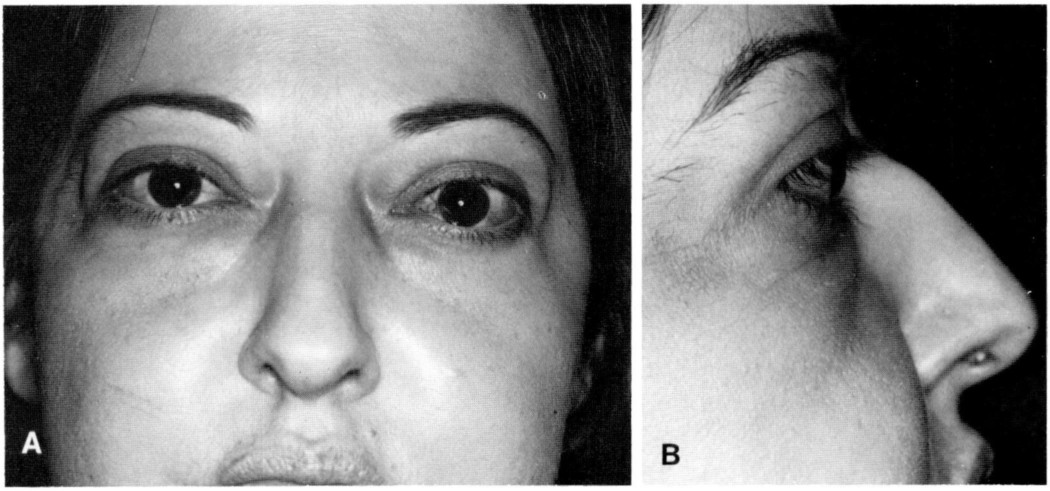

Figure 11.9 Postoperative anterior (*A*) and lateral (*B*) views of the same patient subsequent to antral-ethmoid orbital decompression.

References

1. Schultz, R. C.: Frontal sinus and supraorbital fractures from vehicle accidents. *Clin. Plast. Surg.*, *2*:93, 1975.
2. Newman, M. H., and Travis, L. W.: Frontal sinus fractures. *Laryngoscope*, *83*:1281, 1973.
3. Gross, C. W., Teague, P. F., and Nakamura, T.: Reconstruction following severe nasofrontal injuries. *Otolaryngol. Clin. North Am.*, *5*:653, 1972.
4. May, M., Ogura, J. H., and Schramm, V.: Nasofrontal duct in frontal sinus fractures. *Arch. Otholaryngol.*, *92*:534, 1970.
5. Donald, P., and Bernstein, L.: Compound frontal sinus injuries with intracranial penetration. *Laryngoscope*, *88*:225, 1978.
6. Shaw, R. C., and Thering, H. R.: Reconstruction of cranial defects. *Clin. Plast. Surg.*, *2*:539, 1975.
7. Dickinson, J. T., Cipcic, J. A., and Kamerer, J. B.: Principles of frontal reconstruction. *Laryngoscope*, *79*: 1019, 1969.
8. Longacre, M. D.: Reconstruction of cranial defects

with split rib. *Plast. Reconstr. Surg.*, *19:*186, 1957.
9. Olsen, N. R., and Newman, M. H.: Acrylic frontal cranioplasty. *Arch. Otolaryngol.*, *89:*774, 1969.
10. Sessions, R. B., Wolfe, S. K., Moiel, R. H., and Cheek, W. R.: Wire mesh foundation for methyl methacrylate cranioplasty. *Laryngoscope*, *84:*1020, 1974.
11. Calcaterra, T. C., Riley, C., and Jarek, B. W.: Forehead reconstruction with silicone elastomer sponge. *Arch. Otolaryngol.*, *98:*382, 1973.
12. Calcaterra, T. C., Moseley, J. I., and Rand, R. W.: Cerebrospinal rhinorrhea: Extracranial surgical repair. *West. J. Med.*, *127:*279, 1977.
13. Dandy, W. D.: Pneumocephalus (intracranial pneumatocele or aerocele). *Arch. Surg.*, *12:*949, 1926.
14. Calcaterra, T. C., and Strahan, R.: Osteoplastic flap technique for disease of the frontal sinus. *Surg. Gynecol. Obstet.*, *132:*505, 1971.
15. Calcaterra, T. C., and Rand, R. W.: Current adjuncts in surgery of the sphenoid sinus. *Laryngoscope*, *86:*1692, 1976.
16. Lewis, J. S., and Castro, E. B.: Cancer of the nasal cavity and paranasal sinuses. *Laryngoscope*, *86:*255, 1972.
17. Sessions, R. B., and Larson, D. L.: En bloc ethmoidectomy and medial maxillectomy. *Arch. Otolaryngol.*, *1032:*195, 1977.
18. Tabb, H. G., and Barranco, J. S.: Cancer of the maxillary sinus. *Laryngoscope 81:*818, 1971.
19. Saunders, W. H., and Miglets, A.: Surgical techniques in far advanced carcinoma of orbital-ethmoid maxillary areas. *Trans. Ophthalmol. Otolaryngol.*, *71:* 426, 1967.
20. Shaw, J. B., and Galicicj, J. H.: Craniofacial resection for malignant tumors of the ethmoid and anterior skull base. *Arch. Otolaryngol.*, *103:*513, 1977.
21. Beumer, J., and Calcaterra, T. C.: Prosthetic rehabilitation of large midfacial defects. *Laryngoscope*, *86:* 280, 1976.
22. Calcaterra, T. C., and Hepler, R. S.: Antral-ethmoidal decompression in Graves' disease: Five-year experience. *West. J. Med.*, *124:*57, 1976.

CHAPTER 12

The Eye

Andrew E. Choy, M.D.

This chapter is a discussion of common ophthalmologic problems the reconstructive surgeon may encounter. It reviews basic diagnostic steps useful in determining the extent of ocular and/or orbital pathology, and outlines common ophthalmic surgical procedures for orbital and ocular pathology.

The reconstructive surgeon is confronted by ocular and/or orbital pathology associated with congenital defects, tumors, and acquired lesions. While innumerable specific types of diseases and lesions are associated with any of the above three general categories, the *primary* ophthalmic procedure is *always* to obtain an accurate description of the visual acuity of each eye. This may vary from the typical Snellen chart recording of 20/20 to a written observation that an infant prefers fixating on an interesting toy with one eye than with the fellow eye. The visual acuity measurement is basic information necessary for the treating physician and has frequent medicolegal implications in aquired lesions related to on-the-job injuries. Figure 12.1 demonstrates methods of assessing visual acuity.

CONGENITAL CONDITIONS

The various craniofacial disorders discussed in Chapters 14 and 15 are congenital conditions with associated ophthalmic pathology. The primary concerns with these patients are the prevention of amblyopia (poor visual acuity in an eye), treatment of any strabismus and blepharoptosis, and the resolution of any epiphora resulting from nasal lacrimal duct pathology. Our recommended course of treatment has been previously reviewed.[1]

Hemangiomas are a congenital problem which may affect the orbit causing proptosis, the retina and choroid resulting in serous retinopathy, the iris insertion angle resulting in glaucoma, and the eyelid causing an occlusion amblyopia (Fig. 12.2). Fortunately, most hemangiomas of the eye and orbit can be treated with careful observation and often have a self-resolution. Surgery, sclerosing solutions or steroids may be necessary on rare occasions such as in massive eyelid involvement causing an occlusion amblyopia.

Sturge-Weber syndrome presents ocular, orbital and systemic health problems to the team of physicians managing a patient with this disease. The principal ocular concerns are the effects of choroidal hemangiomas affecting the development of good visual acuity and the increased incidence of glaucoma associated with these patients.

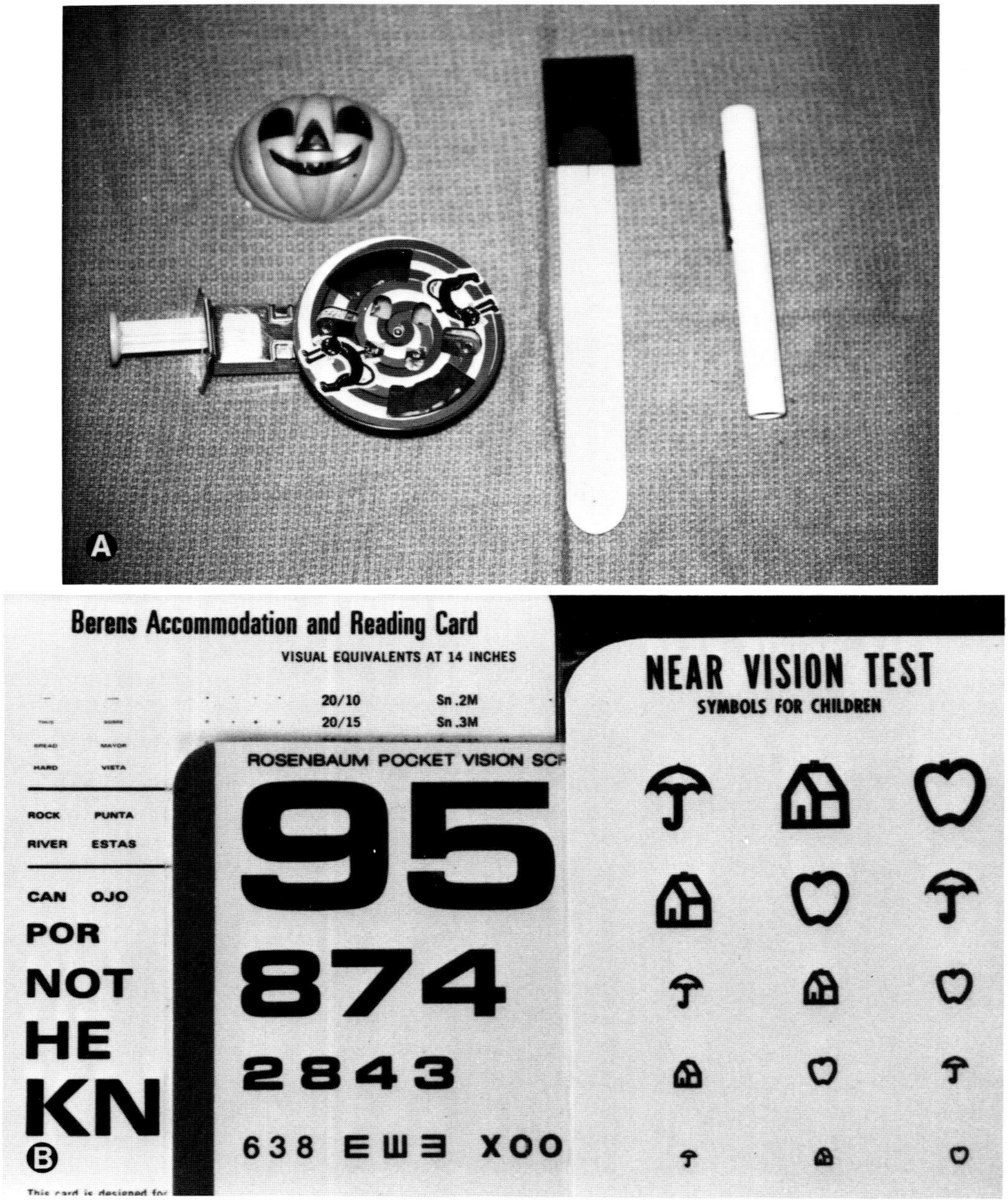

Figure 12.1 (*A*) Interesting toys, a light and/or a light with a red filter can be used to assess visual acuity in the infant and young child. (*B*) Different types of graded visual acuity charts are available. These include pictures, the "E" game, numbers and letters. (*C*) Fixation preference determines if amblyopia is present in the infant or young child. (*a*) Child is content to fixate on an interesting toy with the preferred eye. (*b*) Child cries or attempts fixation with the *nonamblyopic preferred eye* when forced to use the *amblyopic nonpreferred eye.*

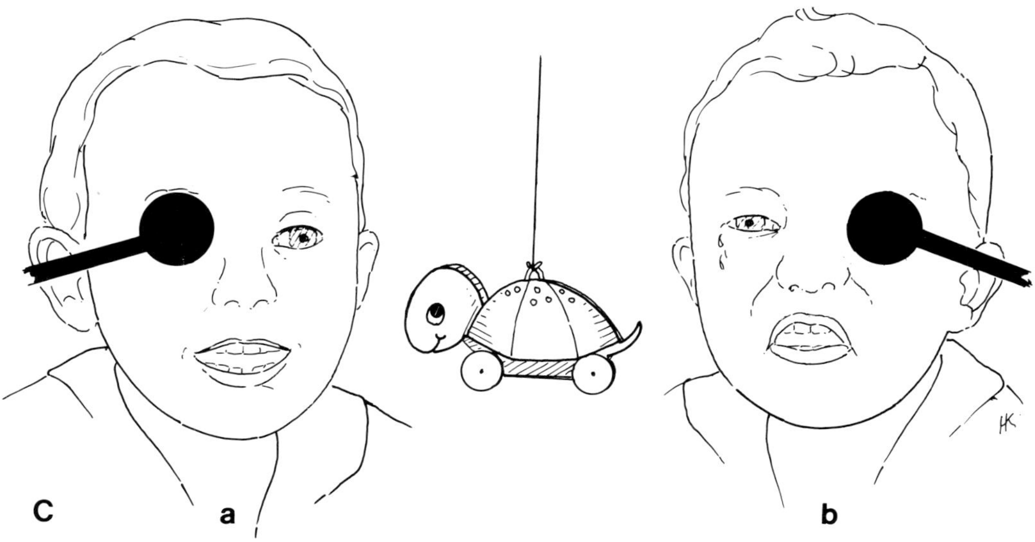

Figure 12.1 (*C*)

Another congenital ophthalmic problem frequently encountered is *blepharoptosis*. The primary concern is prevention of amblyopia in the involved eye from upper eyelid occlusion. A frontalis sling type of operation is the treatment of choice when such poor levator palprebrae muscle function threatens occlusion amblyopia in the infant or child.

In the child under the age of 3, Supramid or silicone is the recommended material to use in the sling. Another very suitable material is preserved homologous fascia lata available from the University of Toronto Department of Ophthalmology or preserved homologous sclera which is often available from a local eye bank.[2] While we have had success with the preserved homologous tissue, we have also encountered two cases of reaction to the tissue which required subsequent reoperation. In the patient over the age of 3 with poor to absent levator muscle function, autologous fascia lata is the material of choice to use in the sling. Over the age of 3, very adequate amounts of fascia lata may be obtained. Crawford has recently modified his fascia lata stripper for use in the much younger patient.[3]

Most ophthalmic reconstructive surgeons agree that aesthetic blepharoptosis repair should be performed some time between the age of 3 and the start of school if the visual acuity is not threatened or an undue head posture is present.[4–6] Deferring the ptosis repair to this older age often results in better patient cooperation and a more accurate assessment of levator muscle function (Fig. 12.3). A levator resection is the procedure of choice in patients with fair to moderate levator function. Those patients with a minimal to absent levator muscle function should have a sling procedure. Tables on the amount of resection, where to set the upper eyelid margin, and other details are in the textbooks cited above.

The levator palpebrae superioris muscle and the superior rectus develop from a common embryologic anlage. It is not surprising that an associated superior rectus underaction is commonly found in the ptotic eye. The resulting hypotropia (involved eye is lower than the nonptotic eye) may be subtle and may require good patient cooperation to measure the deviation. In these cases of dual pathology, the strabismus is repaired prior to blepharoptosis surgery. Finally, deferring ptosis surgery until an older age if possible allows the orbit and the surrounding soft tissues to further develop and thus somewhat simplify the reconstructive surgeon's task.

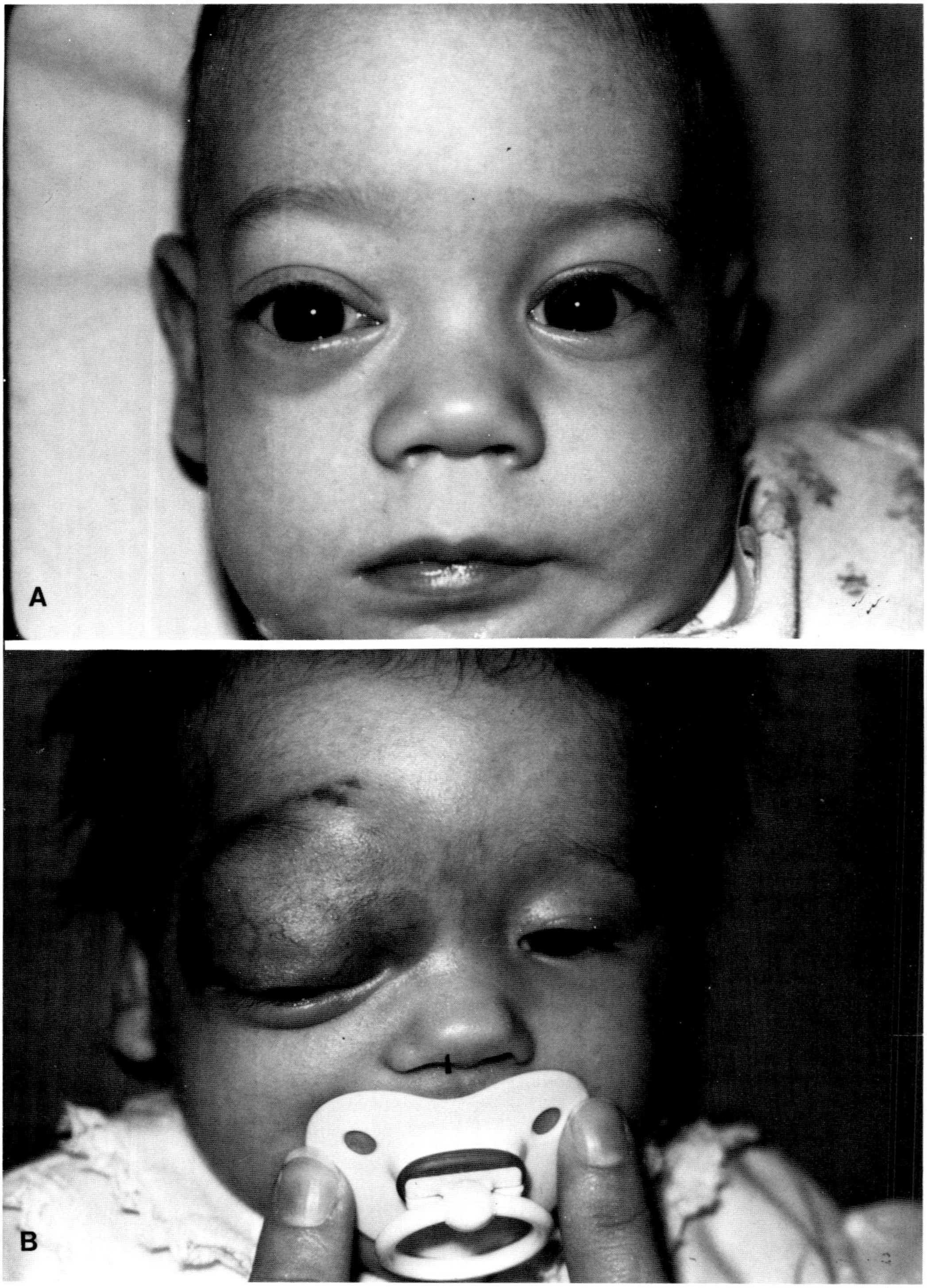

Figure 12.2 (*A*) Proptosis from deep orbital hemangioma, right eye. (*B*) Capillary hemangioma causing an eyelid deformity which may lead to an occlusion amblyopia.

The following congenital ophthalmic problems are less common than the ones previously reviewed. These lesions my occur in conjunction with other deformities or as an isolated problem.

A *dermoid cyst* may arise in the orbit, brow, lid, diploe of the skull or in the paranasal sinuses. The dermoid arises from ectoderm where the fetal cleft closes. The most common site of origin is the temporal angle of the superior orbit margin followed by the superior nasal orbit angle (Fig. 12.4). These cysts are usually superficial and may be resected by an anterior skin incision. The entire cyst wall must be excised with care taken not to spill any of the contents lest any of the remaining tissue act as a nidus of foreign body reaction resulting in a recurrence of a cyst. A large dermoid cyst may be deep and involve the cranial fossa. Careful radiologic studies are indicated and neurosurgical assistance may be required.

Colobomas are usually situated in the nasal half of the superior eyelid. The next favored site is the temporal half of the inferior eyelid. Lid colobomas are a frequent finding in the Treacher Collins syndrome (ocular-facial-mandibular dyostosis). Colobomas of the eyelid occur in various shapes. The most common is triangular with the base at the lid margin. Repair of congenital lid colobomas does not differ from techniques used for colobomas of traumatic and post-tumor excision origin.

Primary congenital entropion is a rare entity. Entropion seen in youngsters is usually secondary to mechanical problems and/or due to a lack of eyelid margin support from a small or absent globe. The primary ophthalmologic concern is mechanical corneal injury caused by the inversion of the eyelid margin and eyelashes.

Epiblepharon is characterized by an enlarged pretarsal skin fold which may extend over the lid margins pushing the eyelashes against the globe particularly on down gaze. This condition is different from congenital entropion where the entire length of the eyelid margin is inverted like a senile entropion. Epiblepharon is relatively more common than congenital entropion. Unlike congenital entropion, epiblepharon may spontaneously resolve within the first few years of life and the cilia on the cornea seem to cause few signs and symptoms such as increased lacrimation and ocular injection. Surgical intervention should be delayed for as long as the cornea can be kept intact.

Anomalies of the canthus are often associated with changes in palpebral fissure size and obliquity. *Telecanthus* (lateral displacement of the medial canthi) presents as an increased intercanthal distance. This may be an isolated clinical finding, a part of the ptosis, blepharophimosis and epicanthus inversus syndrome, or in association with telorbitism.

Blepharophimosis indicates a decrease in the normal size of the palpebral aperture. This clinical finding is usually associated with other congenital anomalies. Blepharophimosis may be confused with epicanthus. An epicanthal fold hides some of the palpebral aperture but does not shorten its length. There is a physical decrease in the palpebral fissure dimensions in blepharophimosis.

Surgical repair of blepharophimosis usually involves the medial and lateral canthi and is often performed in conjunction with blepharoptosis and epicanthus inversus surgery. In contrast, epicanthus is normally found in Orientals and also may be seen in children of other races. The epicanthus tends to fade in non-Orientals as the child grows and the nose bridge develops. Surgical correction for epicanthus is best delayed until the age of 10 and performed if the condition has remained stationary for several years. Telecanthus repair involves shortening of the medial canthal tendon plus repair of the epicanthus. When telecanthus is found in association with teleorbitism, orbital translocation surgery is performed in addition to the soft tissue reconstruction.

Canthal anomalies may also exaggerate the normal upward temporal slant of the palpebral aperture (mongoloid obliquity) or result in the opposite down and outward slant of the palpebral fissure (antimongoloid obliquity). These anomalies have been attributed to the abscence or malformation of the lateral canthal ligaments plus the malformation and malposition of the orbital bones seen in several of the craniofacial disorders.

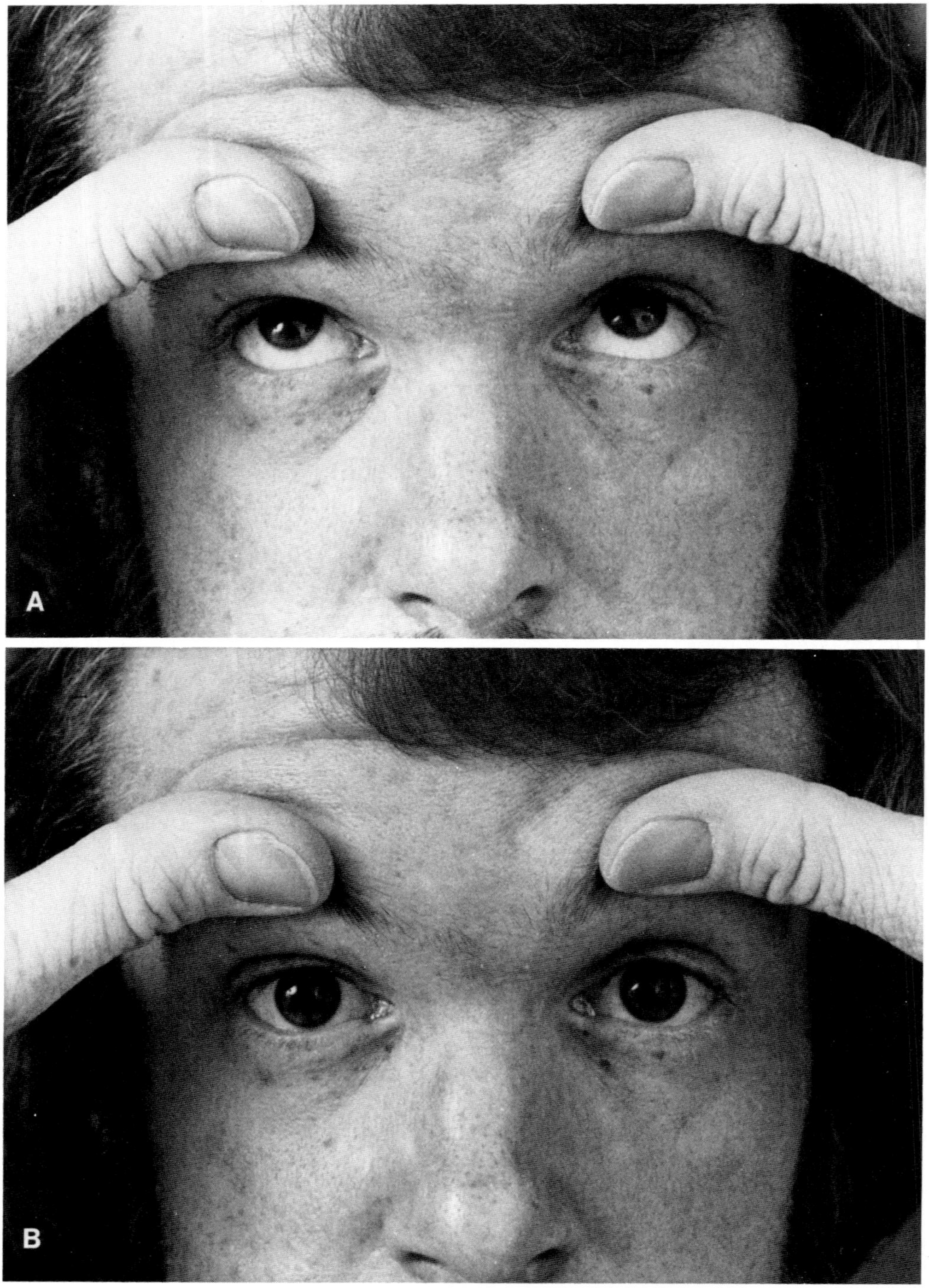

Figure 12.3 (*A*) Upward gaze
(*B*) Primary position:
Note palpebral vertical height
Note eyelid position on the globe
(*C*) Downward gaze

↑ Excursion from downward to upward gaze while splinting the orbicularis determines the amount of levator function.

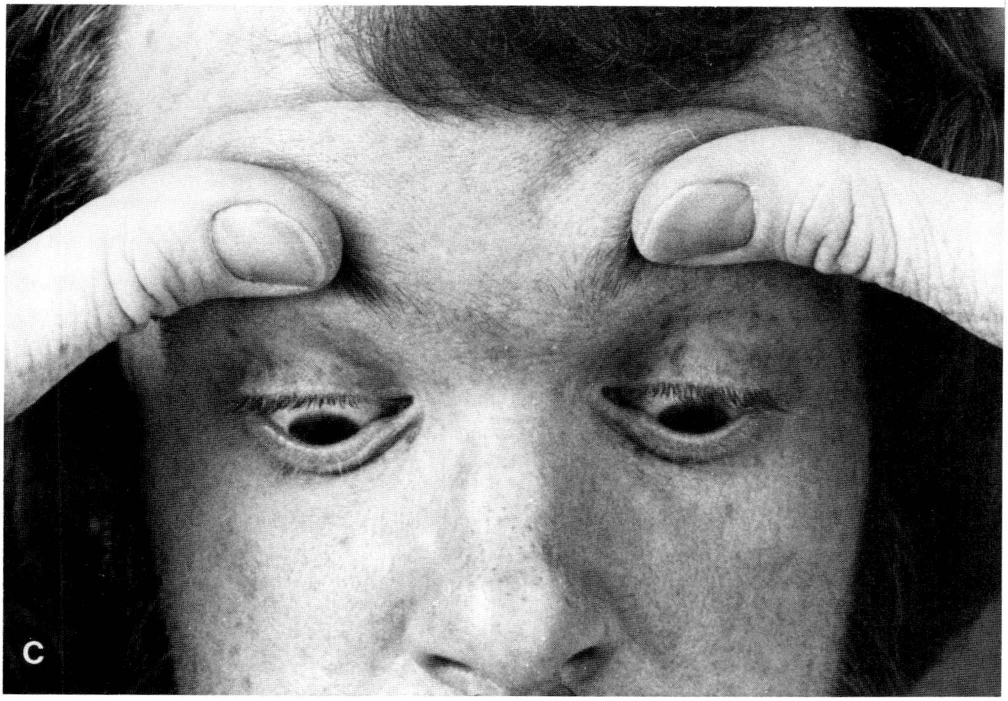

Figure 12.3 (*C*)

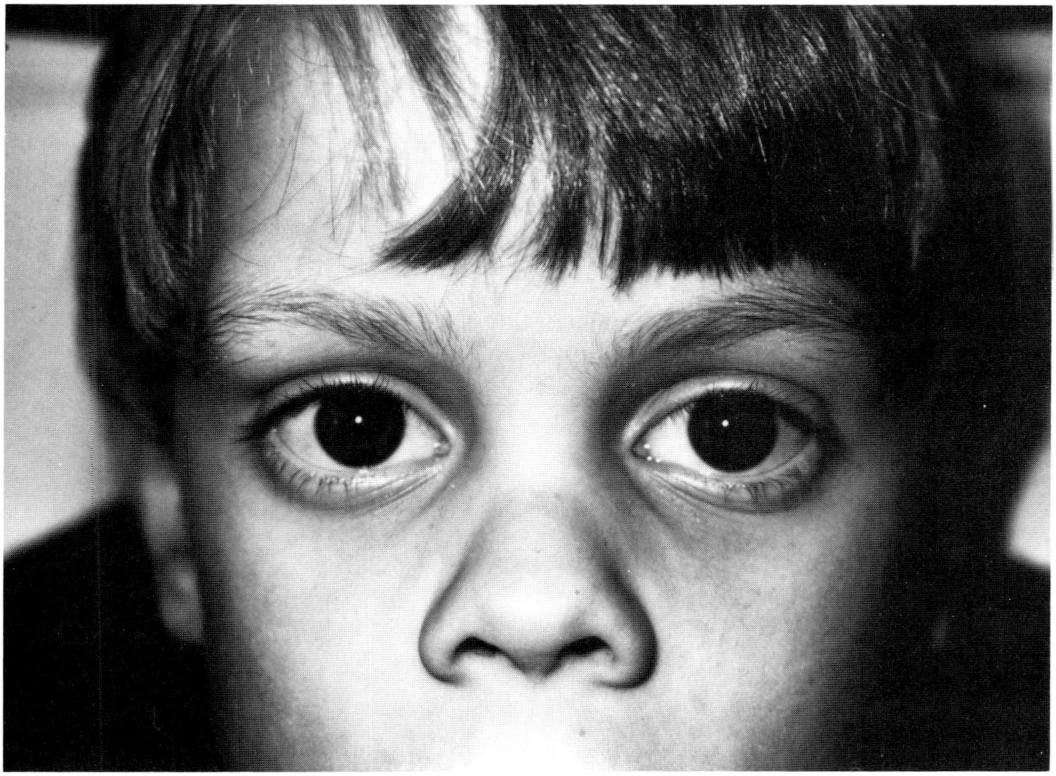

Figure 12.4 Superior temporal orbit dermoid cyst of right eye.

ACQUIRED LESIONS

Acquired lesions of the eye, surrounding tissues and orbit may be divided into mechanical and nonmechanical. Nonmechanical trauma includes thermal, chemical, electrical, ultrasonic, radiation and stress injuries. Ophthalmic problems of thermal and chemical etiology are most likely to confront the reconstructive surgeon.

While hypothermia can be deleterious to the eye and surrounding tissue, burns to the face and eyes are more commonly encountered. It is stressed again that an accurate determination of visual acuity is necessary in these unfortunate victims.

Thermal Burns

The globe is rarely directly involved by *flame burns*. The rapid reflex closure of the eyelids protects the globe while the eyelashes and eyebrows are scorched. The eyelid skin may be deeply burned and even widespread injury occur to the face and/or body. Occasionally the corneal epithelium may be damaged (Fig. 12.5). Fortunately, the epithelium regenerates within 48 hours.

When the heat is intense and prolonged, the globe may be severely damaged. However, these patients rarely survive. A delayed loss of vision associated with optic nerve pallor can occur in severe body burns. This finding has occurred primarily in infants, children and young adults.[7]

In superficial eyelid burns, the eyelashes and eyebrows are singed, the skin is hyperemic, and edema may cause complete lid closure over the eye. The edema of the eyelid and the entire face may be massive in partial thickness skin loss. This swelling usually peaks at 36–48 hours and then slowly subsides. Infection may occur on the raw surfaces as the eschar sloughs off. Orbital cellulitis follows if the infection spreads inward.

Granulation and then fibrosis follow the eschar slough. This slow healing process may endanger the eye if the degree of cicatricial ectropion is severe. When the eyelids are drawn away from the globe, injected and hypertrophic palpebral and bulbar conjunctiva plus exposure keratitis develop. This condition can lead to corneal ulceration, perforation of the globe, and ultimate loss of useful vision if left unattended.

Aberrant regrowth of the eyelashes may irritate the eye causing a keratoconjunctivitis. Discomfort and epiphora may result from meibomian gland duct obliteration and metaplasia of the mucocutaneous junction permitting the skin to contact the conjunctiva. Severe epiphora follows damage to the lacrimal puncta and canaliculi with subsequent cicatrization.

Contact burns from hot bodies or scalds may directly involve the globe as well as the lid and adenexa. Eyelid involvement from scalding is often superficial. A partial thickness skin

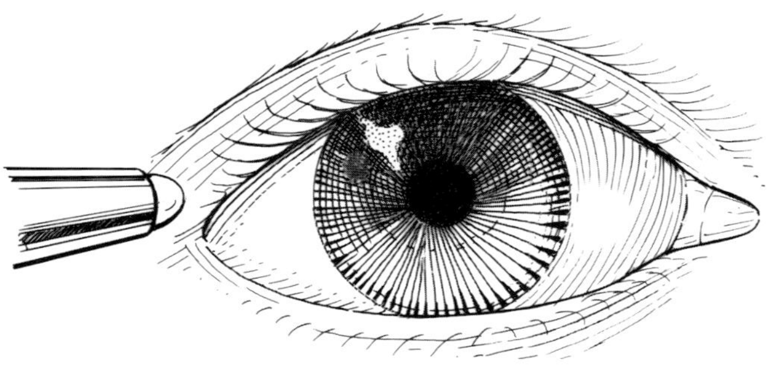

Figure 12.5 Fluorescein dye stains devitalized corneal epithelium in an abrasion. A cobalt blue or bright pen light readily highlight the stain.

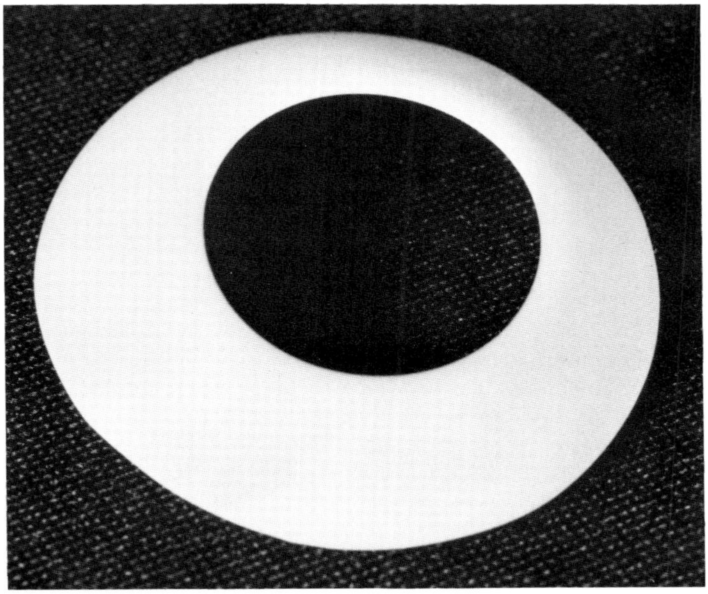

Figure 12.6 Conjunctival cul-de-sac conformer with a central opening facilitates examination and monitoring of the visual axis.

loss from scalding can result. The blink reflex usually protects the globe. It is unusual to have corneal erosion and/or conjunctival symblepharon formation resulting from a scald.

Hot bodies have a greater incidence of globe injury. Very hot bodies traveling at a high rate of speed frequently lead to severe eyelid skin burns, conjunctival destruction, corneal scarring and even loss of the eye. If the eye survives the initial insult and damage to the surrounding tissues, subsequent cicatricial contraction can result in a number of deformities. These problems include pseudopterygium, entropion with trichiasis, symblepharon, restricted extraocular movements, ankyloblepharon, epiphora from displaced and/or obstructed lacrimal puncta, and/or ectropion with its problem of exposure keratitis.

Treatment of skin and eyelid burns is aimed at the prevention of sepsis and the restoration of an adequate globe covering before a cicatricial deformity develops. When the cornea is severely exposed and threatened, a tarsorraphy or transplantation of a full thickness skin flap from the temple or forehead may be necessary. Eyelid reconstruction is discussed in Chapter 4.

The acute care of burn injuries to the eye involves the use of topical and systemic antibiotics for possible sepsis. Cycloplegic drops alleviate the ciliary body spasm of iritis and prevents the development of a constricted, bound-down pupil. Topical anesthetics are avoided because of the unfavorable effects upon epithelialization and possible serious injury to visual acuity.[8] Systemic analgesics and sedatives are best for comfort maintenance. The risk of symblepharon formation is decreased by inserting the conjunctival sac conformer with a central opening which permits continuous monitoring of the cornea and posterior structures of the eye (Fig. 12.6).

The chronic injuries of ocular burns include leukomas and symblepharon. A penetrating or lamellar keratoplasty may be the initial and only major surgical treatment necessary when a corneal opacity which hinders good visual acuity remains unvascularized. If the cornea is highly vascularized, careful preparation of the entire globe as well as the cornea is required prior to any keratoplasty attempt.

Symblepharon which causes eyelid deformities and/or extraocular motility restrictions is improved by mucous membrane grafting. The best source of mucous membrane is extra conjunctival tissue. Buccal mucosa is satisfactory and certainly preferred to genital mucosa which is a poor match and desquamates unpleasantly. In cases of massive symblepharon and a limited amount of mucous membrane harvested, the use of a fine Supramid or silicone sheet stent is helpful.[9]

Electrical injuries are more commonly the result of domestic or industrial electrocutions than from lightning. There is little clinical difference between electrical and thermal burns to the eyelids and skin. Electrical burns tend to be painless, dry, aseptic and circumscribed when compared to the usual heat burn. These characteristics are likely due to the very high temperature and short duration of electrical burns.

The conjunctiva often becomes hyperemic with varying degrees of chemosis. Corneal lesions range from transient interstitial opacities and edema which clear within several days to deeper injuries that may cause scarring or necrosis with perforation. The degree of iris and ciliary body irritation depends upon the severity of the electrical injury. A miotic pupil is typical though instances of mydriasis associated with compromised accommodation are occasionally seen. Retina, choroid and vitreous lesions are infrequent. These may include retinal edema, cystoid changes, hyper- and hyporetinal pigment changes, and vitreous opacities.

Cataract formation is the most common electrical injury. The extent of lenticular change has no definitive relationship to the strength of the electrical current. There is also a great variation between the time of electrical injury and when cataract changes become clinically observeable. Industrial accidents usually result in a cataract on the side of injury while lightning more commonly causes bilateral cataract changes. The cataract changes are characteristically found in the lens capsule and the cortex directly below.

Radiation Injuries

Radiation injuries are the result of direct tissue absorption. A latent period will elapse between the absorption of energy and the appearance of its biological effects. The latency period varies with the wavelength employed, the intensity of the exposure, and the vulnerability of the particular tissue. In general, the reaction to thermal radiation (hertzian and infrared) tends to be immediate, while the latency to ultraviolet radiation is measured in hours. Ionizing radiation effects are generally observed over weeks or months.

Shortwave diathermy may produce thermal lesions. It has been reported that chronic exposure to microwave diathermy contributes to cataract formation.[10]

Enormous amounts of infrared radiation may be released with ultraviolet radiation in a flash burn. A flash burn is similar clinically to the ordinary thermal burns previously discussed. The clinical findings associated with chronic, subliminal exposure to infrared radiation are hyperemic blepharitis, failure of accommodation and/or corneal opacification. The well known heat cataract described as occurring in long time glassworkers and furnacemen is thought to result from chronic infrared radiation exposure. So-called sun blindness, photoretinitis, or eclipse blindness is the result of a solar chorioretinal burn injury. Industrial sources such as electric or oxyacetylene welding produce infrared radiation that may cause temporary retinal edema.

The ultraviolet spectrum produces abiotic lesions of which solar (snow blindess) or industrial photophthalmia is the most frequent clinical problem. The patient presents with an acute keratitis with foreign body sensation, pain, photophobia, tearing and blepharospasm. Ultraviolet effects upon the skin include the typical sunburn. It is thought that chronic exposure to ultraviolet radiation contributes to senile keratosis.

Ionizing radiation (x-ray) to the eye and adjacent structures is the major cause of globe and adenexal injuries. Complications and side effects of therapeutic radiation usually arise sometime after the completion of treatment. Side effects occur from radiation treatment of purely ocular conditions as well as radiation treatment of adjoining structures such as the pituitary fossa, maxilla, nasopharynx and paranasal sinuses. All of the structures of the eye have been cited as becoming involved with radiation side effects and its complications. The most serious of postradiation complications is the development of malignant changes.

Radiation effects to the skin, bone and cartilage, and the external eye are of primary concern to the reconstructive surgeon. The acute skin lesion is erythema which either heals completely or progresses to a chronic lesion. The chronic lesions include loss of hair-bearing areas, a brownish induration, hyperkeratosis or a smooth, dry and atrophic appearance. The skin may become pigmented or depigmented with devascularization or heavily marked telangiectatic areas. Shrinkage of the eyelid tissue may cause a secondary ectropion or entropion.

The harmful effects of radiation upon the orbital bone and cartilage include bone necrosis, growth disturbance and malignant degeneration. Bone necrosis is caused by vascular ischemia and is seen usually in adults. The growth disturbance affects the growing bones of youngsters. This is often associated with soft tissue atrophy and results in various degrees of facial and skull asymmetry (Fig. 12.7).

Conjunctival injuries from ionizing radiation correspond to the reaction seen in other mucous membranes of the body. The later side effects include persistent conjunctival injection for months to years and the appearance of spider-like telangiectatic vessels. Extensive scaring may result in fornix obliteration, symblepharon development and the restriction of extraocular movements. The conjunctival injuries may become interwoven with eyelid shrinkage deformities. These include entropion or ectropion, scarring and contracture of the skin, puncta obliteration, chronic blepharitis, and/or loss of the eyelashes. Eyelid necrosis with tissue loss is unusual with present improved treatment methods.

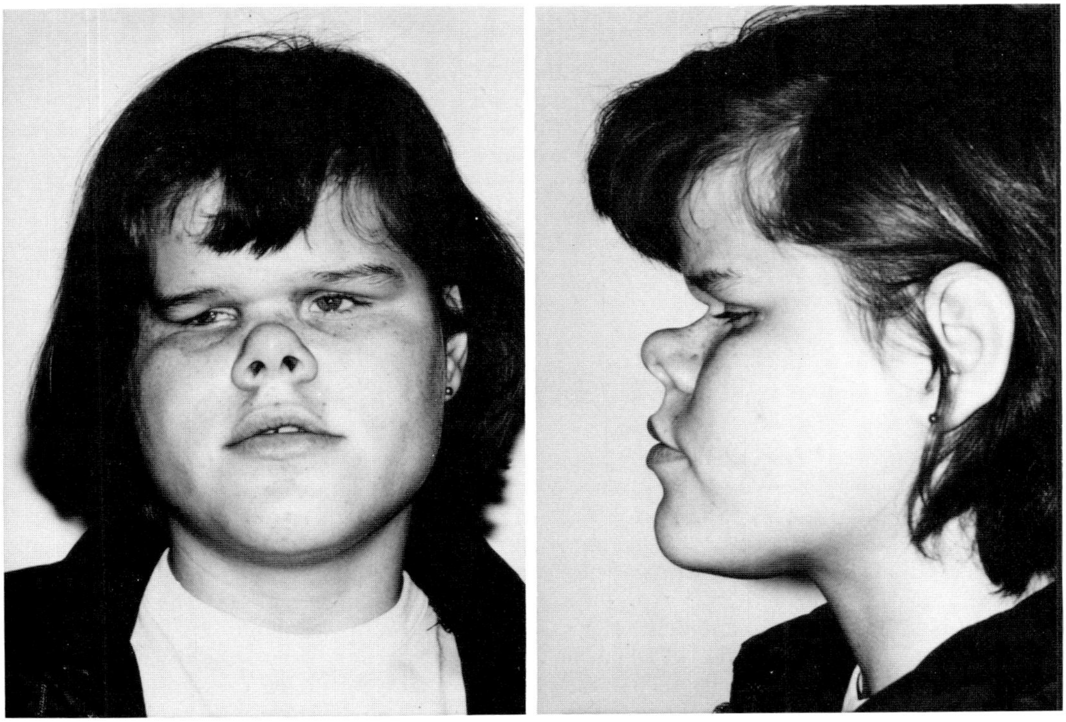

Figure 12.7 Asymmetry of the facial features resulting from early enucleation of both eyes and radiation therapy for retinoblastoma (frontal and lateral).

Other therapeutic radiation complications involve the sclera, cornea, choroid and uveal tissues, the lens, vitreous and retina. These ocular structures are in the area of expertise of the ophthalmologist and beyond the scope of this text or chapter to cover in any detail.

Chemical Injuries

Chemicals are the other common source of nonmechanical injury to the eye and surrounding tissues. The extent of injury is dependent upon the duration of contact, the physical properties of the chemical which determine penetration and chemical reaction with the involved tissues, and the reversibility of the chemical reaction. Chemical injuries to the eye occur as a solid particle in the conjunctival sac acting as a foreign body, as an airborne contaminant, or most commonly as a splash from a liquid.

The particular mechanism of chemical injury to the tissue proteins is as diverse and varied as there are chemicals. However, little distinction can be made on clinical examination of the patient among the various modes of injury. Acid and alkali injuries which most commonly involve the reconstructive surgeon do have characteristic clinical pictures.

Strong acids denature and coagulate tissue proteins forming insoluble acid proteinates. The clinical lesion tends to be sharply limited to the area of contact with nonprogression because the precipatated protein forms a dense barrier. Further chemical activity is neutralized by the buffering action of the tissues.

In contrast, alkali burns spread widely with continued tissue reaction for several days. The reason is alkalis dissociate and saponify the fatty acids. This destroys the cell membrane structure of tissues allowing penetration of the alkali. The hygroscopic nature of the alkalis draws water from the cells leading to further tissue softening, spread of destruction, and total necrosis.

The late complications of acid and alkali burns involve the reconstructive surgeon. Skin and eyelid deformities are the areas of principal concern. Symblepharon formation is frequently associated with these eyelid deformities (Fig. 12.8). Treatment for symblepharon has been reviewed in this chapter and the details of eyelid management are covered in Chapter 4.

Other possible complications from chemical injuries include corneal opacification, neovascular membranes, and recurrent ulcerations. Scleral thinning with staphyloma may occur. Secondary intraocular changes of uveitis, glaucoma and cataract may present as late sequelae. All of these ocular problems are best managed in conjunction with the ophthalmology consultant.

Mechanical Injuries

We are constantly reminded of the mechanical injuries which result from our mechanized, industrialized and often violent modern environment. These injuries may embarass the bony orbital structures, the eyelids and adenexal tissues including the lacrimal drainage system, the extraocular muscles, the globe and its particular tissues, the optic nerve, and/or the vascular supply to all of the previously mentioned structures.

The bony skeleton of the orbit provides protective case for the globe. The eye is further encased in a cushion of fat and other soft tissues. Blunt trauma and high impact injuries such as vehicular accidents are the most common source of orbital fractures and displacements (Fig. 12.9). The orbit, orbital injuries and their treatment have been previously discussed in this text. In this section, we will concentrate on the mechanical injuries to tissues other than the bony orbital structures.

The eyelids and adenexal structures may become edematous, boggy and echymotic from

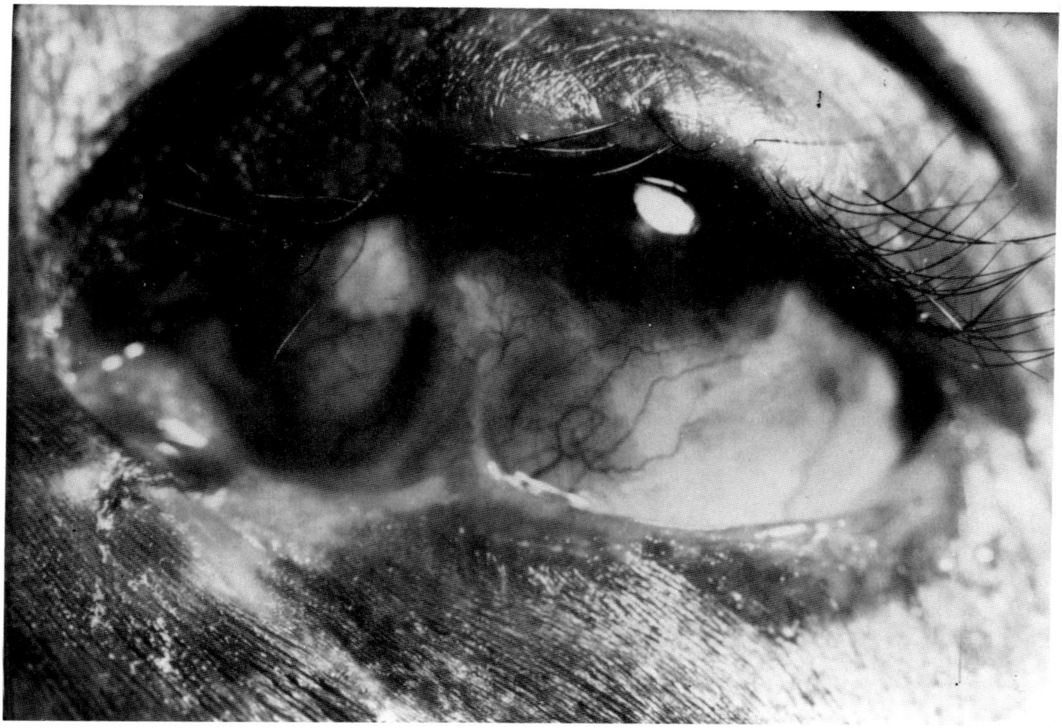

Figure 12.8 A chemical injury to the globe and eyelids causing partial corneal opacification, symblepharon formation, eyelid deformity and increased epiphora from malposition and damage to the punctum.

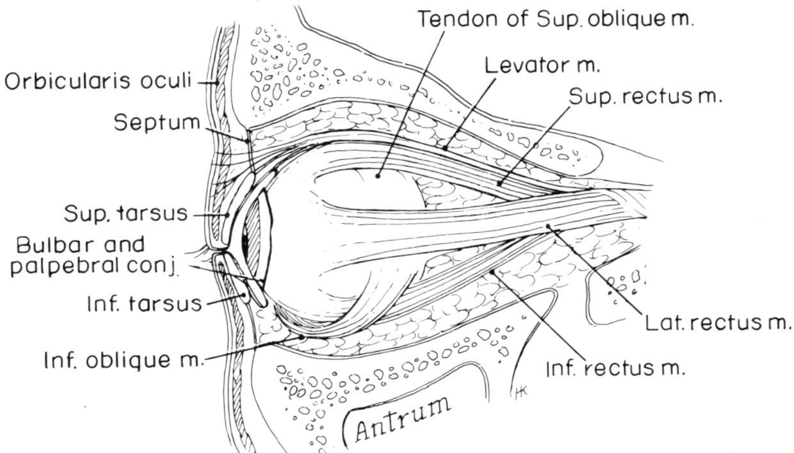

Figure 12.9 Within the protective bony shell of the orbit and its connective tissue contents lies the eye.

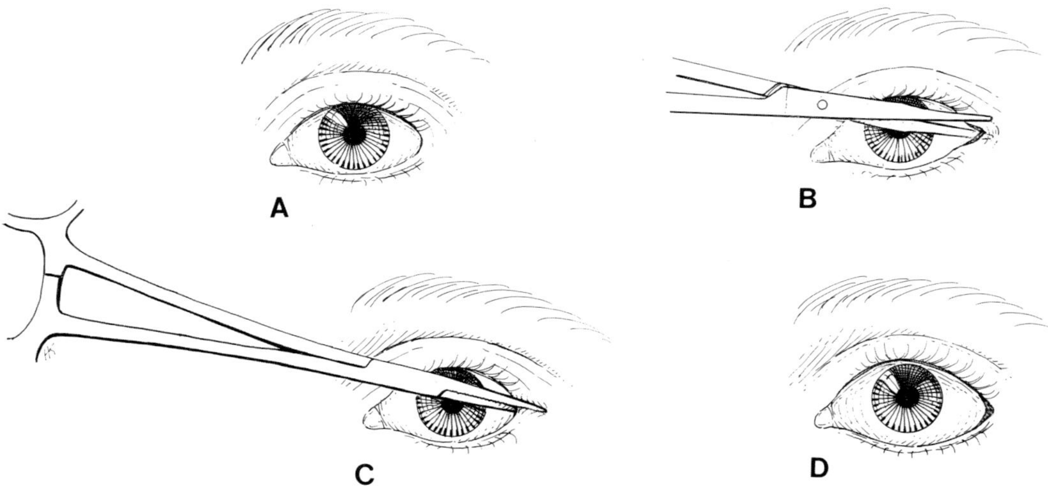

Figure 12.10 (*A*) Proptotic globe presses tightly against the eyelids. (*B*) A mosquito clamp crushes the tissues and provides hemostasis. (*C*) The canthotomy is created by cutting along the crush line with scissors. (*D*) The palpebral aperture expands permitting expansion of the swollen orbital contents.

any type of mechanical injury. This is usually a self-limited problem which resolves without compromising the eye or producing any unaesthetic side effect.

The edema may occasionally cause an inward turn of the eyelashes (trichiasis) or an entropion. This results in a mechanical corneal irritation. Liberal use of artificial tear ointments and topical antibiotic coverage is usually sufficent to protect the cornea. A protective shell, such as a bandage or soft contact lens, may occasionally be necessary for further protection. Unattended mechanical irritation of the cornea can lead to decreased or loss of vision due to extensive scarring or infection developing in the traumatized cornea.

A rare but real threat is glaucoma caused by massive edema which compresses the globe. Optic nerve compression could also result if the edema is extensive. Some of the pressure from the eyelid edema can be relieved by a lateral canthopexy (Fig. 12.10). An orbital decompression procedure must be performed if the edema is to such an extent that vision is threatened from the globe and/or optic nerve compression. Careful monitoring by the ophthalmologist is essential to help determine when to proceed with further surgical intervention.

Sharp and high velocity blunt trauma can cause lacerations, tears and avulsion injuries of the eyelids and adenexa. These injuries and their treatment have been reviewed in Chapter 4, but here we will review tears and *lacerations to the medial eyelid* area which involve the *puncta* and *canaliculi*. The trauma physician must be alert and vigilant for their occurrence. It is easy to overlook this area in a massive injury as well as to pass over a seemingly harmless nick. Careful attention in both instances will help avoid a prolonged course of constant epiphora and discomfort followed by more extensive drainage system surgery and follow-up care.

Disruption of the canaliculi requires immediate surgical repair. This should be performed within 24 hours of the injury. Only if the patient is too seriously ill to undergo the reparative procedure should a delay of more than 48 hours be tolerated. The treatment of choice is to intubate the cut ends of the canaliculi with the Quickert probes and silicone tubing.[11]

Various techniques have been described to aid the surgeon's search for the cut nasal end of the canaliculus. One suggestion has been to observe the flow of injected sterile milk through the cut distal portion of the canaliculus. Others have recommended the use of fluorescein dye or methylene blue instead of the sterile milk. We have found these dyes more of a hinderance than help, because they tend to stain not only the involved canaliculus but all the surrounding structures. The operating microscope has been most helpful in the search for a difficult-to-find cut canaliculus end. Another trick is to infiltrate the surrounding tissues with local anesthetic containing 1:100,000 or 1:200,000 epinephrine. The pinker canaliculus lumen often becomes apparent in the blanched surrounding tissue. The operating microscope is a very helpful adjunct at this point.

The other key to sucessful reapproximation of the cut canaliculus is to resuture the ends with 10-0 or 9-0 nylon or Prolene suture. The operating microscope facilitates this portion of the surgery. The surrounding tissues will come into their former anatomical positions once the cut canaliculus is resutured. These adjacent soft tissues may be reapproximated with interrupted 6-0 absorbable suture. The eyelid margin and skin wounds are carefully closed with silk suture. I prefer silk over nylon or Prolene on the skin near the eye because it is less rigid and therefore less likely to cause mechanical irritation to the globe.

The skin sutures are removed 5 days after surgery. The silicone tube remains in the canalicular-lacrimal drainage system as a closed loop for a minimum of 3 months. The closed loop is created by tying the two loose ends of the silicone in the inferior turbinate region of the nares and reinforcing it with silk suture. We remove the silicone tubing about 6 months after surgery though the tubes have been in place for as long as 9 months without any adverse effects. The tubing is removed by cutting the closed loop in the medial cul-de-sac and having the patient blow the silicone tube out through the nose. The silicone can also be withdrawn from the nose with a bayonnet foreceps.

The Veirs rod is my second choice for canalicular intubation and reapproximation. The surgical procedure is similar to that described for silicone tube intubation. The disadvantages of the Veirs rod compared to the silicone tube are: it is inflexible; a closed loop is not formed; and the rod is anchored into place with exposed sutures. The exposure of the anchor suture to the eyelid skin surface places the rod in greater jeopardy of being lost.

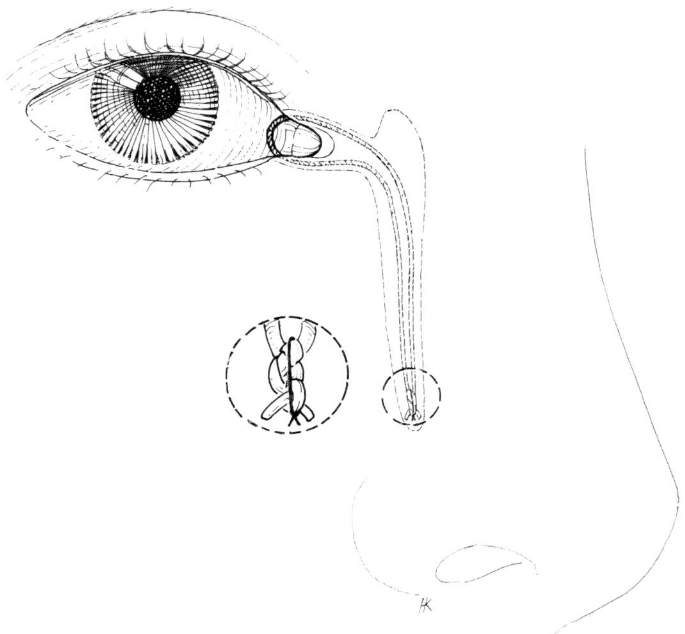

Figure 12.11 The silicone tubing in position with multiple knots and reinforcement with 4-0 silk suture.

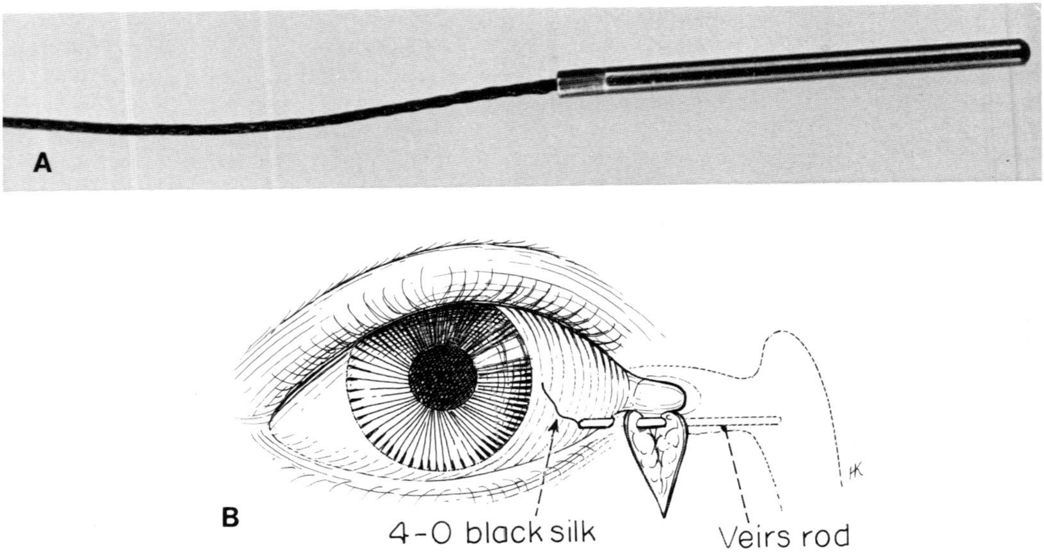

Figure 12.12 (*A*) Veirs canalicular rod with the swedged-on 4-0 silk suture. (*B*) Intubation through the inferior punctum to join the two lacerated ends of the canaliculus facilitating repair and providing reinforcement support during healing.

Another method of reapproximating the lacerated canaliculus is the use of the pigtail probe. The pigtail probe frequently facilitates finding the lacerated distal end of the canaliculus. However, false passages can and are created.[12] A silicone tube is recommended for intubation. Heavy silk suture is sometimes substituted for the silicone though it does not appear to work as well. The surgical repair is similar to previously described and illustrated procedures for the Quickert probes and silicone or the Veirs rods.

Extraocular muscle dysfunction may be uncovered in a patient shortly after an injury. The patient may voluntarily complain of diplopia or diplopia recognition may be easily elicited from the patient when the eyes are dissociated with a red glass filter (Fig. 12.13). The diplopia is frequently temporary. This may be due to muscle or periorbital edema, a slight injury to the muscle or to its innervation. These relatively minor problems will resolve in conjunction with the healing of the injured adjacent tissues. It is the chronic extraocular muscle restrictions causing diplopia because of entrapment, cicatricial leashes and paresis that concern the reconstructive surgeon.

The entrapped and restricted extraocular muscles from an orbital floor "blow-out" fracture is a familiar problem. The typical patient provides a history of blunt trauma to the eye and orbit, physical findings of restricted elevation of the involved eye, enophthalmos and hypesthesia along the inferior orbital nerve distribution, and radiologic confirmation of the fracture. Putterman, Stevens, and Urist[13] have stimulated controversy by recommending long periods of observation before surgical repair of the blow-out fractures or no repair. Review articles have pointed out that the surgical exploration and repair of these orbital floor fractures is not free of significant morbidity.[14, 15] The initial enthusiasm which followed Converse and Smith's article has been tempered.[16] Most surgeons now wait 2–4 weeks after the injury before attempting a surgical repair.

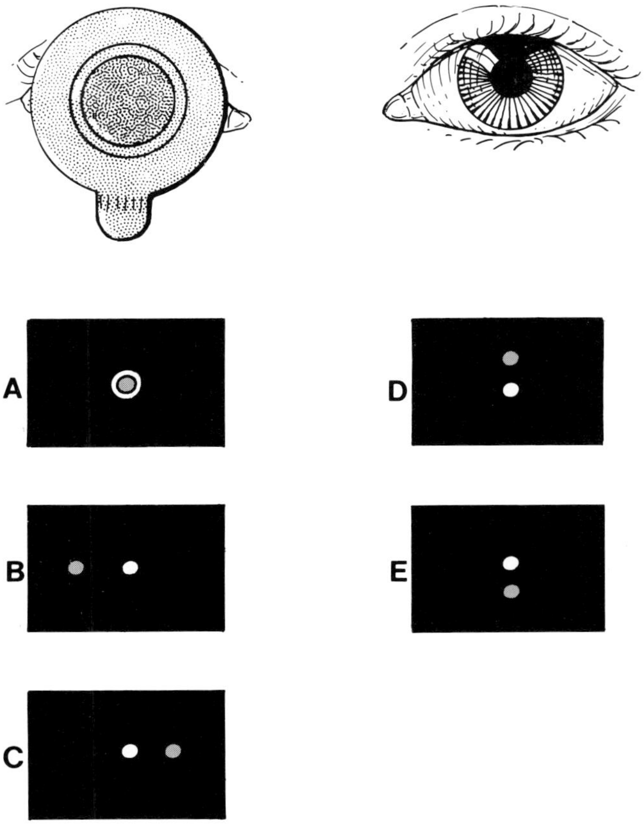

Figure 12.13 A red lens is placed before the right eye. The patient fixates on a bright white light directly before him. (*A*) If the two eyes are in normal alignment, the red image from the right eye and the white image from the left eye are *fused together*. (*B*) The image reported by the patient if the right eye is crossed inward (esotropia). (*C*) The image reported by the patient if the right eye is deviated outward (exotropia). (*D*) The image reported by the patient if the right eye is below (hypotropia) the plane of the left eye. (*E*) The image reported by the patient if the right eye is located above (hypertropia) the horizontal plane of the left eye.

This waiting period permits the acute effects of the injury to subside. Occasionally, the previously demonstrated diplopia disappears. Whether to proceed with surgery if there is no longer diplopia is left to other authors and journals to resolve. Obviously, however, surgical intervention is indicated if a positive forced duction test persists.

In the case that an operation is planned, an ophthalmologic consultation should be obtained prior to surgery. The ophthalmologist pays particular attention to any retina, optic nerve, lens and/or iris angle pathology which will have long term implications regarding visual acuity, color perception, cataract formation, and glaucoma. The patient will frequently blame the surgeon and the reparative surgery for these later ocular problems if pre-existing conditions are not pointed out to the patient prior to surgery.

A traction or forced duction test may confirm the presence of an entrapped muscle. The test must be performed following the arc of the globe and the patient must be relaxed in order for it to be valid. The traction test will occasionally "pop" free the entrapped muscle. The forced duction or traction test in experienced hands can also help differentiate between superior and inferior extraocular muscle restrictions. A superior extraocular muscle restriction is indicated if a more free excursion occurs with retroplacement of the eye while rotating the eyeball upward. An inferior extraocular muscle restriction is indicated if unusual resistance is encountered by the same maneuver.[17]

The active forced generation test will also help to differentiate between a paretic versus a restricted extraocular muscle (Fig. 12.14). The saccadic velocity is a more sophisticated test to differentiate between a palsied or paretic and a mechanically restricted muscle.[18] Most orbital injuries result in a mechanical restriction of the extraocular muscle though finding a paresis is not rare.[19] It is therefore extremely helpful in the physician-patient relationship if the patient can be told beforehand whether the repair of the orbital fracture and freeing the extraocular muscles will relieve diplopia and enophthalmos or if additional strabismus surgery is likely because the involved muscle is palsied.

Mechanical trauma can cause cicatricial problems similar to those associated with chemical injuries to the eye and orbit. A common problem would be poor eyelid apposition which could lead to exposure keratopathy, epiphora and globe injection. Malposition of the puncta would be another cause of epiphora. A scarred and shortened conjunctiva could result in diplopia in certain fields of gaze.

Penetrating and perforating injuries to the eye are managed by the ophthalmic surgeon. These injuries must be repaired as quickly as possible in order to preserve as much vision and the eye. The details concerning this area of patient management are beyond the scope of this chapter. However, it is extremely important for all the surgical specialist involved in the management of such a seriously injured patient to remind the anesthesiologist to NOT USE SUCCINYLCHOLINE during the intubation process of general anesthesia. The use of such a polarizing agent will result in further extrusion of intraocular contents through the wound when the extraocular muscles go into tetany and raise the intraocular pressure.

The iris and its insertion into the trabecular meshwork-ciliary body complex are very prone to injury from blunt trauma. The most obvious and frequent injury is a *hyphema.* Prompt ophthalmological care is necessary. Such measures as hospitalization, strict bedrest with the head elevated, bilateral eye patching, frequent monitoring of the intraocular pressure, systemic and topical medication to control an elevated intraocular pressure, and/or intraocular removal of the hyphema clot may be required.

Other injuries may include iris dialysis, disinsertion of the iris root, and/or angle recession. Diagnosis and determination of the extent of these injuries often require special gonioscopic and slit lamp examination. A hyphema or these other injuries may not cause any immediate detrimental effects to the eye or visual acuity. However, these patients should be advised to have regular ophthalmologic care as their injured eyes are more prone to glaucoma, lens, vitreous and retinal problems in later years.

An obvious result of an iris injury is the dilated or mydriatic pupil. This may be temporary or become a permanent defect due to an iris sphincter tear. Amblyopia may develop in the child under the age of 9 with an injured eye which has a mydriatic pupil. Full maturation of formed vision does not occur until age 8–9. An injured eye with mydriasis may have diminished focusing ability and a child is prone to ignore the use of this affected eye. Such a child will need regular monitoring of the visual acuity and amblyopia therapy if this proves necessary.

A sphincter tear as previously described will cause anisocoria or unequal pupils. This contrast in pupil size is more readily noticeable in patients with light colored irides. If the pupil diameter is large and/or the iris loss is marked, disabling photophobia may result. A tinted contact lens can often alleviate the symptoms of photophobia and mask the anisocoria.

Dislocation or subluxation (partial dislocation) of the lens can occur with mechanical trauma. Decreased visual acuity accompanies either condition. An ophthalmic consultant with close follow-up care is necessary.

Vitreous hemorrhage, intraretinal bleeding and/or surface retinal hemorrhage may be discovered following mechanical trauma. Retinal detachment solely from trauma has a low incidence.[20] However, traction retinal detachment from fibrotic bands due to previous hemorrhage is a definite later complication of trauma.

The eye, in all its glorious delicacy needs an astute clinician to salvage its anatomy.

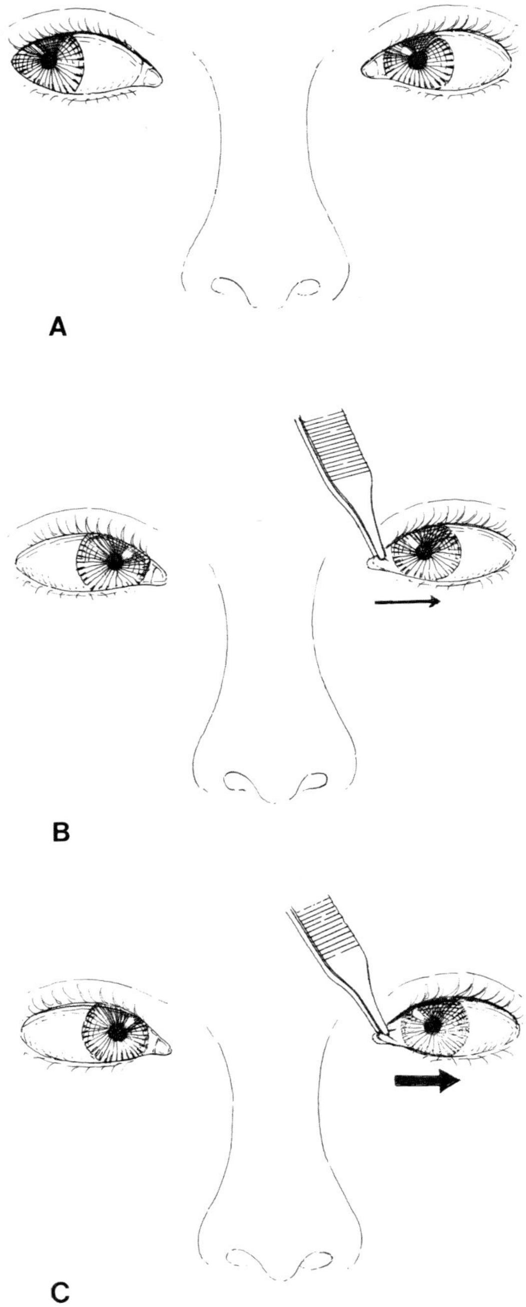

Figure 12.14 Active forced generation test. The patient has difficulty abducting (lateral movement) the left eye. This test helps determine if the etiology is a paresis or a mechanical restriction. (*A*) Both eyes gaze to the right without difficulty. A fine tooth foreceps (e.g. Bishop-Harmon) grasps the globe and conjunctiva securely near the limbus (junction of the cornea and conjunctiva). The patient is asked to gaze to the *left* quickly. (*B*) In a paresis, there is little tugging on the forecep as the eye "floats" to the left in abduction. (*C*) On the other hand, mechanical restrictive problems characteristically generate a strong abduction (lateral) movement creating a firm tug on the foreceps.

References

1. Choy, A. E., Marglis, S., Breinin, G. M., and McCarthy, J. G.: Analysis of preoperative and postoperative extraocular muscle function in surgical translocation of bony orbits; a preliminary report, in *Symposium on Diagnosis and Treatment of Craniofacial Anomalies, Vol. XX*, p. 128. C. V. Mosby, St. Louis, 1979.
2. Crawford, J. S.: Preserved Fascia Lata Bank, Department of Ophthalmology, Hospital for Sick Children, University of Toronto, Toronto, Canada.
3. Crawford, J. S.: A new instrument to help separate and obtain fascia lata. *American Society of Ophthalmic Plastic and Reconstructive Surgery, 10th Annual Scientific Symposium*, 1979 (in press).
4. Beard, C.: *Ptosis*, p. 139. C. V. Mosby, St. Louis, 1976.
5. Fox, S. A.: *Ophthalmic Plastic Surgery*, p. 364. Grune & Stratton, New York, 1976.
6. Callahan, A.: *Surgery of the Eye: Diseases*, p. 25. Charles C Thomas, Springfield, Ill., 1956.
7. Walsh, F. B., and Hoyt, W. F.: *Clinical Neuro-opthalmology, Vol. III*, pp. 2480–2482. Williams & Wilkins, Baltimore, 1969.
8. Burns, R. P., Foster, R. K., Laibson, P. K., and Gipson, I. K.: Cronic toxicity of local anesthetics on the cornea, in *Symposium on Ocular Therapy, Vol. X*, p. 31, edited by I. H. Leopold and R. P. Burns. John Wiley & Sons, New York, 1977.
9. Choy, A. E., Asbell, R., and Taterka, H.: Symblepharon repair using a silicone sheet implant. *Ann. Ophthalmol.*, *9:*197, 1977.
10. Kurz, C. H., and Einaugler, R. B.: Cataract secondary to microwave radiation. *Am. J. Ophthalmol.*, *66:* 866, 1968.
11. Quickert, M. H., and Dryden, R. M.: Probes for intubation in lacrimal drainage. *Trans. Am. Acad. Ophthalmol. Otolaryngol.*, *74:*431, 1970.
12. Saunders, D. H., Shannon, G. M., and Flanagan, J. C.: The effectiveness of the pigtail probe method of repairing canalicular lacerations. *Ophthalmic Surg.*, *9:* 33, 1978.
13. Putterman, A. M., Stevens, T., and Urist, M. J.: Nonsurgical management of blowout fractures of the orbital floor. *Am. J. Ophthalmol.*, *77:*232, 1974.
14. Milauskas, A. T.: *Diagnosis and Management of Blowout Fractures of the Orbit with Clinical, Radiological and Surgical Aspects.* Charles C Thomas, Springfield, Ill., 1969.
15. Emery, J. M., von Noorden, G. K., and Schlernitauer, D. A.: Management of orbital floor fractures. *Am. J. Ophthalmol.*, *74:*299, 2972.
16. Converse, J. M., and Smith, B.: Enophthalmos and diplopia in fracture of the orbital floor. *Br. J. Plast. Surg.*, *9:*265, 1957.
17. Scott, A. B.: The superior oblique tendon sheath syndrome. Differential diagnosis of deficient elevation in adduction. In *Orthoptics—Past, Present, Future*, pp. 463–485, edited by S. Moore, J. Mein and L. Stockbridge. Symposia Specialists, New York, 1976.
18. Metz, H. S., Scott, W. E., Madson, E., and Scott, A. B.: Saccadic velocity and active force studies in blowout fractures of the orbit. *Am. J. Ophthalmol.*, *78:* 665, 1974.
19. Scott, W. E.: Differential diagnosis of vertical muscle palsies, in *Symposium on Strabismus, Transactions of the New Orleans Academy of Ophthalmology*, pp. 118–134. C. V. Mosby, St. Louis, 1978.
20. Duke-Elder, S., and Dobree, J. H.: Diseases of the Retina. In *Systems of Ophthalmology, Vol. X*, p. 784. Henry Kimpton, London, 1967.

CHAPTER 13

Surgical Procedures for Diseases of the Neck

Fred R. Eilber, M.D., F.A.C.S., and
F. Kristian Storm III, M.D., F.A.C.S.

Diseases of the head and neck range from local infections to malignant tumors. Within this range are the congenital malfunctions and the benign tumors. Some of the infections, and malfunctions and nearly all of the tumors will require complex surgical procedures. Although malignant tumors do arise in the head and neck, most operative procedures in this area are the result of metastases from other primary sites. This chapter will briefly discuss the more insidious infections and malfunctions that can require surgical techniques and will illustrate the location and procedures for the radical dissections required for treatment of neoplasia of the head and neck.

ANATOMY

The anatomy of the neck is often confusing because so many vital structures are contained in such a small area. This fact leaves little margin for error, and makes a sound understanding of the normal neck anatomy absolutely mandatory for accurate diagnosis and treatment.

A key to the understanding of neck anatomy rests in the "triangles" from which the location of vital structures can be related (Fig. 13.1). The "anterior triangle" is bordered by the strap muscles, the posterior belly of the digastric, and the sternocleidomastoid, and contains the internal jugular vein, carotid artery and vagus nerve. The "posterior triangle" is bordered by the sternocleidomastoid, the trapezius and clavicle, and contains the accessory nerve, phrenic nerve and brachial plexus. The "digastric triangle" is bordered by the anterior and posterior bellies of the digastric muscle and horizontal ramus of the mandible, and contains the marginal mandibular branch of the facial nerve, lingual nerve and hypoglossal nerve. All congenital and acquired diseases, infectious and neoplastic processes occurring within the neck can be related to these landmarks.

These investigations were supported by grant CA12582 from the National Cancer Institute (DHEW) and Medical Research Service of the Veterans Administration.

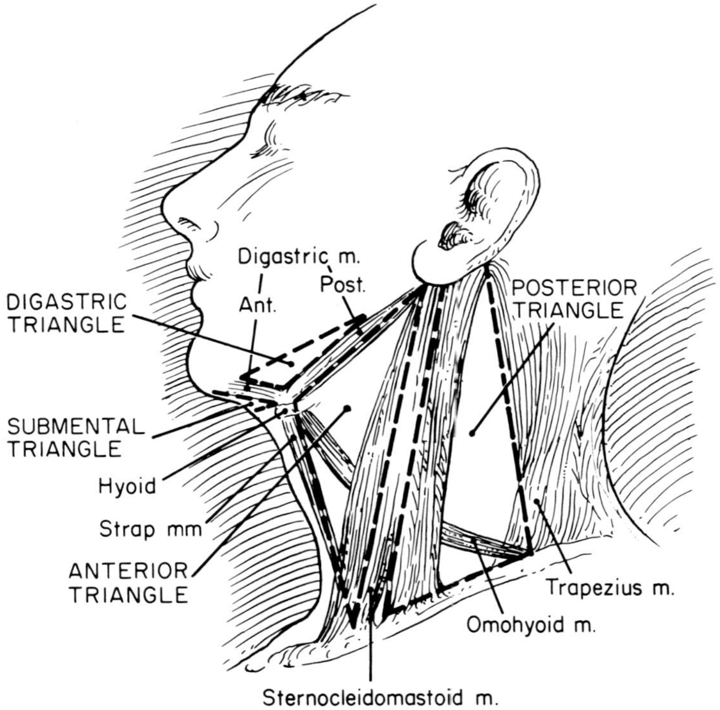

Figure 13.1 The "triangles" of the neck anatomy.

Lymphatics

Rouviere subdivided the cervical lymph nodes into 10 basic groups and described their lymphatic tributaries. These groups may be conceptualized as a superior horizontal chain about the base of the skull and mandible, a vertical chain in the mid-neck, and a horizontal chain in the supraclavicular region, resembling the capital letter "I." The major areas of lymphatic shed to the various lymph node groups and chains must be appreciated before undertaking a primary tumor workup, as nodal metastases generally follow a predictable route of spread (Fig. 13.2).

The *superior horizontal chain* contains the submental, submandibular, parotid, posterior-auricular and occipital groups of lymph nodes. These nodes receive drainage from all cutaneous areas of the head, the parotid gland, gums, anterior floor of the mouth and anterior tongue.

The *internal jugular chain* receives afferent lymphatic shed from the superior horizontal chain, and is also the direct lymphatic shed of the nasal fossa, middle ear, pharynx, palate, posterior tongue, larynx, cords, all major salivary glands, thyroid and parathyroid glands.

The *transverse cervical chain* lays at the base of the neck and contains the "scalene nodes," named for their proximity to this muscle. These nodes receive lymphatic drainage from the internal jugular chain and may eventually become diseased from progressive metastatic spread of any head and neck neoplasm. However, isolated involvement of these lymph nodes is most often from primary disease located below the base of the neck, from the upper extremities, breast, lung, esophagus, stomach and pancreas.

CONGENITAL DISEASES OF THE NECK

Abnormal development of the branchial arches may result in cysts, sinuses or fistulas within the neck. Remnants of the first branchial arch may result in a small *preauricular sinus* or *fistula* extending into the temporomandibular joint or nasopharnygeal cavity. An undeveloped second arch may result in a branchial *cyst* or *fistula* commonly found along the anterior border of the sternocleidomastoid muscle in the mid- or low-neck. Simple cysts can be easily excised because they seldom adhere to surrounding tissue. However, deep sinuses or fistulas often require long and tedious dissection for complete removal. Branchial fistulas presenting within the suprasternal notch may extend between the internal and external carotid arteries before reaching the oropharynx.

A persistent *thyroglossal duct* or *cyst* may result from abnormal development of the median thyroid anlage. These remnants present in the midline, at or below the hyoid bone, and may extend to the base of the tongue. Resection of the mid-third of the hyoid bone is almost always required for complete excision. Since the rare lingual thyroid also may present as a small mass in the area of the vestigial foramen cecum, a thyroid scan is recommended prior to resection of masses in this area to ensure adequate thyroid tissue in the neck.

Congenital vascular or lymphatic anomalies also may appear as neck masses. Immature "strawberry" hemagiomas appear in infancy and may undergo marked enlargement over the first several months of life. However, these lesions usually regress spontaneously and surgical therapy is rarely, if ever, warranted. Conversely the *cavernous hemangioma* is often fully developed

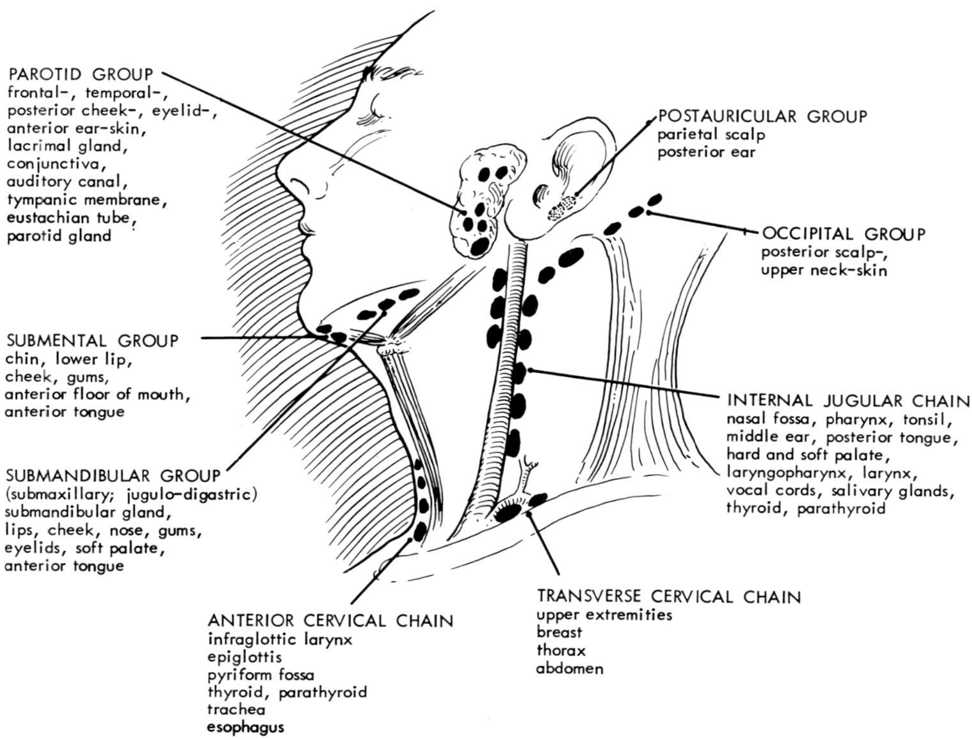

Figure 13.2 The lymph node groups and chains.

at birth and is not subject to dramatic growth changes. These lesions often involve deep structures, such as muscle or nerves, and may contain lymphangiomatous elements. They may regress on prednisone therapy although wide surgical excision may be required.[4] The *cystic hygroma* is a benign overgrowth of lymphatic channels and multilocular cysts formed during fetal development. These masses are soft and can be transluminated. Although surgical excision may be the most expedient form of therapy, particular care must be exercised in order to avoid sacrifice of normal tissue.

ACQUIRED DISEASES OF THE NECK

Several acquired diseases most commonly of pharyngoesophageal or vascular origin may present as neck masses.

Zenker's diverticulum presenting as a mid-neck mass, more often on the left, is probably caused by incoordinated ataxic muscular contractions during swallowing. The sac protrudes between the inferior pharyngeal constriction and cricopharyngeus muscles, and may achieve great size. Surgical intervention is warranted in cases of dysphagia, hoarseness, regurgitation and aspiration. In general, one-stage diverticulectomy is preferred for larger lesions, and cricopharyngeal myotomy for smaller lesions. In critically ill and malnourished patients, diverticulopexy may be considered.

Rare *vascular anomalies* also may account for a mass in the neck, and can include aneurysms of the carotid or vertebral systems, and tortuosity of the internal carotid artery. These patients usually seek medical attention for symptoms related to embolic or thrombotic cerebral compromise. These masses are often pulsatile with a bruit, and are best defined by angiography.

Trauma is the most frequently acquired disease of the neck. Blunt trauma may cause fracture of the larynx or massive hematoma with attendant upper airway obstruction. In these cases, tracheostomy may be lifesaving. Penetrating trauma, in the form of stab wounds or gunshot wounds, are becoming ever more common in urban society. In general, any wound that penetrates the platysma muscle should be explored in the operating room with the patient intubated under general anesthesia. Minor wounds may be explored initially under local anesthesia in the emergency department; however, once it is determined that the platysma muscle has been penetrated, the wound should be covered and the patient transported to a complete operating facility. In unusual cases, arteriography, venography, radiography with water-soluble contrast material and triple endoscopy may be helpful in determining the extent of injury.

INFECTIOUS DISEASES OF THE NECK

Cervical Adenitis

Inflammatory involvement of the cervical lymph nodes was once the most common abnormality in the head and neck region. Today, however, it accounts for less than 10% of the neck masses in patients presenting for treatment. Even so, persistent, firm and tender cervical lymph nodes should alert the physician to the possibility of staphylococcus or tuberculous adenitis. Correct diagnosis and treatment require needle aspirate or incisional biopsies for culture and sensitivity. A history of tuberculosis or possible exposure to nonpasteurized milk or infection of the oral pharynx should alert the physician to a possible diagnosis of tuberculosis.

Lugwig's Angina

Flagrant cellulitis about the head and neck from a primary source of infection in the submental peritonsillar retropharyngeal space has been classified as Lugwig's angina. Although this condition is rare today, it presents as a frightening, rapidly progressive swelling associated with speech difficulty and airway problems. The condition is most often caused by an anaerobic infection, and most commonly *Fusobacterium necrophorum.* This infection is dangerous because the swelling or direct extension of the submental space involving the epiglottis, or in the retropharyngeal space can cause evident mediastinitis. Prompt treatment with antibiotics or, in some instances, incision and drainage through the upper neck is required. Occasionally intubation or tracheostomy may be necessary.

Glandular Infection

Acute suppurative parotitis is most commonly observed in the newborn or in debilitated and dehydrated elderly patients.[6] The diagnosis is usually self-evident—marked swelling, tenderness and elevated temperature. Its cause is the common pathologic organism, *Staphylococcus aureus*. Prompt treatment includes efforts at improved oral hygiene with irrigations, adequate hydration, culture and sensitivity tests of any exudate from Stensen's duct. If the disease is detected early (less than 12 hours after onset) external irradiation therapy at low dose has been of some use. However, since most cases are seen at later stages in development, radiation therapy is of little or no value and incision and drainage may be required for control of infection. Multiple incisions made through the facial skin parallel to the facial nerve branches or elevating the usual parotid incision and subsequent deeper incisions parallel to the facial nerve may be required. Chronic parotitis is rare and some authors advocate superficial parotidectomy for this condition.[3]

Submandibular Infections

Infections of the submandibular gland usually manifest as chronic sialadenitis. Soft tissue x-rays of the neck often reveal calcifications. The proper management of this condition is biopsy and in most instances complete surgical excision of the entire submaxillary gland is the preferred method of therapy. The patient should be assured that this condition is benign.

BENIGN TUMORS OF THE NECK

Lipomas

The most common benign tumor of the head and neck region is the lipoma. This has never been known to metastasize. However, it is imperative to differentiate it from the malignant liposarcoma. Complete surgical excision of lipomas results in a cure rate of 95% even for very large tumors. On presentation, if the tumor is firm, an incisional biopsy should be performed to obtain a histologic diagnosis prior to definitive therapy.

Neuroma

Neurofibromas can and do occur in the neck and are treated by complete surgical removal of the tumor. Myelograms to rule out extension into the cervical *foramina* and spinal canal are advisable prior to surgical excision.

Chemodectoma

This is a nonchromaffin paraganglioma tumor which is termed a carotid body tumor. This tumor often presents as an asymptomatic painless mass in the neck and the tumors in the area of the jugular bulb should be considered as possibly being chemodectoma. Angiogram is diagnostic. Metastases are rare and the tumors are usually benign. The disease may be familial and also bilateral. Subadventitial surgical approach excision of this lesion is the preferred method of therapy.

Paragangliomas

The glomus jugularity is a paraganglionic tumor involving the vagus nerve. In some instances high epinephrine or norepinephrine levels have been reported. The difficulty in management of these tumors is the intervascular extension and danger of tumor thrombus in the jugular vein and extension into the middle cranial fossa. This tumor should be considered in patients who present with impairment of cranial nerves IX, X and XI. Weakness of cranial nerves VII, VIII and XII indicate probable intracranial extension. Surgical resection of these tumors is sometimes warranted and requires a combined cranial and cervical approach.

TREATMENT TECHNIQUES

Biopsy

Biopsy is a prerequisite to treatment of tumors of the head or neck. Various methods and techniques are available for the biopsy of cervical lymph nodes or cervical masses. Accurate diagnosis is impossible without a nondistorted tissue sample for histologic examination. There are three common techniques, the needle, the incisional, and the excisional biopsy. Thin needle biopsy can provide accurate diagnosis of many of the neck masses. However, this technique requires a pathologist who has experience with specimens. The other two techniques, the incisional and the excisional biopsy, require a physician who is very familiar with all the operative procedures of the head and neck in order to plan for and to place the incision within the area of future excision. The biopsy scar must be excised with the definitive procedure. The excisional biopsy should not be considered unless the mass is less than 2 cm in size. Excisional biopsy of the larger masses often results in extended local procedures, hematomas, and wound contamination, all of which complicate subsequent definitive management.[8]

Clinical Evaluation

When evaluating patients who present with cervical lymph node enlargement, it is important to relate the exact location of the lymph node enlargement in the neck to the cervical triangles. The location of the lymph nodes and the areas of primary drainage are shown in Figure 13.2. With this knowledge a careful search for the primary can be undertaken. In general, enlarged lymph nodes in the lower one-third of the neck or the supraclavicular area are indicative of tumor below the clavical that could include metastases from a primary malignant tumor in the lung, stomach, pancreas, or kidney. For midline masses, a thyroid scan is indicated. Enlarged lymph nodes in the higher cervical chains, either anteriorly or posteriorly, require a search for a primary tumor of head or neck.

This search includes a meticulous inspection of the oral cavity, hypopharynx and larynx by indirect laryngoscopy. Nasopharyngeal examination either with a mirror or preferably with a nasopharyngoscope also is indicated. If a mass or lesion is visualized in this area, a biopsy should be performed. If no lesion is visualized by careful head and neck examination, it is reasonable to perform an incisional biopsy of the neck node. After histologic evaluation and if the pathologist determines the cause as lymphoma or cervical adenitis, then the examination is complete. However, if the diagnosis is squamous cell carcinoma, additional evaluation of the primary by direct laryngoscopy must be carried out. This examination includes careful visualization and palpation of the oral cavity, hypopharynx and larynx. If no lesion can be visualized, blind biopsies of the nasopharynx, tonsil and base of the tongue are indicated as these are the most common sites of occult primary carcinomas.

Staging of Nodal Metastases in the Neck

The surgeon will find that knowledge of the stage of the lymph node involvement in the cervical region is useful. The classification devised by the M. D. Anderson Tumor Institute is easily performed and provides useful information.[5] The standard nomenclature and classification is given in Table 13.1. The classification system is based on the pathologic observation that if a lymph node has enlarged to 3 cm then tumor is no longer confined to the node but has invaded the perinodal tissue. Furthermore, these observations have shown that multiple lymph node involvement or fixed nodes indicate a poor prognosis.

RADICAL NECK DISSECTION

Principles

The radical neck dissection removes the cervical lymphatic channels and glands in order to eradicate regional metastatic disease. As originally described by Crile, the dissection was

Table 13.1
Clinical Staging of Cervical Lymph Node Metastases

N_0 =	negative
N_x =	single node excised
N_1 =	single node <3 cm
N_{2A} =	single node >3 cm (not fixed)
N_{2B} =	multiple unilateral nodes
N_{3A} =	unilateral fixed nodes
N_{3B} =	bilateral nodes

usually performed after the primary tumor was controlled by radiation therapy. However, theory today dictates that resection of the primary cancer and neck dissection occur simultaneously either *incontinuity* or *en bloc*. Parotidectomy combined with cervical lymph node dissection, composite resections and *commando operations* are examples of such treatment. Radiation therapy, either pre- or postoperatively, has become an adjuvant to surgical therapy.

The neck dissection, as usually performed, begins with ligation of the internal jugular vein at the *base of the neck*, and proceeds from inferior to superior. However, we have found that this procedure often results in unnecessary hemorrhage during dissection due to venous engorgement from outflow obstruction. As an alternative, we prefer early ligation of the internal jugular vein at the *base of the skull*, and a dissection carried out from superior to inferior. The latter approach markedly decreases intraoperative bleeding and transfusions have been rarely, if ever, required. This method will be described.

PROCEDURE

In order to achieve adequate exposure of the operative area, the patient is placed in a 15° semi-Fowler position to lessen venous engorgement and attendant blood loss. Care must be used because the greater head elevations increase the risk of an air embolus. The "head-drape" exposes the tip of the ear lobe. The corner of the mouth also may be exposed if extensive dissection of the facial nerve is expected in order to allow assessment of nerve continuity by "nerve stimulation" if required.

Several types of incisions have been used for the radical neck dissection (Fig. 13.3). As with any flap subject to necrosis, efforts must be directed toward the creation of pedicles with the widest possible base and the fewest acute angles. The procedure becomes critical when

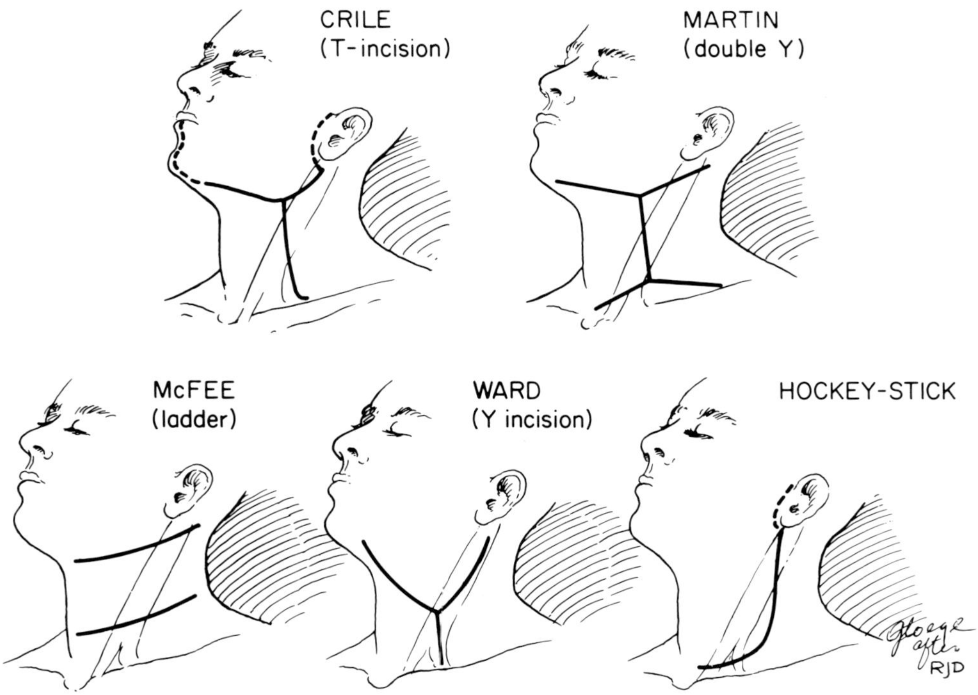

Figure 13.3 Various incisions used for radical neck dissections.

dissection is done after the tissue has been subject to irradiation. Should necrosis occur within the neck flap, the resultant exposure of the carotid artery may well result in death of the patient. For this reason, we prefer the "hockey stick" or "MacFee" incisions. The "hockey stick" incision is particularly useful when bilateral neck dissections are indicated, or when neck dissection is combined with parotidectomy or thyroidectomy (Fig. 13.4). The incision is carried through skin, subcutaneous tissue and platysma muscle. Flaps are created by sharp dissection in the loose areolar tissue plane immediately underneath the platysma: superior to the mandible, anterior to the strap muscles, posterior to the trapezius and inferior to the clavicle.

The deep dissection is begun by incising the fascia overlying the anterior and posterior bellies of the digastric muscle, and dividing and ligating the facial artery and posterior facial vein. This fascia, containing the marginal mandibular branch of the facial nerve, is swept superiorly and out of the field of dissection (Fig. 13.5). The submandibular gland is separated from the posterior border of the mylohyoid muscle, and with this muscle retracted, resection of all contents of the digastric triangle is performed with care to preserve the lingual and hypoglossal nerves lying on the floor of the triangle. The dissection is continued posteriorly across the tail of the parotid gland to include the lower parotid lymph nodes. The sternocleidomastoid (SCM) muscle is divided at the mastoid process by cautery, using the deeper splenius muscle with its abrupt change in muscle fiber direction as a guide to completion of transection. The accessory nerve and internal jugular vein are then divided and ligated near the base of the skull. The dissection is carried inferiorly along the border of the trapezius muscle by incising the superficial and deep layers of the deep cervical fascia. The omohoid muscle and SCM muscle are divided by cautery near the clavicle, and the internal jugular vein is divided and ligated one centimeter from its junction with the subclavian vein (Fig. 13.6).

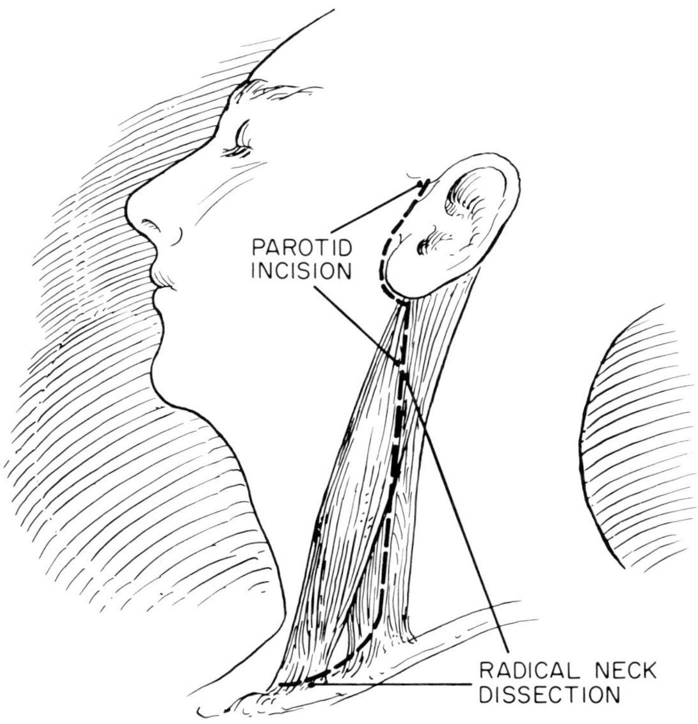

Figure 13.4 The "hockey stick" incision for parotidectomy and neck dissection.

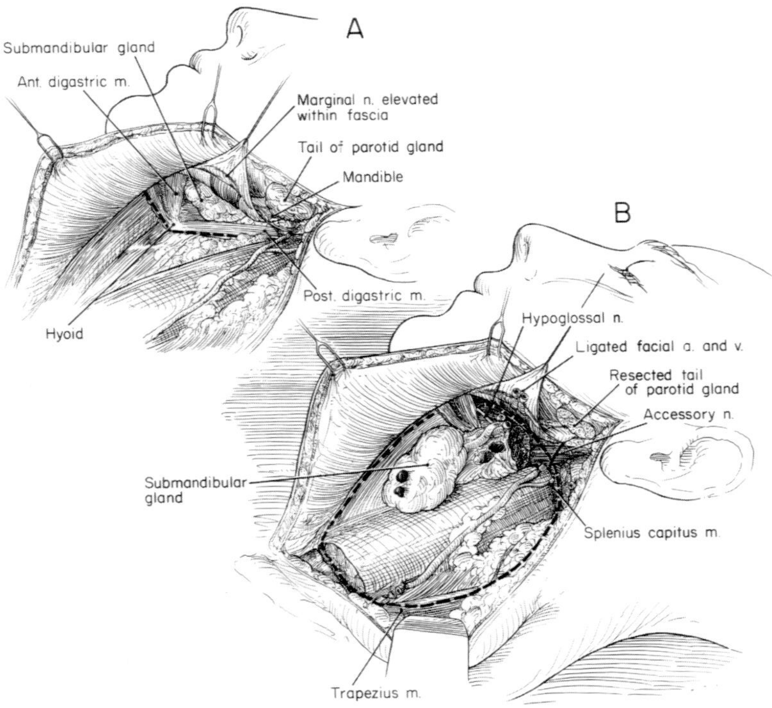

Figure 13.5 The deep dissection—the fascia is swept from the field.

This procedure can be modified to preserve the SCM muscle, jugular vein and accessory nerve, particularly if no clinically evident nodal metastases are present. This modification may be accomplished easily, but will result in some prolongation of the operative time. Rather than transect these structures, the fascia of the SCM muscle is incised and dissected from the muscle which then is retracted from the field. The deeper fascia surrounding the jugular vein is likewise incised in a subadventitial plane and allowed to remain with the specimen. The accessory nerve is identified either at the border of the trapezius or over the proximal jugular vein, is dissected free and preserved (Fig. 13.7). With this "modified neck dissection," all fascia and node-bearing tissue may be adequately resected while preserving function and adding to the cosmetic result.

The resection is completed by placing the specimen on tension and dissecting from posterior to anterior in the plane just superficial to the levator muscle and brachial plexus. The phrenic nerve is identified and the several cervical sensory branches sacrificed. The dissection is continued to the carotid artery. The vagus nerve is identified and preserved; however, the ansa cervicalis may be sacrificed. Continuing medially, the omohyoid muscle is divided at the hyoid bone and the specimen is resected from the strap muscles, completing the dissection (Fig. 13.6).

One or two closed suction drains are left in place and the wound is closed in two layers. The drains are removed when output becomes serous and is less than 50 ml per day.

Combined Superficial Parotidectomy and Neck Dissection

Removing the parotid lymph nodes is an integral part of staging and therapy for many highly malignant cutaneous neoplasms of the face, ear and scalp.[9] These lymph nodes can be

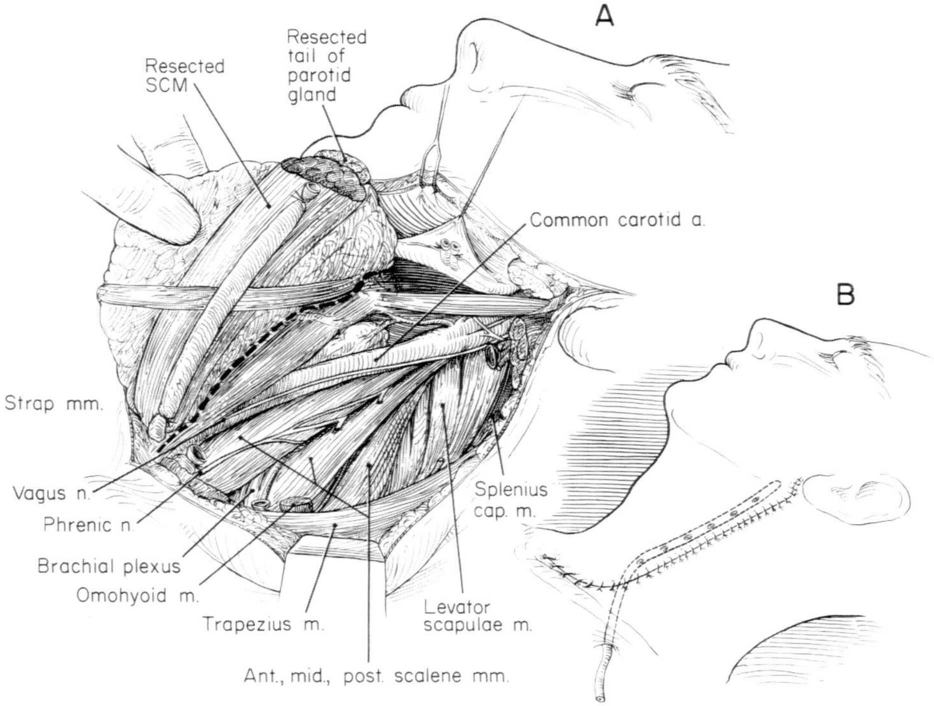

Figure 13.6 The internal jugular vein is divided and ligated 1 cm from its junction with the subclavian vein.

removed by performing a superficial parotidectomy in combination with the radical neck dissection.[1]

PROCEDURE

A reverse "J" incision is made anterior to the ear, from above the tragus to below the ear lobe, which may be extended into the "hockey stick" incision used for neck dissection. Sharp and blunt dissection is used just anterior to the tragus until the junction of the cartilaginous and bony portions of the external auditory canal is identified. The common facial nerve is located just inferior and anterior to this point. Each branch of the nerve is serially identified and preserved as the superficial parotid lobe is resected, proceeding from posterior to anterior (Fig. 13.8). Alternatively, the common facial nerve may be found by first identifying its marginal mandibular branch as it passes *under* the posterior facial vein at the border of the mandible, then dissecting in a retrograde manner to the main nerve trunk.

The marginal mandibular nerve is always at risk of injury during these procedures. While the course of this nerve varies, it is *always* above a line drawn between the external auditory canal and the inferior border of the posterior belly of the digastric muscle. It should be remembered that this nerve is usually located more inferiorly than expected, often as low as 1 cm below the horizontal ramus and angle of the mandible. Extreme caution therefore should be used in this area.

Once the gland is resected from the facial nerve, an in continuity neck dissection may be combined as described.

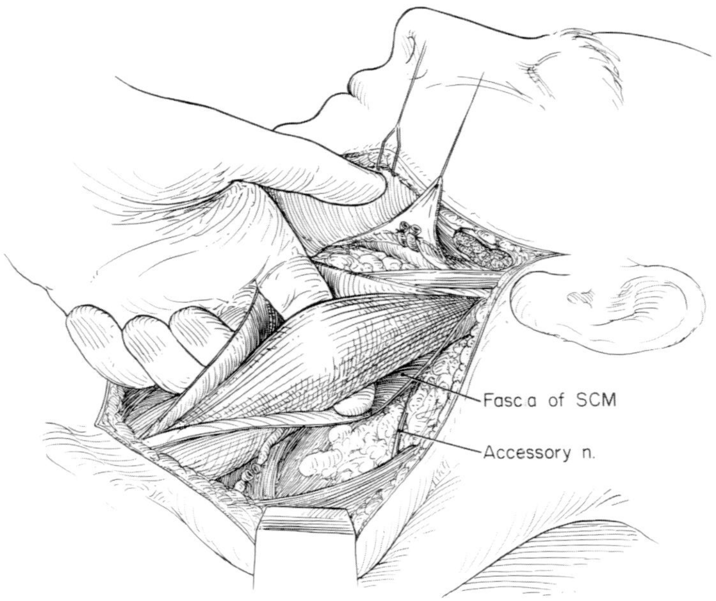

Figure 13.7 The accessory nerve is identified, dissected free and preserved.

Partial Neck Dissections

In selected cases, less than a standard neck dissection may be warranted. These *partial* neck dissections are designed to remove only the first eschelon lymph nodes draining a particular site and are most often used for disease staging.

The "subdigastric" neck dissection removes the entire contents of the digastric triangle (Fig. 13.4), and is useful for staging lesions that drain to the submandibular group of lymph nodes. A subdigastric dissection often is combined with a "submental" dissection for lesions that drain to the submental lymph nodes.

The "supraomohyoid" neck dissection removes the contents of the digastric triangle, and anterior and posterior triangles above the omohyoid muscle to include the submandibular and upper internal jugular lymph nodes. The dissection provides staging of lesions draining to the superior horizontal chain.

The "anterior" neck dissection removes the contents of the digastric and anterior triangles, as far back as the internal jugular vein, and often is combined with superficial parotidectomy for staging lesions draining to the parotid group of lymph nodes. This dissection does not remove the anterior cervical lymph node chain, although it can be combined with such a dissection bilaterally for malignant lesions of the thyroid, the so-called "jugular-to-jugular" neck dissection.

The "posterior" neck dissection removes the contents of the posterior triangle, and is useful for staging posterior ear and scalp lesions. It often is combined with an "occipital" dissection for lesions of the occipital scalp.

Results of Cervical Lymph Node Dissection

Numerous factors must be considered in evaluating the efficacy of the standard or modified radical neck dissection for neoplastic disease of the head and neck. The ability to control

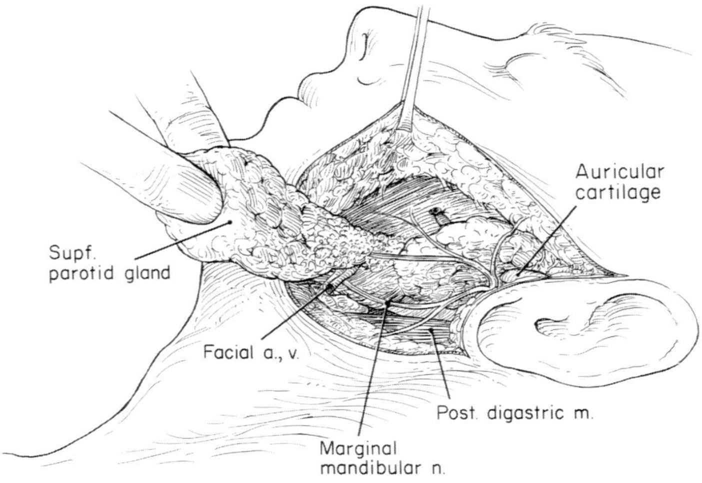

Figure 13.8 The common facial nerve is identified and preserved as the parotid lobe is resected.

tumor if this is the primary site is of paramount importance. However, the histologic type of the neoplasm is of major import as well. For example, several large series indicate that the results achieved with neck dissections for patients with squamous cell disease who have multiple lymph node involvement, lymph nodes that are greater than 3 cm in size or fixed nodes have from 40 to 60% local recurrence in the neck.[2, 5, 7] Furthermore, 20% of these patients may have recurrence in the opposite neck with stage N_2 or N_3 disease. The results of primary radiation therapy for stage N_2 or N_3 cervical disease are equally disappointing in that a 50 or 60% local recurrence rate is reported. However, recent studies for N_2 or N_3 cervical disease have shown that the combination of surgery and radiation to the involved neck has reduced the local recurrence to 10–20%.[7] The advantages derived from pre- or postoperative radiation seem to be equivalent. Postoperative radiation certainly is more appealing from a surgical standpoint because the incisions can be done in unaltered skin. As stated earlier, if the neck dissections must be performed on previously irradiated patients, extreme care must be taken to ensure coverage of the carotid artery as exposure of this artery almost surely will result in carotid rupture, which has a 95% mortality. Originally, the rationale for the radical neck dissection was based on the hypothesis that en bloc removal of the cervical lymph nodes, jugular vein, and SCM muscle would eliminate local recurrence in the neck. It now is clear that the local recurrence rate with N_2 or N_3 squamous cell carcinoma of the neck is extremely high. Many authors have advocated modified neck procedures which either preserved the SCM muscle or nerve XI and the jugular vein or any combination thereof feeling that the cosmetic and functional results are far superior to a radical neck dissection. This surgical approach would seem reasonable for squamous cell disease if lymph node involvement is minimal and pre- or postoperative radiation is contemplated. This modified procedure also may be applicable for neck dissections for thyroid cancer, as the results appear to be equal with those from radical neck dissection.

Finally, in elective dissections for melanoma with nonpalpable disease, the reported results appear to be equivalent to those from the radical neck dissections. It is most important to recognize that patients treated with the modified neck dissections must have either radiation therapy or, in the case of thyroid disease, hormonal therapy, in addition to the modified surgical procedure.

References

1. Ballantyne, A. J.: Malignant melanoma of the skin of the head and neck. *Am. J. Surg.*, *120*:425, 1970.
2. Barrie, J. R., Knapper, W. H., and Strong, E. W.: Cervical nodal metastasis of unknown origin. *Am. J. Surg.*, *120*:466, 1970.
3. Costerline, P. F., and Jaques, D. A.: The surgical management of recurrent parotitis. *Surg. Gynecol. Obstet.*, *146*:419, 1978.
4. Edgerton, M. T.: The treatment of hemangiomas. *Ann. Surg.*, *183*:517, 1976.
5. Jesse, R. H.: The philosophy of treatment of neck nodes. *Ear Nose Throat J.*, *56*:58, 1977.
6. Kaban, L. B., Mulliken, J. B., and Murray, J. E.: Sialadenitis in childhood. *Am. J. Surg.*, *135*:570, 1978.
7. Perez, C. A., Jesse, R. H., and Fletcher, G. H.: Metastatic carcinoma in cervical lymph nodes: Unknown primary site, in *Neoplasia of the Head and Neck*, pp. 289–302, Year Book, Chicago, 1974.
8. Razack, M. S., Sako, K., and Marchetta, F. C.: Influence of initial neck node biopsy on the incidence of recurrence in the neck and survival in patients who subsequently undergo curative resectional surgery. *J. Surg. Oncol.*, *9*:347, 1977.
9. Storm, F. K., Eilber, F. R., Sparks, F. C., and Morton, D. L.: A prospective study of parotid metastases from head and neck cancer. *Am. J. Surg.*, *134*:115, 1977.

CHAPTER 14

Classification of Craniofacial Anomalies

Henry K. Kawamoto, Jr., M.D., D.D.S.

CONGENITAL CRANIOFACIAL ANOMALIES

The striking impact of a congenitally deformed face is undeniable. The initial emotional and psychological stress borne by the parents is perpetuated for years to come by the afflicted child. Fortunately, vast strides have been made in reconstructive surgery that have softened the blow and have brought new hope to the disfigured child.

Despite the great advances made in the understanding and the treatment of congenital malformations, the ultimate goal of prevention appears no where in sight. At blame for this state is the complexity of the problem and the immense nature of the field.

Incidence

Being the most common congenital facial anomaly, the best studies of frequencies are those concerning clefts of the lip and palate. Estimates of occurrence range from 0.60 to 2.13 per thousand births.[1, 2] Racial and ethnic backgrounds and sex influence the incidence. The frequency is low in blacks, somewhat higher in Caucasians, and highest in Orientals.[3–5] Clefts of the lip with or without an associated cleft of the palate are seen more frequently in males. On the other hand, females experience a higher incidence of isolated clefts of the palate.[6]

Hemifacial (craniofacial) microsomia (1st and 2nd branchial arch syndrome) is the next most frequent congenital facial anomaly. The incidence is far less than that of clefts of the lip and palate. The frequency has been estimated to be between 0.18 and 0.33 per thousand births.[7, 8]

The rate of occurrence of the remaining congenital facial malformations falls off rapidly. Their incidence is not well documented. Even when lumped together as a group, the number is small. A rough estimate of 0.014–0.048 per thousand births provides an idea of their rarity.[9]

Etiology

The diversity of congenital malformations is matched by their causes. In some an inheritance pattern is well known. Environmental factors have been suggested in others. A great number occur in a sporadic fashion without any apparent cause.

Treacher Collins (mandibulofacial dysostosis[10–12] and Crouzon's syndrome[13–15] are examples of malformations with well known patterns of inheritance. The mode of transmission is autosomal dominant with a variable degree of penetration and expression. Repetition of these anomalies through several generations has been documented. Numerous other anomalies are also perpetuated on a genetic basis.

Many teratogenic agents have been shown to cause facial malformations in animals; not all have been shown to have the same effect in humans. Pollution of the intrauterine environment of the embryo by these agents can produce devastating deformities.[16–18] As an example, diphenylhydantoin (Dilantin)[19, 20] and diazepam (Valium)[21, 22] have been implicated in producing clefts of the lip and palate in humans.

In some cases the term multifactorial is applicable to describe the etiology of an anomaly. A genetically susceptable embryo may escape disfigurement if the intrauterine environment remains undisturbed. However, the introduction of a teratogenic agent can trip the balance and the anomaly can be expressed in its full form. This schema is felt to be at play in the formation of the common clefts of the lip and palate.

Lastly, there exists a vast number of malformations without any known cause. The anomalies appear in a sporadic manner. A small sampling would include frontal nasal dysplasia, encephalocele, craniofacial microsomia, and oro-ocular clefts.

With the wide range of etiologic agents at play, genetic counseling becomes an important component of the treatment.

Classification

A workable classification system is highly prized but, unforunately, has yet to be devised. Part of the problem lies in determining how one should describe a malformation. Also contributing to the task is the wide variety of craniofacial anomalies. Many attempts at classifications have been made using several approaches.

The earliest efforts to sort the craniofacial anomalies were based on descriptions of the anatomic defect. When a recognizable pattern of malformations was found to occur with regular frequency, the term malformation syndrome was applied. Often the syndrome became known by an eponym in honor of those who succeeded in focusing attention to the entity. With a greater understanding of the ultrastructure, a small fraction of the malformations could be precisely identified by an enzymatic or chromosomal aberration. Each nonmenclatural method has its inherent limitations. All too frequently an unmanageable tangle, linking a string of various proper names or ajdectives, was arbitrarily given.

The volume and the overlap of malformations also pose a difficult hurdle. Over 150 facial cleft syndromes have been described[23] and it is estimated that 25–50 new syndromes a year are being identified and finding their way into print.[24] To compound the issue, several competing names can be used for the same syndrome.

Craniofacial malformations have attracted the attention of many disciplines in the health sciences. The needs of the various specialties differ. The particular designation that might suit the needs a geneticist and a syndromologist might be lacking for a craniofacial microbiologist. Similarily, a surgeon might prefer a convenient label that conveys the constellation of anatomic defects.

To highlight the pathologic anatomy is desirable. Therefore, recognizing the fact that no classification is complete and infallible, the malformations will be described in terms of *craniofacial clefts* and *craniosynostosis* in this chapter.

CRANIOFACIAL CLEFTS

In 1976, a complete description of the Tessier classification of craniofacial clefts appeared in the literature.[9, 25] The pioneering efforts of Tessier in the field of craniofacial surgery attracted patients from all parts of the world. Examining an unrivaled number of patients and collating the findings, he categorized the malformations into well defined clefts. The classification is a working classification. It correlates clinical appearance with surgical anatomy. Being informative and practical, the classification is of particular value for the surgeon.

Classification Schema

The orbit is considered as a key structure. Its strategic location allows it to serve as a buffer zone by separating the cranium from the face (Fig. 14.1). A horizontal line drawn through the canthi is used as an equator to denote the cranial portion of the cleft from that of the facial component.

From the horizontal orbital reference, vertical "time zones" can be drawn which correspond to the location of the various clefts. Starting at the midline and progressing around the orbit, the clefts are numbered 0 to 14. The *facial* clefts numbered 0 to 7 are found caudal to the orbital equator. Cleft No. 8 coincides with the equator and passes laterally from the lateral canthus. The *cranial* representations of the cleft are numbered 9 through 14.

The concept of the "time zones" is an important one. The *facial* clefts (Nos. 0–7) and the *cranial* clefts (Nos. 9–14) can occur independently or in combination with one another to form a *craniofacial* cleft. When a craniofacial cleft is seen it *tends* to follow the same vertical "time zone." Thus, the following combinations are often seen: 0–14, 1–13, 2–12, 3–11, 4–10.

With the "time zone" concept in mind the clinician is forced to look up and down the entire axis and the immediate neighboring zones. Unexpected and often overlooked malformations will be discovered if this pattern of examination is used.

Corresponding to the surface location of the soft tissue cleft is its underlying bony counterpart (Fig. 14.1). The extent of involvement of each component is variable. Seldom are they affected with equal severity. As a general rule, the bony deformation is greater in those facial clefts located lateral to the infraorbital foramen. Conversely, in clefts found medial to the foramen, disorganization of the soft tissue is generally greater. A frequent exception to this rule is the Cleft No. 3.

Although bilateral representation of craniofacial clefts occurs, unilateral forms are the most common. Multiple clefts of different types can also be seen in the same individual.

CLEFT NO. 0

The axis of the Cleft No. 0 coincides with the facial midline (Fig. 14.2). Being midline in nature, the deformity is symmetrical. Prolongation of the cleft into the cranial region is represented by Cleft No. 14.

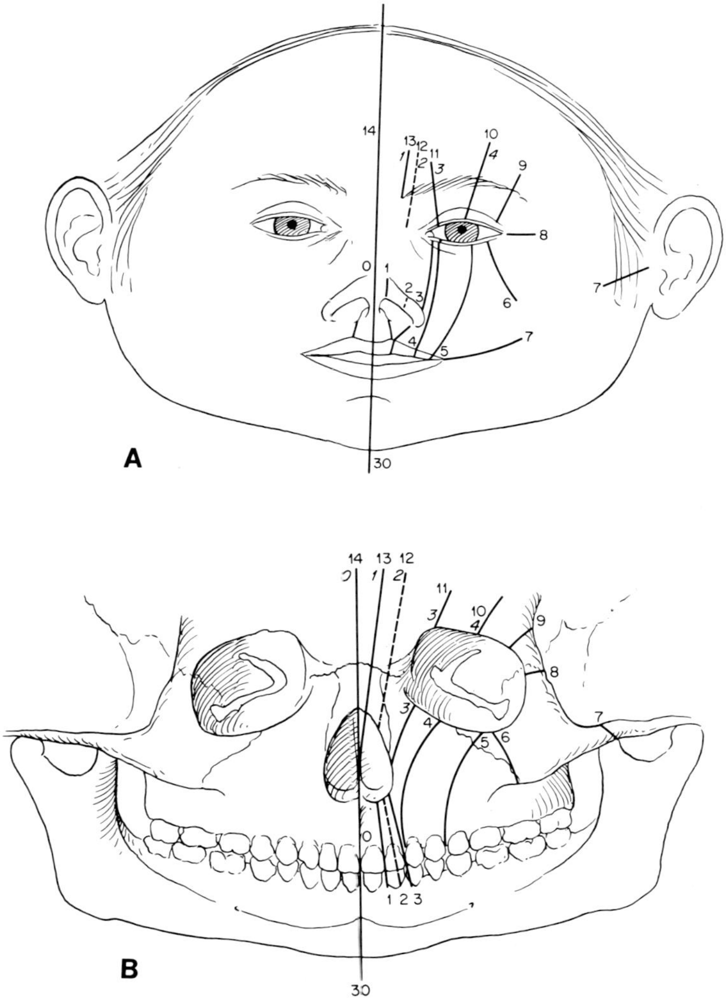

Figure 14.1 Tessier classification. (*A*) Topographic location of soft tissue component of craniofacial clefts. (*B*) Path of clefts through underlying skeleton. (Reproduced with permission from H. K. Kawamoto, Jr.: *Clinics in Plastic Surgery*, *3*:529, 1976.[9])

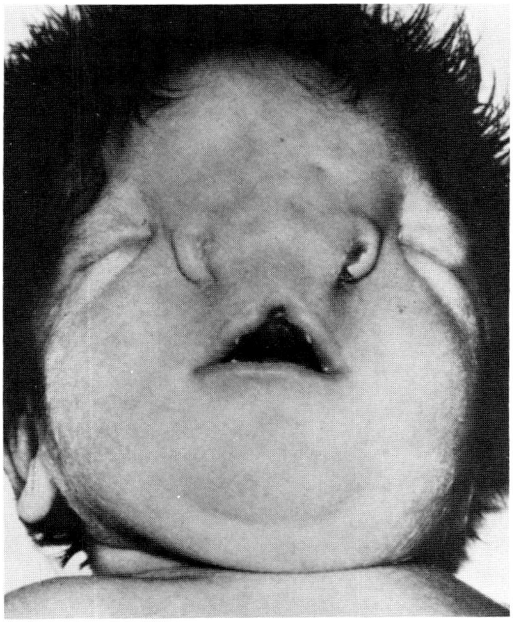

Figure 14.2 Cleft No. 0. Cleft through derivatives of frontonasal process producing a true midline cleft of the lip, bifid nose with broadened columella and telorbitism.

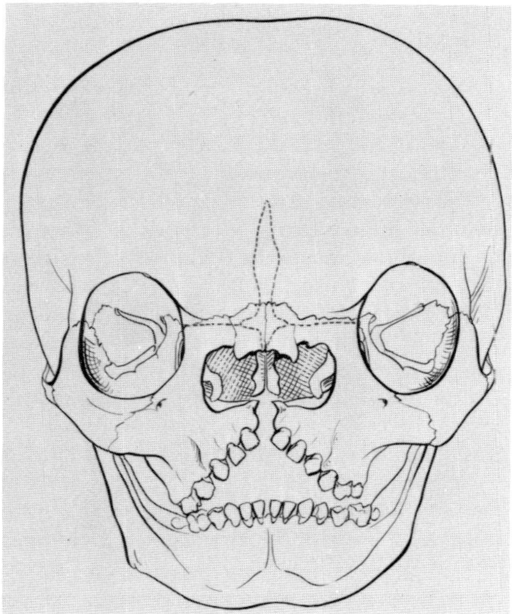

Figure 14.3 Cleft No. 0. Skeletal component with cleft through midline of premaxilla, widened nasal septum and nasal bones, broadening of frontonasal process of maxilla, and telorbitism. (Reproduced with permission from H. K. Kawamoto, Jr.: *Clinics in Plastic Surgery*, *3*:529, 1976.[9])

Included in the Cleft No. 0 group are malformations such as a true median cleft of the upper lip, bifid nose, medial facial clefts,[26] frontonasal dysplasia,[27] and median encephalocele. Although not included in the original Tessier classification, the holoprosencephaly group of anomalies fits well into this cleft pattern.[9, 28]

Soft tissue features (Fig. 14.2). The midline location of clefts of the upper lip distinguishes it from the common "harelip." The presence of the philtral ridges and the peaks of cupid's bow identifies the defect as a *true* median cleft lip. In contrast, the entire prolabial segment is absent in a *false* median cleft lip that is associated with the holoproscencephaly of malformations.

The entire nose is excessively wide. The nostrils are intact and are laterally displaced. A midline groove in the columella and the nasal tip is often seen (bifid nose). When the deformity is continued into the cranium as a Cleft No. 14, telorbitism (hypertelorism) accompanies the deformity.

Intraorally, the labial frenulum can be duplicated. A midline cleft of the palate is sometimes present.

Osseous features (Fig. 14.3). Deformation of the supporting structures can be variable. The nasal septum is thickened, duplicated, or occasionally absent. The nasal bones range from being hypoplastic or excessively large. The nearby frontal processes of the maxilla are, however, broadened and contribute to the telorbitism.

Intraorally, a diastema separates the central incisors. The palate can be split along the midline.

CLEFT NO. 1

Prior to the Tessier classification, the facial clefts in the No. 1 time zone escaped recognition as a discrete entity. They had been lumped together with the malformation described in the preceding section. Although rare in occurrence, a distinct pattern is recognizable which distinguishes the group.

Soft tissue features (Fig. 14.4). The unique characteristic of this cleft is the notch in the dome of the nasal tip. The midline structures such as the columella are intact.

The upper lip can be divided in the paramedian location of the "common" cleft lip, that is, through the philtral ridge.

When the cleft involves the interobital region, the nasal bridge is widened on the ipsilateral side. The medial canthus is not involved per se, but is displaced laterally and inferiorly. The cranial extension corresponds to Cleft No. 13.

Osseous features (Fig. 14.5). In its complete form, the cleft passes between the central and lateral incisors and into the pyriform aperture. The fault lies just lateral to the anterior nasal spine and does not encroach upon the nasal septum.

In the region of the nasal bone, the cleft continues in one of two directions. The most common is through the nasal bone. The alternate route is located at the junction of the nasal bone with the frontal process of the maxilla.

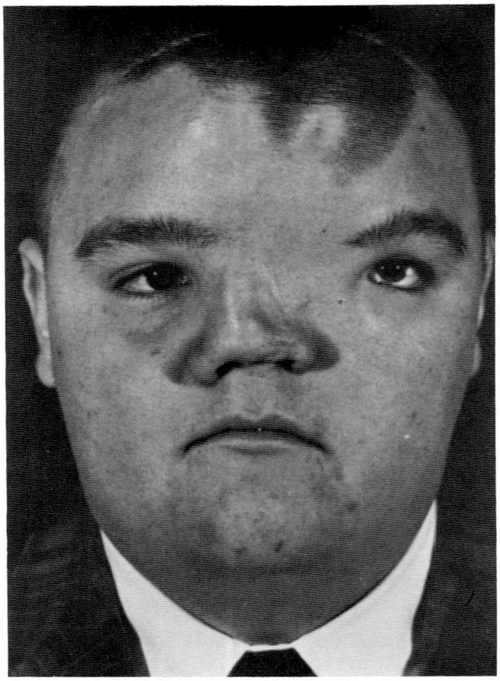

Figure 14.4 Cleft No. 1. Paramedian cleft starting at nasal dome and continuing up the nose to produce telorbitism. Continuing cephalad as a Cleft No. 13, a peculiar omega-shape frontal hairline disturbance is seen. (Reproduced with permission from J. M. Converse: *Reconstructive Plastic Surgery*, Ed. 2. W. B. Saunders, Philadelphia, 1977.)

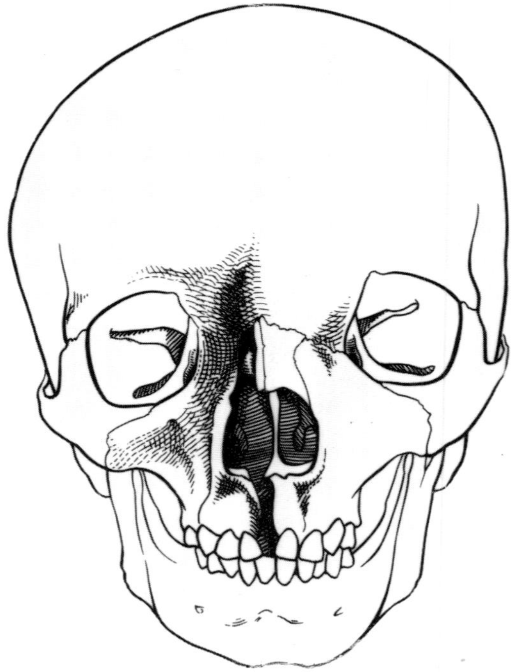

Figure 14.5 Cleft No. 1. Path coursing through paramedian osseous structures of maxilla, pyriform aperture, nasal bones, and cephalad as No. 13 cleft. (Reproduced with permission from H. K. Kawamoto, Jr.: *Clinics in Plastic Surgery*, 3:529, 1976.[9])

CLEFT NO. 2

Like the Cleft No. 1, this No. 2 cleft was not recognized as a separate entity. Although it closely resembles a paramedian Cleft No. 1, it is located slightly more laterally. The cleft is extremely rare.

Soft tissue features (Fig. 14.6). The key distortion of this cleft is the hypoplastic middle third of the alar rim of the nose. It continues cephalad on the lateral aspect of the nose but remains medial to the medial canthus.

When the lip is involved, the cleft is found in the same area as the "common" cleft of the lip. This location is shared with Clefts Nos. 1 and 3.

Osseous features (Fig. 14.7). In the dental arch, the cleft passes through the region of the lateral incisors and into the pyriform aperture. The nasal septum is left intact but may be deviated by the neighboring distortion. A notch at the junction of the nasal bone and frontal process of the maxilla is seen when the cleft extends into the interorbital region.

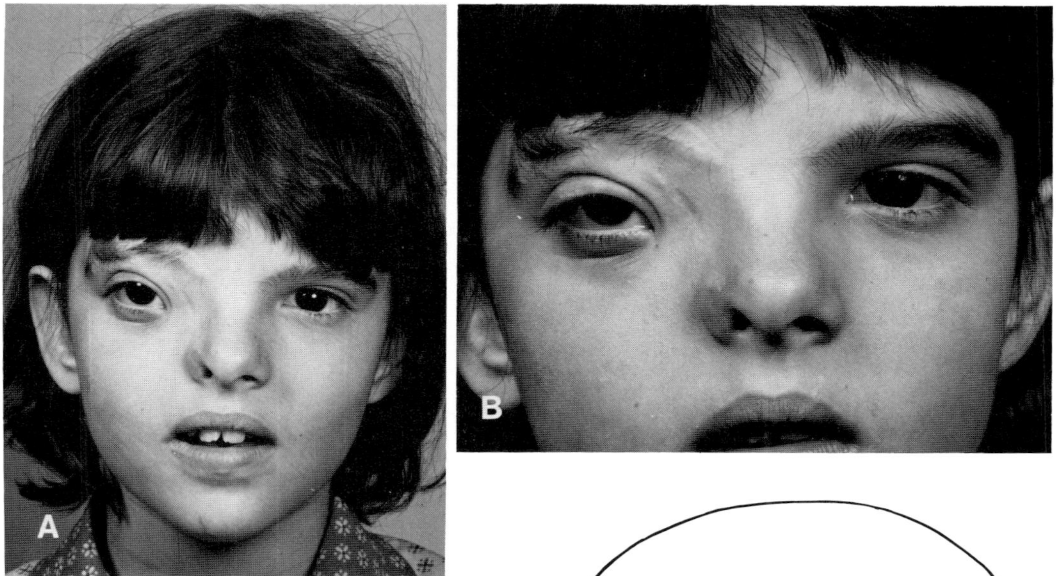

Figure 14.6 Cleft No. 2. Hypoplastic middle third of alar rim and lateral displacement of medial canthus by the ipsilateral widening of the frontonasal process of maxilla. (Reproduced with permission from J. M. Converse: *Reconstructive Plastic Surgery*, Ed. 2. W. B. Saunders, Philadelphia, 1977.)

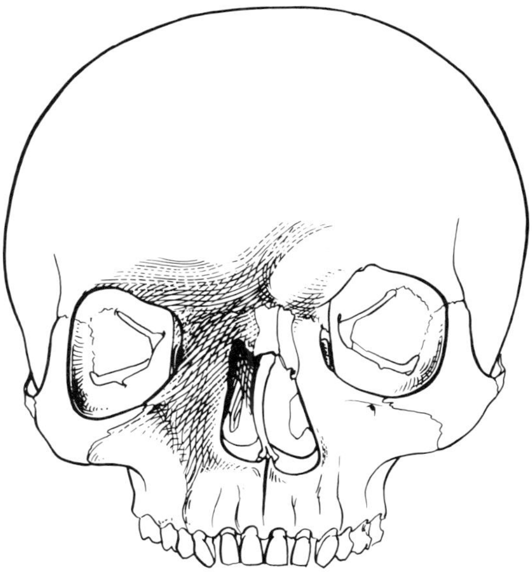

Figure 14.7 Cleft No. 2. Osseous cleft of a broadened frontonasal process of maxilla. Increased interorbital distance as a cleft is continued into cranium as Cleft No. 12. (Reproduced with permission from H. K. Kawamoto, Jr.: *Clinics in Plastic Surgery*, *3*:529, 1976.[9])

CLEFT NO. 3

This cleft is a well known anomaly. It is recognized by several names: nasomaxillary cleft,[29] oblique facial cleft,[30] naso-ocular cleft,[31] and oro-naso-ocular cleft.

The location of the cleft coincides with the embryologic interface between the frontonasal and maxillary processes. If one includes the incomplete form, this cleft is not as rare as reported in the literature.

Soft tissue features (Fig. 14.8). Characterizing the malformation are the nasal and orbital findings.

The cleft undermines the alar base. In severe forms, the coloboma of the nasal ala can extend up to the medial canthal area. The distance between the alar base and the medial canthus area. The distance between the alar base and the medial canthus is foreshortened.

The embryologic tubing of the naso-optic groove is disturbed. The nasolacrimal system is thus malformed. The blocked nasolacrimal duct and the sac are prone to repeated infections[29] and the inferior canaliculus is beyond repair.[32] Total extripation of the system and reconstruction is the treatment of choice.

The medial canthus and its tendon are distorted and inferiorly displaced. A coloboma of the lower eyelid is located medial to the punctum. Because of the lack of the underlying skeletal support, the entire globe settles in a caudal direction. Microphthalmia is occasionally associated with the deformity.

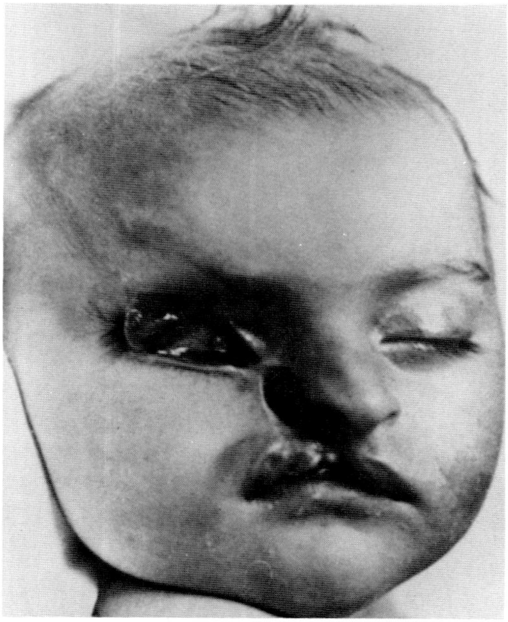

Figure 14.8 Cleft No. 3. Severe unilateral form with "common" cleft lip, undermined nasal alar base, gaping naso-optic groove with involvement of medial canthal area and ocular contents. (Reproduced with permission from H. K. Kawamoto, Jr.: *Clinics in Plastic Surgery*, *3*:529, 1976.[9])

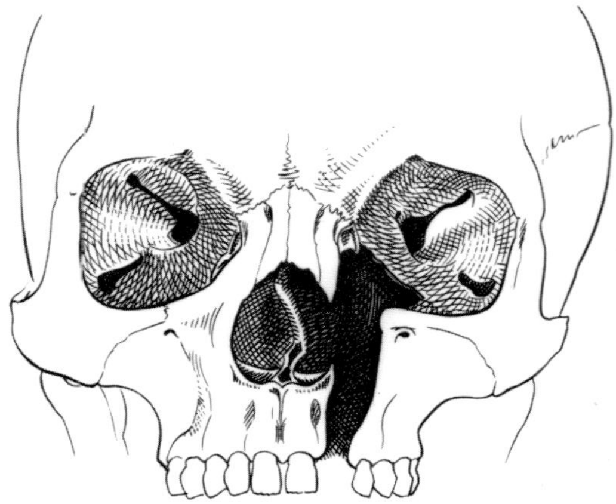

Figure 14.9 Cleft No. 3. Destructive osseous path involving lateral-cuspid region, medial wall of maxillary sinus, inferomedial orbital wall and lacrimal groove. Mouth, nasal cavity, maxillary sinus and orbit are confluent. (Reproduced with permission from H. K. Kawamoto, Jr.: *Clinics in Plastic Surgery*, *3*:529, 1976.[9])

The upper lip is split in the same location as the "common" cleft lip. As mentioned earlier, the Clefts Nos. 1 and 2 are also found in this area. In a study by Whitaker, Katowitz, and Randall,[33] a high incidence of nasolacrimal anomalies was shown to be associated with clefts of the lip. It, therefore, behooves the clinician to closely inspect the so called "common" cleft lip. Doing so might uncover occult forms of major facial clefts.

Osseous features (Fig. 14.9). The skeletal disorganization of Cleft No. 3 is the most vicious of all the facial malformations.

In the alveolar region the cleft passes between the lateral incisor and the canine. It then courses through the lateral portion of the pyriform aperture to undermine the alar base.

In full expressions of the cleft, the septation between the nasal cavity and the maxillary sinus is absent. The frontal process of the maxilla is also disrupted as the defect terminates in the medial aspect of the orbital floor and the lacrimal groove. Thus, the mouth, nasal cavity, maxillary sinus, and the orbit are confluent.

CLEFT NO. 4

A shift away from the median structures is seen beginning with facial Cleft No. 4. Structures derived from the frontonasal process of the embryo are spared. Thus, the nose and the philtral region of the lip are not directly involved but are distorted only by their proximity to the cleft.

The cleft has been called an oro-ocular cleft,[31] vertical facial cleft,[32] oculofacial I cleft (Morian II),[34] and oblique facial cleft. Confusion is raised by the use of these designation for similar but distinctly different facial clefts. This overlap is avoided in the Tessier numbering system.

Soft tissue features (Fig. 14.10). The cleft of the lip is now located lateral to that of the "common" cleft of the lip. It lies lateral to the philtral ridge and cupid's bow. The cleft passes lateral to the nasal ala onto the medial portion of the cheek. It terminates in the region of the inferior puncta of the lower eyelid.

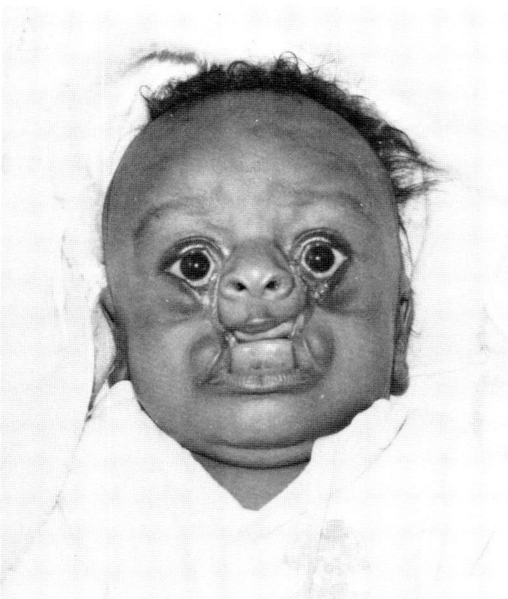

Figure 14.10 Cleft No. 4. Bilateral form. Derivatives of frontonasal process are intact as cleft passes lateral to cupid's bow and nasal complex. Medial most portion of lower eyelids are involved with displacement of the remaining eyelid in an inferior and lateral direction.

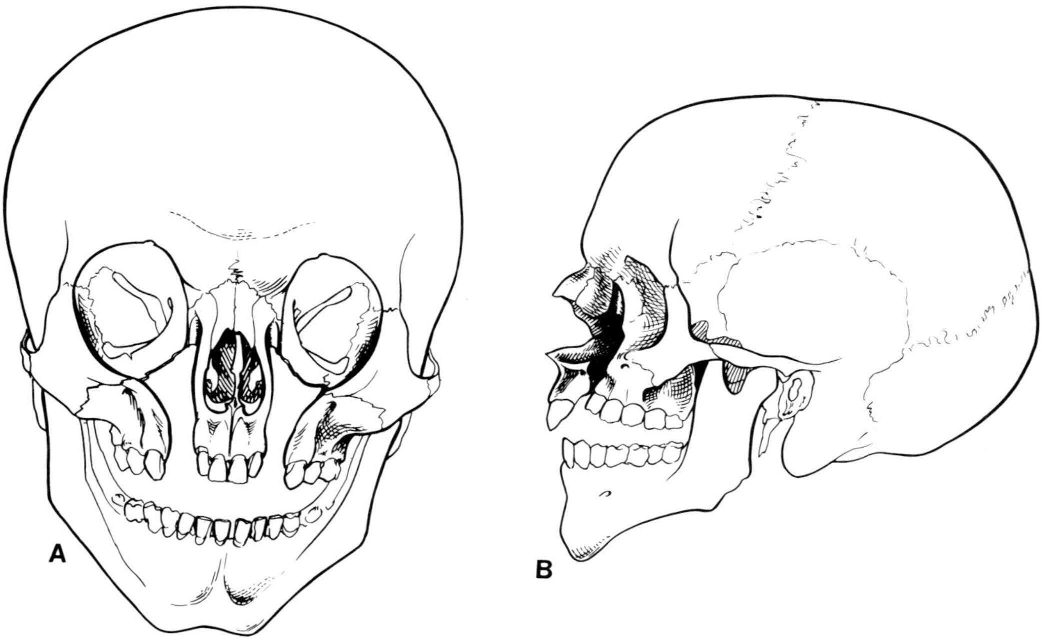

Figure 14.11 Cleft No. 4. (*A*) Bilateral involvement separating premaxilla and nasal complex from rest of facial skeleton. Medial and inferior portion of inferior orbital rim and floor are disrupted. (*B*) Lateral view showing protruding premaxilla, cephalad tilt of nasal complex, and extension of cleft into lacrimal groove. (Reproduced with permission from H. K. Kawamoto, Jr.: *Clinics in Plastic Surgery*, *3*:529, 1976.[9])

The vertical distance between the orbit and the mouth is decreased. The medial canthal structures are inferiorly displaced but the medial canthal tendon is nearly normal. The globe follows the caudal migration of the ocular structures.

Although the nose is not directly involved in the cleft, it appears foreshortened on the ipsilateral side. When the cleft is bilateral in nature, the premaxillary elements protrude and an upward tilt of the nose creates a porcine nasal appearance.

Osseous features (Fig. 14.11). The aveolar cleft passes between the lateral incisor and cuspid. It continues lateral to the pyriform aperture onto the anterior wall of the maxilla. The fault lies medial to the infraorbital foramen and enters the medial portion of the inferior orbital rim and floor. Orbital dystopia is produced by the sinking of the globe into the fissure.

The nasal cavity is not violated by the cleft. Normal septation between it and the maxillary sinus exists. However, posterior choanal atresia is often associated with the malformation.

CLEFT NO. 5

The No. 5 cleft is notably rare. It is the least observed facial cleft. The deformity has been loosely termed an oblique facial cleft and is also called an oculofacial II cleft (Morian III).[34]

Soft tissue features (Fig. 14.12). The cleft of the lip is found medial to the commissure. It

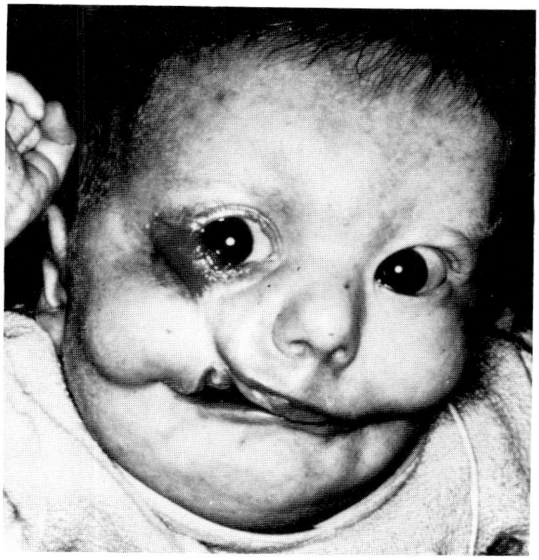

Figure 14.12 Cleft No. 5. Cleft begins medial to the right oral commissure and extends into the medial-lateral third of lower eyelid. Patient also has bilateral Cleft No. 7. (Reproduced with permission from H. K. Kawamoto, Jr.: *Clinics in Plastic Surgery*, *3*:529, 1976.[9])

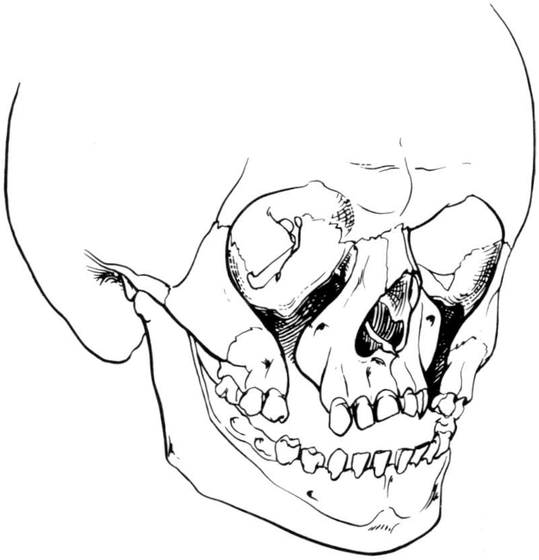

Figure 14.13 Cleft No. 5. Bilateral representation with passage of cleft through premolar area, lateral to infraorbital foramen, and into inferolateral segment of orbital rim and floor. (Reproduced with permission from H. K. Kawamoto, Jr.: *Clinics in Plastic Surgery*, *3*:529, 1976.[9])

traverses the cheek in an upward and lateral direction to end in the region of the medial and lateral thirds of the lower eyelid.

Again, the distance between the ocular structures and the mouth is shortened, drawing the lip and the lower eyelid toward one another. The globe may be normal or microphthalmic.

Osseous features (Fig. 14.13). In the dental arch, the cleft begins in the premolar region. It courses through the anterior wall of the maxilla just lateral to the infraorbital foramen. The cleft enters the inferolateral portion of the orbital rim and floor. The orbital contents are allowed to prolapse into the maxillary sinus.

CLEFT NO. 6

Incomplete expressions of the Treacher Collins (mandibulofacial dsyostosis) syndrome is represented by Cleft No. 6. A zygoma is present but hypoplastic. This is in contrast to the complete form of the malformation (Cleft Nos. 6, 7, and 8 combined) in which the zygoma is absent.

Soft tissue features (Fig. 14.14). The basic clinical characteristics are similar but expressed in a milder form than that of the complete deformity (see Fig. 14.19). The antimongoloid obliquity of the palpebral fissure is less pronounced. A shallow coloboma is seen near the junction of the middle and lateral third of the lower eyelid. Extending from the coloboma and onto the cheek is a shallow groove. The skin contained in this depressed zone appears to be distrophic and is discolored.

The external ear is usually normal or shows only minimal deformation. The middle ear is often involved leaving the patient with a conductive hearing loss.

Osseous features (Fig. 14.15). The hypoplastic zygoma is the hallmark of the cleft. The center of the cleft is located at the zygomaticomaxillary suture line. A palpable notch in the lateral portion of the inferior orbital rim is detectable. The hypoplastic zygoma is responsible for the lowering of the lateral portion of the orbital floor and the caudal displacement of the lateral canthus.

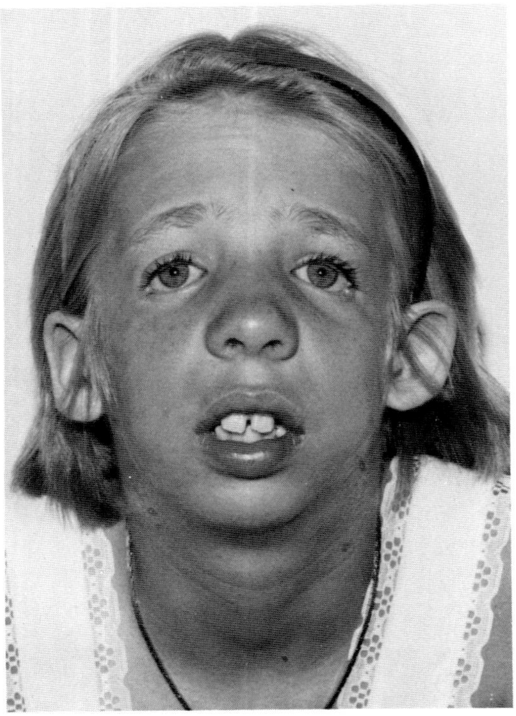

Figure 14.14 Cleft No. 6. Incomplete form of Treacher Collins syndrome. Mild coloboma of lower eyelids which continues inferiorly onto the cheeks. Hypoplastic zygomas fail to support the lateral ocular structures.

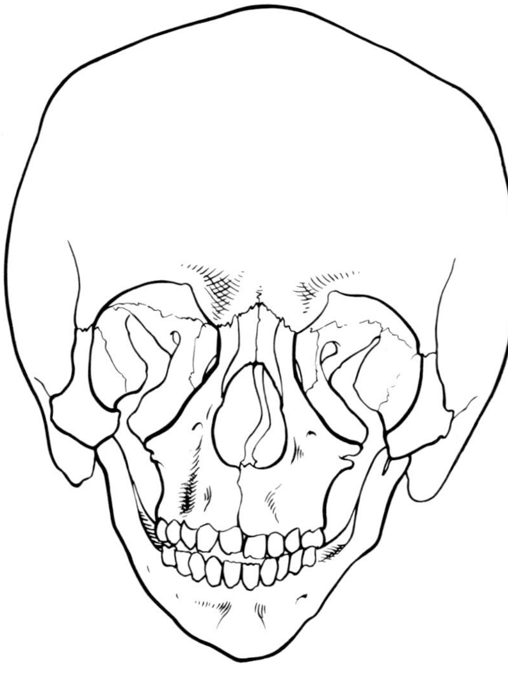

Figure 14.15 Cleft No. 6. Center of fault lies in region of zygomaticomaxillary suture. Maxillary bones are hypoplastic. (Reproduced with permission from H. K. Kawamoto, Jr.: *Clinics in Plastic Surgery*, *3*:529, 1976.[9])

CLEFT NO. 7

Facial Cleft No. 7 is a rather common malformation. It has been known by several names of which the most popular are: first and second branchial arch syndrome,[35] otomandibular dysostosis,[36] hemifacial microsomia,[37] and more recently, craniofacial microsomia.[38]

The malformation is seen at a rate of 0.8–0.33 per thousand births.[7,8] It occurs more frequently in males in a ratio of 3:2.[7] The involvement is usually unilateral but can be bilateral in approximately 10% of the cases.[17,39–41] A genetic component is weak at best.

Soft tissue features (Fig. 14.16). Running across the cheek is a groove extending from the oral commissure to the ear. Ear tags are often located along this line. The external ear is deformed and displays varying degrees of microtia. The cleft radiates from the oral commissure to produce a macrostomia.

The horizontal and vertical dimension of the deformed side are shortened and the chin deviates toward the affected side. The lateral canthus is caudally displaced.

Intraorally the soft palate and the tongue can be hypoplastic on the ipsilateral side. The parotid duct and gland are sometimes absent.

The nerves and muscles of the first and second branchial arch can also be involved. Thus weakness of the muscles of mastication (first branchial arch and trigeminal nerve) and the muscles of facial expression (second branchial arch and facial nerve) can be seen.

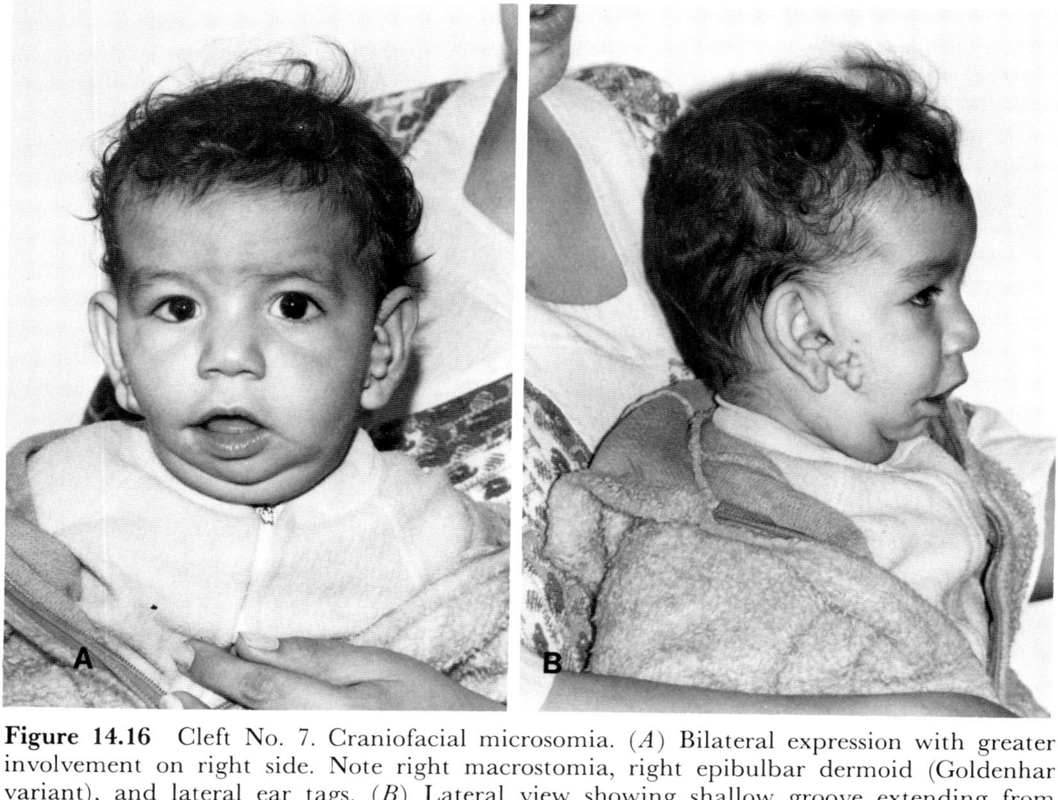

Figure 14.16 Cleft No. 7. Craniofacial microsomia. (*A*) Bilateral expression with greater involvement on right side. Note right macrostomia, right epibulbar dermoid (Goldenhar variant), and lateral ear tags. (*B*) Lateral view showing shallow groove extending from commissure to ear. Ear tags are scattered along the cheek groove.

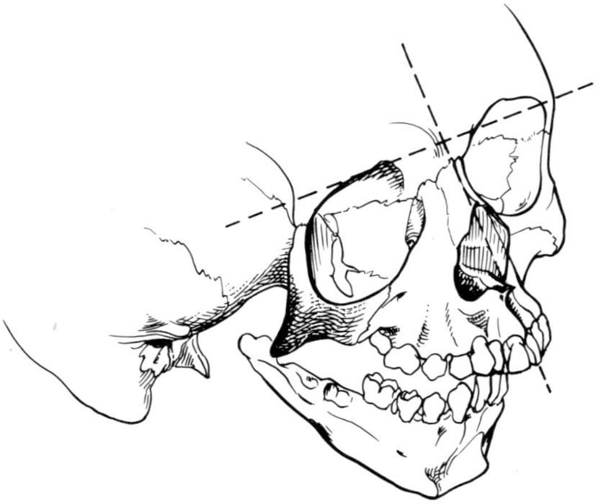

Figure 14.17 Cleft No. 7. Unilateral skeletal involvement with discontinuity of zygomatic arch, near absence of ramus of mandible and inferior displacement of ipsilateral orbit. (Reproduced with permission from H. K. Kawamoto, Jr.: *Clinics in Plastic Surgery*, *3*:529, 1976.[9])

Osseous features (Fig. 14.17). The skeletal center of involvement is near the zygomaticotemporal suture. In the complete form the zygomatic arch is disrupted and is represented by only a proximal and distal stump. The maxilla is hypoplastic and the occlusal plane is elevated on the ipsilateral side.

The malformation of the mandible can be extreme with virtual absence of the ramus, condyle and cornoid process. The formation of the glenoid fossa will vary in direct relationship with the development of the condyle.

In the temporal region, the temporal bone is hypoplastic. The middle ear ossicles that it houses are often malformed and produce a conductive hearing loss.

CLEFT NO. 8

The No. 8 cleft lies in a transition zone between the facial and cranial clefts. Alone, the Cleft No. 8 is infrequently seen. It occurs mainly in combination with Cleft Nos. 6 and 7.

Soft tissue features (Fig. 14.18). The cleft begins in the lateral canthal area and extends horizontally into the temporal hairline. Paucity of hair in the temporal area is often seen. Occasionally the cleft in the lateral canthal region is occupied by a dermatocele.

Osseous features. The cleft is located on the frontozygomatic suture line. When combined with Cleft Nos. 6 and 7, the entire zygoma is apt to be absent.

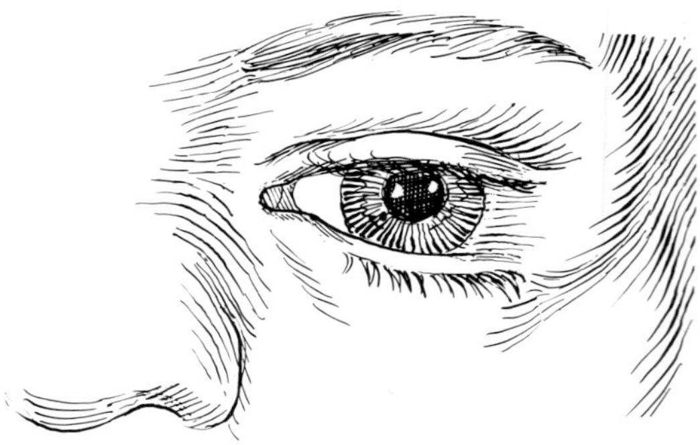

Figure 14.18 Cleft No. 8. Lateral canthus is distorted by the cleft which passes horizontally into the temporal region. (Reproduced with permission from H. K. Kawamoto, Jr.: *Clinics in Plastic Surgery*, *3*:529, 1976.[9])

CLEFTS NOS. 6, 7, AND 8

Bilateral occurrence of this combination of facial clefts is found in patients with the complete form of the Treacher Collins syndrome. The malformation has also been called the Franceschetti-Zwahlen-Klein syndrome and mandibulofacial dystosis.[12, 36] The deformity is well known and the typical facies has been found on a PreColumbian terra cotta statue dating back to the 7th century.[42]

The malformation is inherited in an autosomal dominant manner with variable penetration of the responsible gene. In a review of 200 cases by Rogers,[11] the deformity was found to be transmitted 3 times more frequently by the females of the afflicted families. Although female preponderance for transmission is present, the occurrence of the anomaly is equal between the sexes.

Soft tissue features (Fig. 14.19). The deformity is bilateral and fairly symmetrical in nature. The lateral canthus is displaced inferiorly to give the antimongoloid slant of the palpebral fissures. A coloboma is seen near the junction of the middle and lateral thirds of the lower eyelid. The tarsal plate of the lower eyelid is reduced to a hypoplastic remanent. Eyelashes are absent in the medial two-thirds of the lower eyelid.

A distinct groove of the cheek is found extending from the coloboma toward an accentuated antigonial notch of the mandible. The skin within this facial furrow is atrophic, discolored, and has a sclerodermic quality.

Microtia of a varying degree is seen. A conductive hearing loss is present with malformation of the ossicular chain of the middle ear. In the preauricular area, the sideburns project abnormally forward onto the cheeks.

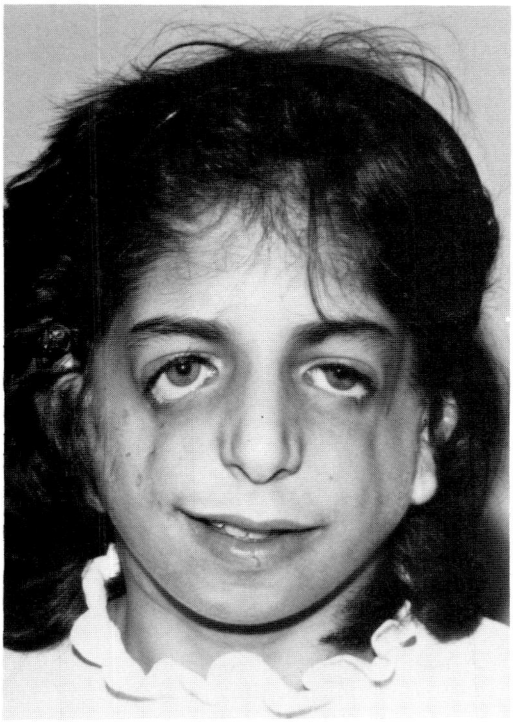

Figure 14.19 Cleft Nos. 6, 7, and 8. Complete form of Treacher Collins syndrome. Note antimongoloid slant of palpebral fissure, severe lower eyelid coloboma with absence of lashes in medial two thirds, and vertical cheek grooves.

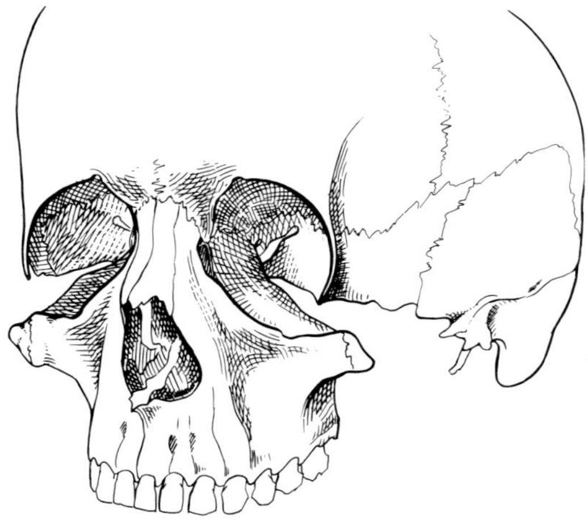

Figure 14.20 Cleft Nos. 6, 7, and 8. Total absence of zygoma. Greater wing of sphenoid serves as lateral orbital rim. (Reproduced with permission from H. K. Kawamoto, Jr.: *Clinics in Plastic Surgery*, *3*:529, 1976.[9])

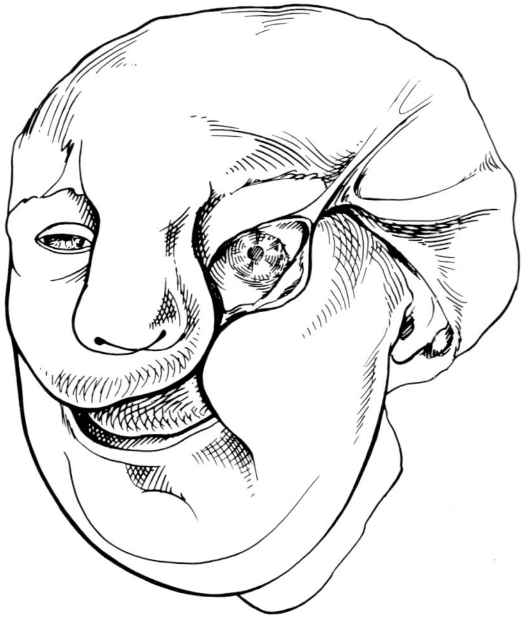

Figure 14.21 Cleft No. 9. Illustration based on patients reported by Morian and Sanvenero-Rosselli. Centered in the lateral one-third of eyelid and orbit. Ipsilateral Cleft No. 5 and contralateral Cleft No. 7 are also shown. (Reproduced with permission from H. K. Kawamoto, Jr.: *Clinics in Plastic Surgery*, *3*:529, 1976.[9])

Macrostomia and clefts of the secondary palate are sometimes present.

Osseous features (Fig. 14.20). The characteristic underlying deformity of the complete form of the syndrome is the absence of the zygoma. The lack of zygomatic support contributes to the eyelid coloboma and antimongoloid slant of the palpebral fissure. The lateral canthal tendon has no place of attachment for the lateral orbital rim is now represented by the greater wing of the sphenoid.

Without the intervening zygoma, the hypoplastic temporalis forms a continuous sheet with the masseter. This abnormal muscle configuration exerts its effect on the mandible. The vertical dimension of the ramus is foreshortened and produces a retrognathic mandible and an open bite. The antigonial notch is accentuated. The small chin adds to the lower third facial deficit.

CLEFT NO. 9

The first of the cranial clefts in the Tessier classification is indeed rare. Only two examples of this cranial cleft have been reported in the literature.[34]

Soft tissue features (Fig. 14.21). The cleft extends from the lateral third of the upper eyelid through the lateral portion of the eyebrow. It continues cephalad into the frontotemporal hairline.

Osseous features. The cleft is centered in the superolateral angle of the orbit. The orbital rim and wall is disrupted in this region as the cleft continues into the frontotemproal cranium.

CLEFT NO. 10

Fronto-orbital encephaloceles are primarily responsible for this cranial cleft. The orbit and its ocular contents are displaced in an inferior and lateral direction.

Soft tissue features (Fig. 14.22). The cleft is located in the middle third of the upper eyelid and eyebrow. The levator apparatus of the upper eyelid is split or attenuated in its midportion. A blepharia of the upper eyelid is occasionally seen.

Osseous features (Fig. 14.23). The central third of the supraorbital rim and the roof of the orbit are involved. The defect continues into the frontal bone lateral to the supraorbital neurovascular bundle. The fault is occupied by the protruding fronto-orbital encephalocele.

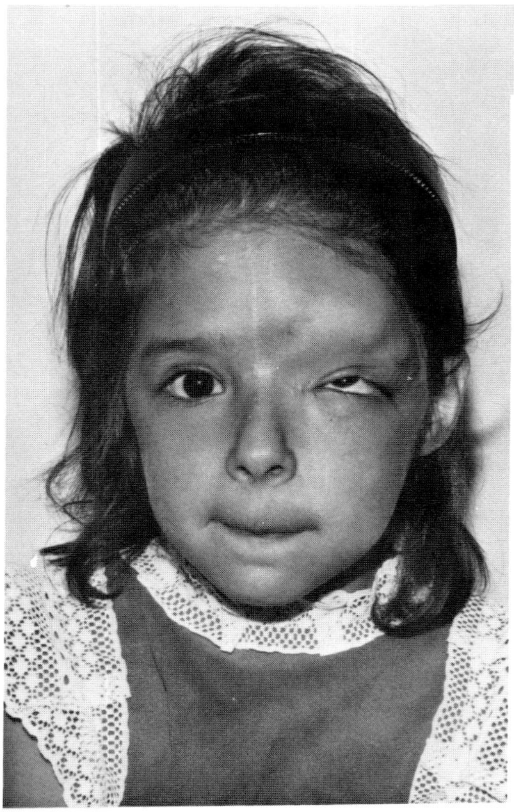

Figure 14.22 Cleft No. 10. Fronto-orbital encephalocele in middle third of orbital rim and roof. Orbital complex is displaced inferiorly and laterally.

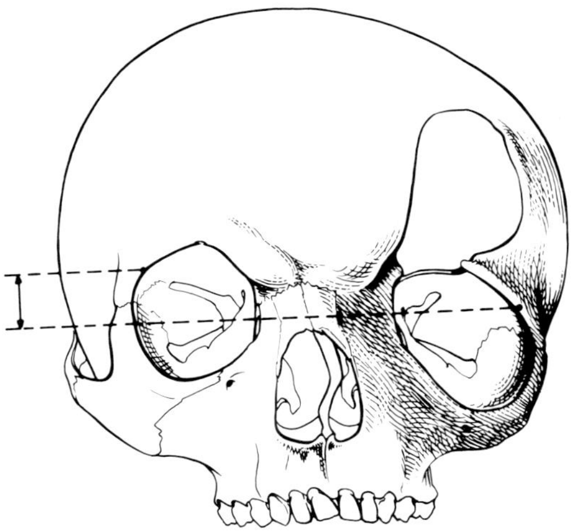

Figure 14.23 Cleft No. 10. Osseous defect and distortion of orbital complex caused by fronto-orbital encephalocele. Dystopic orbit is displaced inferiorly and laterally to produce asymmetrical telorbitism. (Reproduced with permission from H. K. Kawamoto, Jr.: *Clinics in Plastic Surgery*, *3*:529, 1976.[9])

CLEFT NO. 11

As one approaches the midline of the craniofacial skeleton, combinations of cranial clefts with facial clefts are frequently seen. In the case of Cleft No. 11, it is usually found in association with the destructive Cleft No. 3 of the face (see Fig. 14.1).

Soft tissue features (Fig. 14.8). The cleft begins in the medial third of the upper eyelid and the eyebrow. It extends cephalad into the frontal hairline.

Osseous features (Fig. 14.9). The cleft can follow one of two routes on its way into the cranium. Avoiding the interorbital framework, the cleft can pass lateral to the ethmoidal complex. It then continues through the medial third of the orbital rim and into the frontal sinus and frontal bone.

The alternate path traverses the ethmoidal labyrinth, hence is medial to the orbital cavity. Telorbitism is produced by the enlarged ethmoid air cells. The cleft also courses through the frontal sinus and the frontal bone.

CLEFT NO. 12

The cranial extension of the facial Cleft No. 2 is represented by Cleft No. 12. Faulty development of the embryologic frontonsasal process contributes to the malformation.

Soft tissue features (Fig. 14.6). The cleft is located medial to the medial canthus. The canthus itself is displaced inferiorly and laterally by the surrounding turmoil. The trail then continues into the root of the eyebrow and into the frontal hairline.

Osseous features (Figs. 14.7 and 14.24). Beginning with this cleft, the interorbital region is always involved. As a consequence, telorbitism is associated with these malformations.

The cleft passes through the junction of the nasal bone with the frontal process of the maxilla. It also traverses the underlying ethmoid labyrinth to increase the interorbital distance.

Intracranially the cleft is located lateral to the cribriform plate and the olfactory groove (see Fig. 14.24).

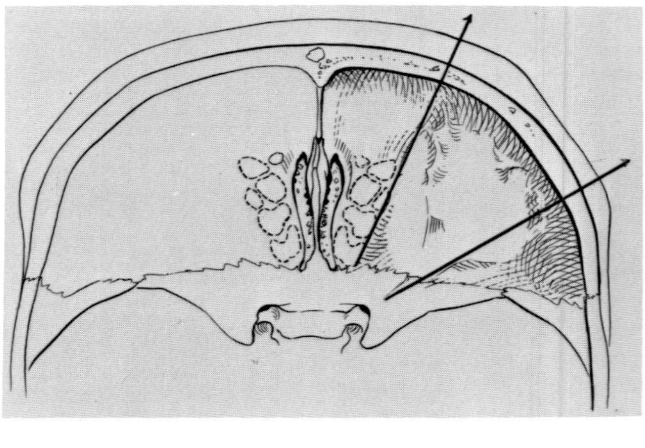

Figure 14.24 Cleft No. 12. Intracranial view of anterior cranial floor. *Arrows* outline walls of orbit. Ethmoid labyrinth is widened by the cleft. Cribriform and olfactory grooves are normal. (Reproduced with permission from H. K. Kawamoto, Jr.: *Clinics in Plastic Surgery*, 3:529, 1976.[9])

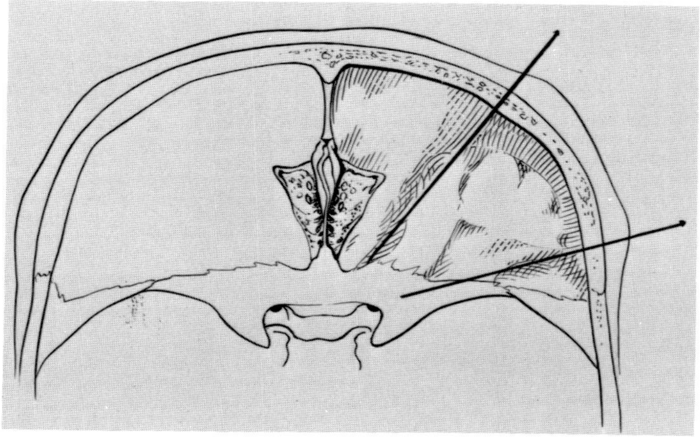

Figure 14.25 Cleft No. 13. Intracranial view of anterior cranial floor. Lateral displacement of orbits as depicted by *arrows* is caused by widening of olfactory grooves by the cleft. (Reproduced with permission from H. K. Kawamoto, Jr.: *Clinics in Plastic Surgery*, *3*:529, 1976.[9])

CLEFT NO. 13

This cranial cleft which is just off the midline can be caused by a paramedian frontal encephalocele or a paramedian frontonasal dysraphia. The facial equivalent of this cleft is Cleft No. 1. When the cleft occurs in a bilateral form, some of the worst examples of telorbitism are produced.

Soft tissue features (Fig. 14.4). Because its paramedial location, the eyelid and eyebrows are not directly violated but can be displaced laterally by the cleft. A distinct feature of the cleft is an omega-shaped disruption of the hairline just off the midline.

Osseous features (Figs. 14.5 and 14.25). The cleft passes through the nasal bone or through the junction of the nasal bone with the frontal process of the maxilla. The ethmoidal labyrinth is involved and extensive pneumatization of the frontal sinus can occur.

On the floor of the anterior cranium, the cleft passes through the olfactory groove (Fig. 14.25). The cribriform plate prolapses into the interorbital space.

CLEFT NO. 14

The trip around the orbit and return to the midline is seen with Cleft No. 14. It coincides with the Cleft No. 0 of the face. Common causes for this malformation are frontonasal dysplasia, frontonasal encephaloceles, or median frontal encephaloceles.

Soft tissue features (Fig. 14.26). A soft, slightly compressible mass that increases on crying is seen when the deformity is due to an encephalocele. This space occupying mass fills the interorbital distance to produce telorbitism.

In cases of frontonasal dysplasia, the nasal bridge is broad and flat. The eyes and eyebrows are widely separated. The widow's peak of the frontal hairline is usually widened and descends abnormally onto the forehead.

Osseous features (Figs. 14.3 and 14.27–14.29). Regardless of the basic etiology, the interorbital distance is increased. The widening can be caused by a large midline bony defect that is occupied by an encephalocele (Figs. 14.27 and 14.28) or by broadening of the nasal bones and the frontal processes of the maxilla (Fig. 14.3).

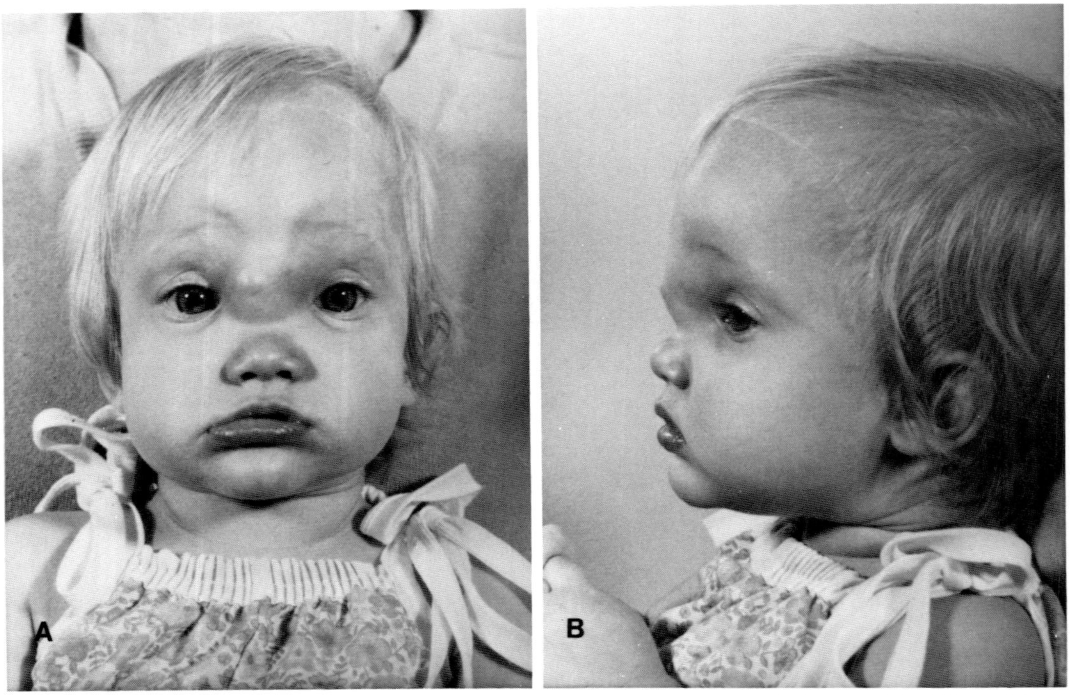

Figure 14.26 Cleft No. 14. Midline cleft due to frontonasal encephalocele. (*A*) Telorbitism caused by protruding encephalocele in orbital region. (*B*) Profile view of encephalocele herniating through region of nasion.

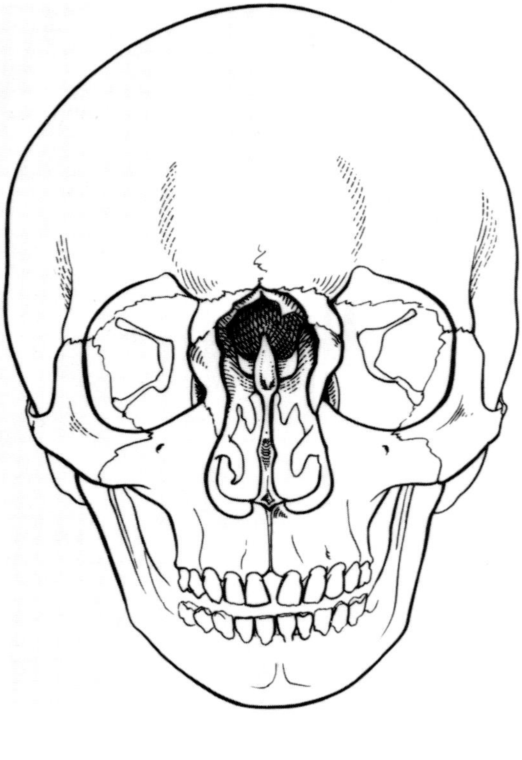

Figure 14.27 Cleft No. 14. Osseous defect caused by frontonasal encephalocele. Note lower position of cribriform plate and lateral displacement of nasal bones and frontonasal processes of maxilla. (Reproduced with permission from H. K. Kawamoto, Jr.: *Clinics in Plastic Surgery*, *3*:529, 1976.[9])

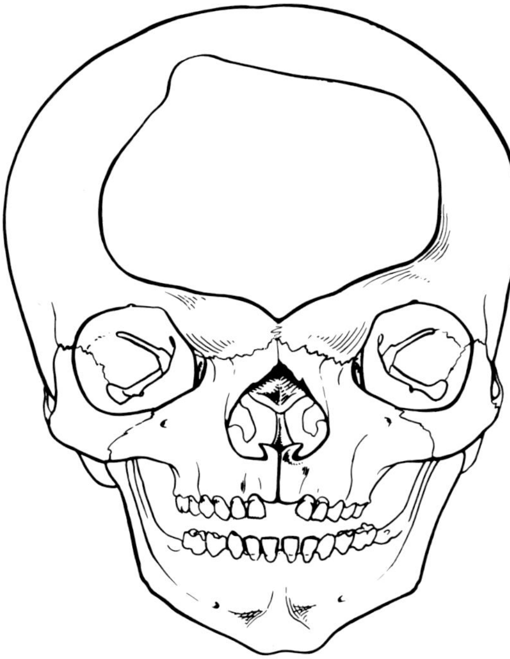

Figure 14.28 Cleft No. 14. Symmetrical telorbitism produced by midline frontal encephalocele. Frontonasal portion of skeleton also increased in width by facial counterpart, Cleft No. 0. (Reproduced with permission from H. K. Kawamoto, Jr.: *Clinics in Plastic Surgery*, *3*:529, 1976.[9])

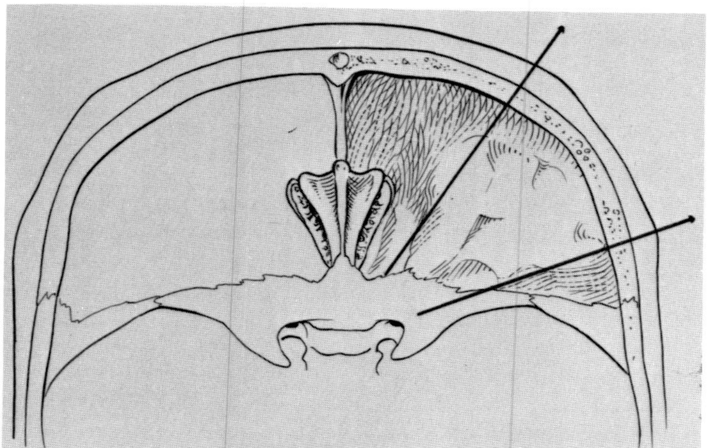

Figure 14.29 Cleft No. 14. Intracranial view of anterior cranial floor. Primary deformity is increased width of midline crista galli. Olfactory grooves are normal. *Arrows* indicate lateral displacement of orbits. (Reproduced with permission from H. K. Kawamoto, Jr.: *Clinics in Plastic Surgery*, *3*:529, 1976.[9])

Intracranially the crista galli is widened or even duplicated (Fig. 14.29). The cribriform plate is also increased in its transverse dimension. Normally, this structure is located 5–10 mm below the level of the orbital roof. With the cleft, caudal displacement up to 20 mm can occur.[44]

CRANIOSYNOSTOSIS

Craniosynostosis anomalies form the second major group of congenital malformations. Unlike the anomalies mentioned in the previous section, they are not the result of a cleft. Instead, a premature closure of one or more cranial sutures is responsible for the deformity.

A wide variety of craniosynostosis malformations exists. The effect on the development of the face will depend a great deal on the specific suture that is involved. Approximately 10% of the cases will show significant facial deformation.[45] Minimal facial consequences are seen, for example, in the premature closure of the sagittal suture (scaphocephaly). Greater facial deformation occurs with the premature closure of the metropic suture (trigonocephaly). Severe disturbances can be created by the involvement of multiple sutures as in kleeblattschädel deformity and the craniofacial dysotosis syndromes.

Incidence

Because of their rarity, the exact incidence of craniosynostosis is unknown. In the United States it has been estimated that approximately 1,200 newborns will be delivered each year with these anomalies.[46] Bertelsen[13] reviewed 219 patients in the Copenhagen area and found 15 patients with Crouzon's syndrome and 5 with Apert's syndrome. The remaining 199 patients had only simple craniosynostosis.

Pathogenesis

Premature closure of the cranial sutures has been thought to be the primary event in the cause of the cranial malformation. This view has been challenged by Moss[47] who feels that the primary fault lies in the malformation of the cranial base with resulting facial disarrangement of the basal attachments of the dura mater. The sutural events are felt to be a secondary phenomenon. An autopsy study of a stillborn with Apert's syndrome adds support to this theory.[48]

Regardless of the primary event, a calvarium with a prematurely closed suture must cope with the rapidly expanding brain which achieves 88% of the adult size during the first year of life. Growth is inhibited in a perpendicular direction to the prematurely closed suture and compensatory over expansion into areas with normal sutures must take place to accommodate the growth of the brain.[49]

It should be recalled that the midfacial mass is attached to the undersurface of the anterior cranial vault. Alterations in growth of the anterior cranium will, therefore, be reflected onto the developing face. Consequently, severe midfacial retrusion can be seen when there is premature closure of the coronal sutures (e.g. Crouzon's and Apert's syndromes). Even greater distortion is seen by premature closure of a hemicoronal suture because of the asymmetries that are introduced (plagiocephaly).

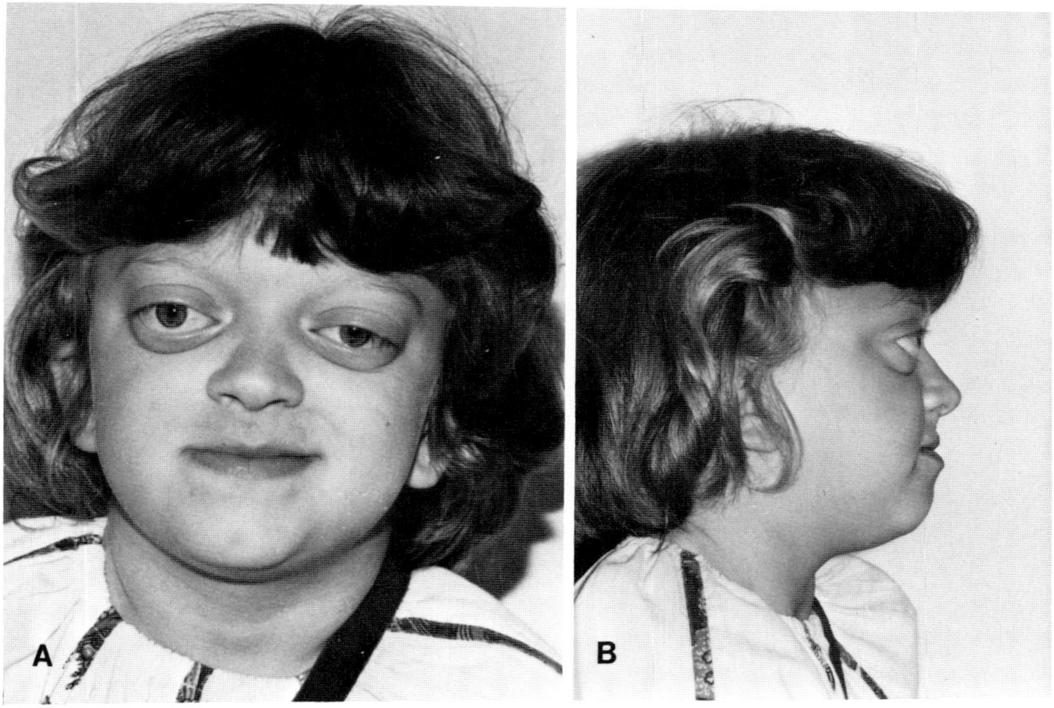

Figure 14.30 Crouzon's syndrome. (*A*) Frontal view showing exorbitism. (*B*) On lateral view of the midface retrusion, exorbitism and forehead can be appreciated.

Optimal treatment would require operative intervention in the early infant period to minimize the distortional impact transmitted to the face.

Classification

The variety of craniosynostosis syndromes can produce a bewildering picture. In an effort to categorize the deformities, Cohen[15] proposed a classification based on clinical similarities and genetic considerations. The anomalies were grouped into 14 major types of which the most common will be discussed in the chapter.

CROUZON'S SYNDROME

The malformation (Fig. 14.30) is characterized by premature closure of the coronal suture. The sagittal and lambdoid sutures can also be involved. The anterior cranial base is foreshortened and the frontal bone is retropositioned.

The midface is hypoplastic and retruded, creating a pseudomandibular prognathic appearance. The orbits are shallow but their contents are normal in volume. Therefore, the globe protrudes well beyond the orbital rim to produce exorbitism. Exposure keratitis can be a

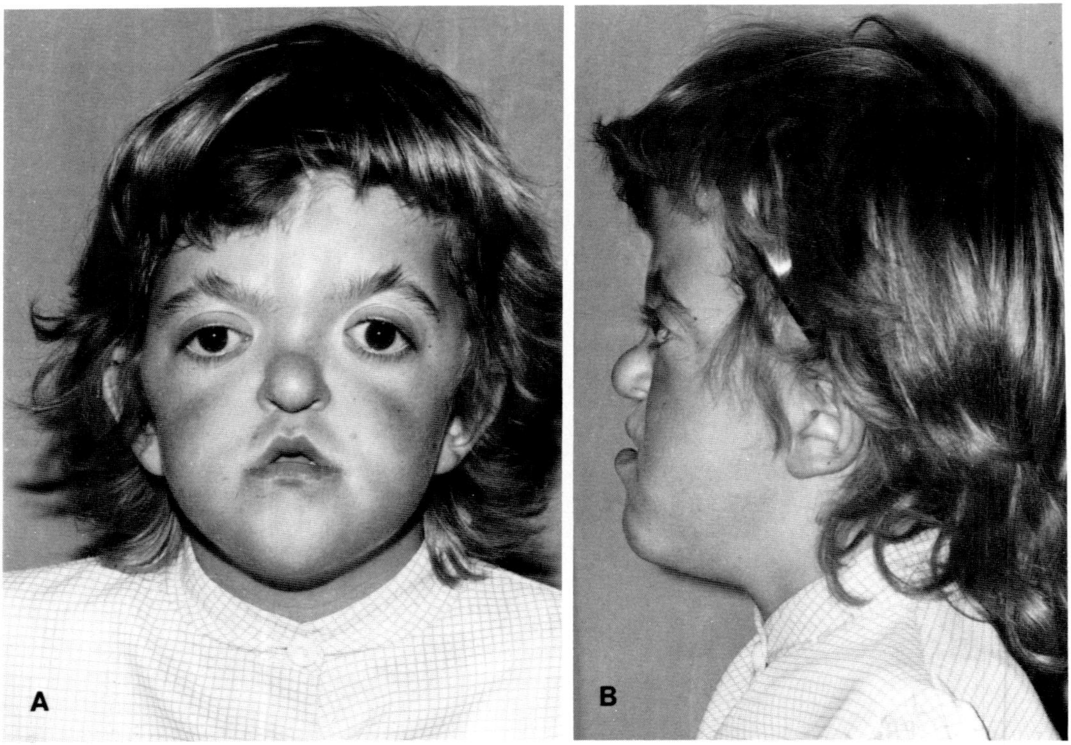

Figure 14.31 Apert's syndrome. (*A*) Width of cranium is increased. Mild telorbitism is exaggerated by the strabismus. (*B*) Profile shows transverse ridge of forehead, exorbitism and midfacial hypoplasia.

problem when the exorbitism is extreme and the eyelids are stretched beyond their means to provide protection. Mild telorbitism is also a feature.

Respiratory difficulties can also be encountered. The retropositioned soft palate fills the oral and nasal pharynx to impair free air exchange.

With regard to the central nervous system, intelligence is generally normal. Increase in intercranial pressure, if not recognized, can cause a deterioration in vision.

The condition is transmitted in an autosomal dominant manner.

APERT'S SYNDROME

Acrocephalosyndactyly is another name given to the syndrome (Fig. 14.31). The calvarium is tower-like, short, and broad (turribrachycephaly). Again the coronal suture is prematurely closed and involvement of the sagittal and lamboidal sutures can contribute to the deformity.

The forehead is flat and high. A transverse ridge is seen in the supraorbital region. The occipital bone is flattened which contributes to the brachycephalic appearance. Most patients have some degree of mental retardation.

Exorbitism is of a milder degree than that seen in Crouzon's syndrome. Mild increase in interorbital distance (telorbitism) is also present. Divergent strabismus and exophoria accentuate the wide spaced appearance of the eyes.

The midface is hypoplastic and is combined with pseudomandibular prognathism. A high arched constricted palate is covered by a Byzantine patterned mucosa. Clefts of the soft palate occur in approximately a third of the cases.

The digits of the hands and the feet are symmetrically deformed. Syndactyly of the middle three digits is the most frequent pattern that is found.

In adolescence, acne vulgaris is commonly noted involving the face, trunk, and the upper extremities.

The mode inheritance is autosomal dominant.

PFEIFFER SYNDROME

The facial features of this malformation resemble those of the previously described craniosynostosis syndromes. The coronal suture is the principal site of premature closure. The hyoplastic midface is suspended from a turribrachycephalic calvarium. Exorbitism and mild telorbitism are associated with the deformity. Intelligence is usually normal.

The malformation is distinguished by its digital anomaly. The thumb and great toe are broad and usually deflected in a varus direction.

The syndrome is inherited in an autosomal dominant pattern.

SAETHRE-CHOTZEN SYNDROME

The coronal suture is again the principal site of involvement (Fig. 14.32). An acrocephalic configuration of the cranium is present. Midfacial hypoplasia is not a feature.

An asymmetrical alteration of the face can be seen with deviation of the nasal septum and

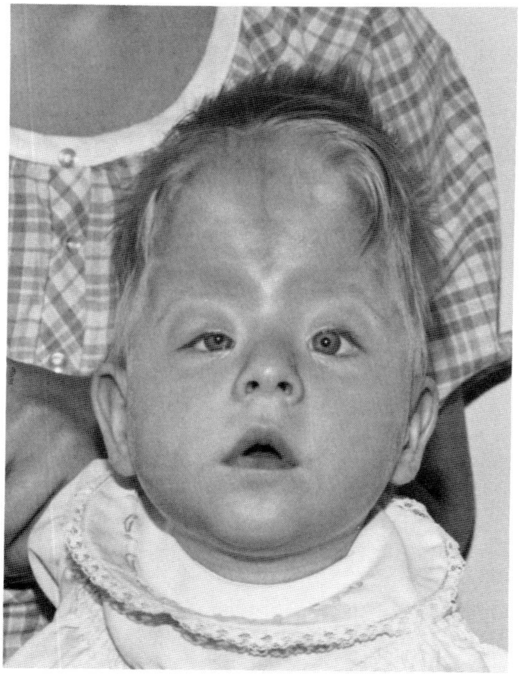

Figure 14.32 Saethre-Chotzen syndrome. Asymmetrical frontal disturbance with eyelid ptosis. Nose deviates away from midline.

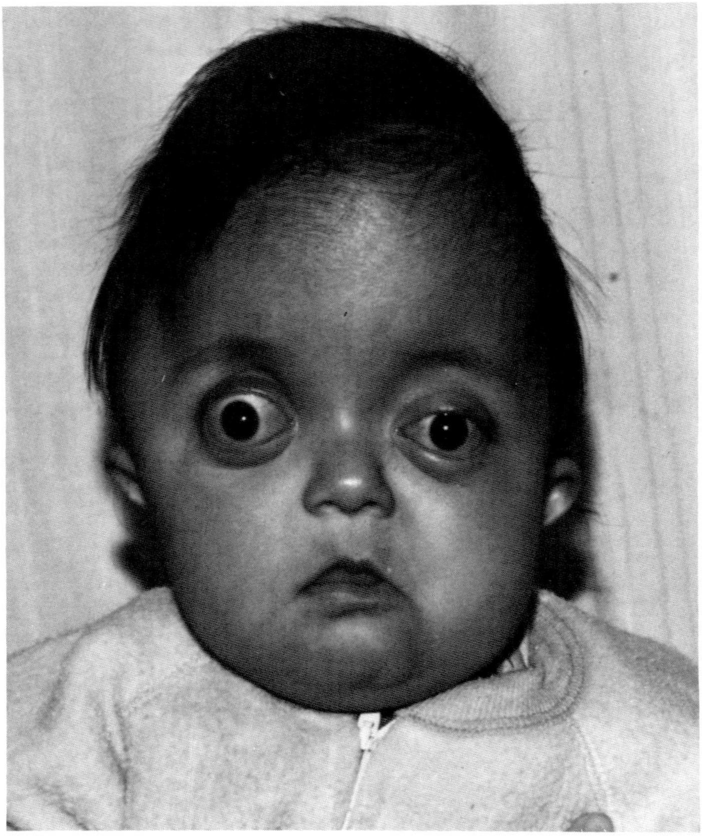

Figure 14.33 Kleeblattschädel anomaly. Mild form with bossing in the temporal region. Exorbitism and midfacial hypoplasia are also features of the anomaly.

unequal levels of the orbits. The frontal hairline is low set and ptosis of the upper eyelid is associated with the malformation. The nose can be beaked or there can be an absence of the frontonasal angle.

The digits can be foreshortened and a partial cutaneous syndactyly is occasionally seen between the index and middle digits.

Transmission of the malformation is by an autosomal dominant means.

CARPENTER SYNDROME

All the coronal sutures can be involved in the malformation which is also known as acrocephalopolysyndatyly. Unequal sutural closure produces an asymmetrical tower-shaped skull.

Polydactyly characterizes this craniosynostosis disorder. Congenital heart malformation can also be present. Those who survive usually have lower levels of intelligence.

The syndrome is transmitted in autosomal recessive pattern.

KLEEBLATTSCHÄDEL ANOMALY

The translation of this German term describes the anomaly: cloverleaf skull (Fig. 14.33). The trilobe configuration is produced by the synostosis of varying combinations of the temporoparietal, coronal, lambdoidal, and the metropic sutures. Hydrocephaly is associated with the deformity. The midface is hypoplastic. Exorbitism may also be seen. The anomaly occurs in a sporadic fashion.

References

1. Stevenson, A. C., Johnson, H. A., Stewart, M. I. P., and Golding, D. R.: Congenital malformation—A report of a study of series of consecutive births in 24 centres. World Health Organization, Geneva, 1966.
2. Neel, J. V.: A study of major congenital defects in Japanese infants. *Am. J. Hum. Genet.*, *10:*398, 1958.
3. Altemus, L. A., and Ferguson, A. D.: Comparative incidence of birth defects in Negroes and white children. *Pediatrics*, *36:*56, 1965.
4. Fogh-Andersen, P.: *Inheritance of Harelip and Cleft Palate.* Nyt Nordisk Forlag Arnold Busck A/S, Coopenhagen, 1942.
5. Fujino, H., Tanaka, K., and Sanui, Y.: Genetic study of cleft lips and cleft palates based upon 2828 Japanese cases. *Kyushu J. Med. Sci.*, *14:*317, 1963.
6. Knox, G., and Braithwaite, F.: Cleft lips and palates in Northumberland and Durham. *Arch. Dis. Child.*, *38:*66, 1963.
7. Grabb, W. C.: The first and second branchial arch syndrome. *Plast. Reconstr. Surg.*, *36:*485, 1965.
8. Poswillo, D. E.: Orofacial malformations. *Proc. R. Soc. Med.*, *67:*13, 1974.
9. Kawamoto, H. K., Jr.: The kaleidoscopic world of rare craniofacial clefts; order out of chaos (Tessier classification). *Clin. Plast. Surg.*, *3:*529, 1976.
10. Rovin, S., Dachi, S. F., Borenstein D. B., and Cotter, W. B.: Mandibulofacial dysostosis, a familial study of 5 generations. *J. Pediatr.*, *65:*215, 1964.
11. Rogers, B. O.: Berry-Treacher-Collins syndrome; a review of 200 cases (mandibulofacial dysostosis; Franceschetti-Zwahlen-Klein syndrome). *Br. J. Plast. Surg.*, *17:*109, 1964.
12. Franceschetti, A., and Klein, D.: Mandibulo-facial dysostosis; a new hereditary syndrome. *Acta Ophthalmol.*, *27:*144, 1949.
13. Bertelsen, T. I.: *The Premature Synostosis of the Cranial Sutures.* Munksgaard, Copenhagen, 1958.
14. Flippen, J. H., Jr.: Cranio-facial dysostosis of Crouzon; report of a case in which the malformation occurred in four generations. *Pediatrics*, *5:*90, 1950.
15. Cohen, M. M., Jr.: A etiologic and nosologic overview of craniosynostosis syndromes. *Birth Defects*, *11:*137, 1975.
16. Kleinsasser, O., and Schlothane, R.: Die Ohrmissbildungen in Rahmen der Thalidomide Embryopathie. *Z. Laryng. Rhinol. Otol.*, *43:*344, 1964.
17. Livingstone, G.: Congenital ear abnormalities due to thalidomide. *Proc. R. Soc. Med.*, *58:*493, 1965.
18. Smithells, R. W., and Leck, I.: The incidence of limb and ear defects since the withdrawal of thalidomide. *Lancet*, *1:*1095, 1963.
19. Smith, J.: Teratogenic effects of anticonvulsants. *Lancet*, *2:*1154, 1972.
20. Spidel, B. D., and Meadow, S. R.: Maternal epilepsy and abnormalities of the fetus and newborn. *Lancet*, *2:*839, 1972.
21. Saxen, I.: Association between oral clefts and drugs taken during pregnancy. *Int. J. Epidemiol.*, *4:*37, 1975.
22. Safra, M. S., and Oakley, G. P.: Association between cleft lip with or without cleft palate and parental exposure to diazepam. *Lancet*, *2:*478, 1975.
23. Gorlin, R. J., Pindborg, J. J., and Cohen, M. M., Jr.: *Syndromes of the Head and Neck*, Ed. 2. McGraw-Hill, New York, 1976.
24. Gorlin, R. J.: Classification of craniofacial syndromes. In *Symposium of Diagnosis and Treatment of Craniofacial Anomalies*, p. 243, edited by J. M. Converse, J. G. McCarthy, and D. Wood-Smith. C. V. Mosby, St. Louis, 1979.
25. Tessier, P.: Anatomical classification of facial, craniofacial and latero-facial clefts. *J. Maxillofac. Surg.*, *4:*69, 1976.
26. De Myer, W.: The median cleft face syndrome. Differential diagnosis of cranial bifidum occultum, hypertelorism, and median cleft nose, lip and palate. *Neurology*, *17:*961, 1967.
27. Sedano, H. O., Cohen, M. M., Jr., Jirasek, J., and Koplin, R.: Frontonasal dysplasia. *J. Pediatr.*, *76:*906, 1970.
28. De Myer, W., Zeman, W., and Palmer, C. A.: The face predicts the brain; diagnostic significance of median facial anomalies for holoprosencephaly (arhinencephaly). *Pediatrics*, *34:*256, 1964.
29. Gunther, G. S.: Nasomaxillary cleft. *Plast. Reconstr. Surg.*, *32:*637, 1963.
30. Sakuri, E. H., Mitchell, D. F., and Holmes, L. A.: Bilateral oblique facial clefts and amniotic bands; a report of two cases. *Cleft Palate J.*, *3:*181, 1966.
31. Harkins, C. S., Berlin, A., Harding, R. L., et al.: A classification of cleft lip and cleft palate. *Plast. Reconstr. Surg.*, *29:*31, 1962.
32. Tessier, P.: Colobomas; vertical and oblique complete facial clefts. *Panminerva Med.*, *11:*95, 1969.
33. Whitker, L. A., Katowitz, J. A., and Randall, P.: The nasolacrimal apparatus in congenital facial anomalies. *J. Maxillofac. Surg.*, *2:*59, 1974.

34. Morian, R.: Ueber die schrage Gesichtsspalte. *Arch. Klin. Chir.*, *35:*245, 1887.
35. Longacre, J. J., DeStefano, A., and Holmstrand, K.: The early versus the late reconstruction of congenital hypoplasia of the facial skeleton and skull. *Plast. Reconstr. Surg.*, *27:*489, 1961.
36. Franceschetti, A., and Zwahlen, P.: Un syndrome nouveau; la dysostose mandibulo-faciale. *Bull. Schweiz. Akad. Med. Wiss.*, *1:*60, 1944.
37. Braithwaite, F., and Watson, J.: Three unusual clefts of the lip. *Br. J. Plast. Surg.*, *2:*38, 1949.
38. Converse, J. M., McCarthy, J. G., Wood-Smith, D., and Coccaro, P. J.: Craniofacial microsomia. In *Reconstructive Plastic Surgery*, Ed. 2, p. 2359, edited by J. M. Converse. W. B. Saunders, Philadelphia, 1976.
39. Converse, J. M., Wood-Smith, D., McCarthy, J. G., Coccaro, P. J., and Becker, M. H.: Bilateral facial microsomia. Diagnosis, classification, treatment. *Plast. Reconstr. Surg.*, *54:*413, 1974.
40. Meurman, Y.: Congenital microtia and meatal atresia. *Arch. Otolaryngol.*, *66:*443, 1957.
41. Dupertius, S. M., and Musgrave, R. H.: Experiences with the reconstruction of the congenitally deformed ear. *Plast. Reconstr. Surg.*, *23:*361, 1959.
42. Poswillo, D.: The pathogenesis of Treacher-Collins syndrome (mandibulofacial dysostosis). *Br. J. Oral Surg.*, *13:*1, 1975.
43. Sanvenero-Rosselli, G.: Developmental pathology of the face and dysraphia syndromes—an essay of interpretation based on experimentally produced congenital defects. *Plast. Reconstr. Surg.*, *11:*36, 1953.
44. Tessier, P.: Orbital hypertelorism; 1. Successive surgical attempts, material and methods, causes and mechanisms. *Scand. J. Plast. Reconstr. Surg.*, *6:*135, 1972.
45. Shillito, J.: Premature craniofacial synostosis—neurosurgical treatment. In *Proceedings of International Conference on Diagnosis and Treatment of Craniofacial Anomalies*, New York, Oct. 25–28, 1971.
46. Christiansen, R. L., and Evans, C. A.: Habilitation of severe craniofacial anomalies—the challenge of new surgical procedures; an NIDR workshop. *Cleft Palate J.*, *12:*167, 1975.
47. Moss, M. L.: The pathogenesis of premature craniosynostosis in man. *Acta Anat.*, *37:*351, 1959.
48. Stewart, R. E., and Kawamoto, H. K., Jr.: Acrocephalosyndactyly (Apert's syndrome); a cause for reconsideration of its pathogenesis. In *Symposium of Diagnosis and Treatment of Craniofacial Anomalies*. p. 258, edited by J. M. Converse, J. G. McCarthy, and D. Wood-Smith. C. V. Mosby, St. Louis, 1979.
49. Virchow, R.: Uber den Cretinismus, namenthlich in Franhen, und uber pathologische Schädelformen. *Verh. Phys-med. Ges. Wurzburg.*, *2:*241, 1851.

CHAPTER 15

Craniofacial Procedures

S. Anthony Wolfe, M.D., F.A.C.S.

HISTORY

The major advances in the surgery of the maxilla made by German surgeons of the 1920s and 1930s (Martin Wassmund—the first Le Fort I osteotomy in 1927,[1] Karl Schuchardt—the first interpterygomaxillary disjunction in 1934[2]) laid the groundwork for the brilliantly innovative British plastic surgeon, Sir Harold Gillies, who performed the first Le Fort III osteotomy in 1949.[3] There was considerable relapse of the advancement Gillies obtained in this patient, and Hugo Obwegeser of Zürich later stressed the importance of autogenous bone grafts placed in the interpterygomaxilliary space and along the anterior maxillary osteotomy lines to maintain the shifted bone segments in their new position.[4] Obwegeser also made a major contribution to mandibular surgery with his popularization of the intraoral sagittal split procedure.[5]

Finally, Paul Tessier of Paris, with a wide background in orbital surgery, synthesized all that had been done before, and made major advances in the treatment of many previously inoperable major craniofacial malformations.[6,7] Singlehandedly, he brought the field of craniofacial surgery into being, and to him we owe the methods of treatment which will be discussed in this chapter for the treatment of:

1. Craniofacial dysostosis (CFD), or the Crouzon-Apert deformities
2. Orbital hypertelorism (hypertelorbitism), orbital dystopia, plagiocephaly, microphthalmia, exophthalmos and enophthalmos
3. The lateral facial dysplasias: hemifacial microsomia, the Treacher-Collins-Franceschetti syndrome
4. Blepharophimosis.

The above congenital conditions, along with applications in the treatment of acquired deformities due to trauma and concer, constitute the bulk of craniofacial surgery.

The underlying principle of craniofacial surgery is the same as that of all other areas of

The author would like to express his thanks to the members of the Craniofacial Anomalies Clinic of the Mailman Center for Child Development of the University of Miami School of Medicine who participated in the treatment of many of the patients shown in this chapter: Drs. Larry Page and Robert Jacobson, Neurosurgery; Dr. Samuel Berkowitz, Orthodontics; Drs. Al Smith, John Flynn and Richard Tenzel, Ophthalmology; Dr. Wilma Maue-Dickson, Craniofacial Research.

The greatest debt of course is to Dr. Paul Tessier. Virtually all patients with craniofacial anomalies the world over can thank him for the methods of treatment now available to them.

reconstructive plastic surgery: "Replace what is normal in normal position and retain it there."[8] This is a much more profound statement than it may seem at first glance, since it presupposes a knowledge of:

1. What composes the normal structure? (anatomy)
2. How does it differ at various ages? (facial growth)
3. What is the normal position of the structure relative to other facial structures? (cephalometry, anthropological and ethnological differences, and artistic taste)
4. How can the structure be moved? (means of wide exposure of all portions of the face, including intracranial structures, with preservation of the vital functions of vision, olfaction, respiration, mastication, facial sensation and movement, but with minimal or no facial scarring)
5. And finally, how to keep the structures there? (methods of autogenous bone grafting and soft tissue reconstruction).

DEFINITION

Various definitions of craniofacial surgery have been put forward—that it should include only those cases which have had a concomitant transcranial approach, or only those cases which have had a complete subperiosteal "stripping" to within 15 mm of the apex of at least one orbit. However, craniofacial surgery, like plastic surgery, of which it is a direct outgrowth, cannot be limited to the treatment of a small number of congenital anomalies. It is, like its parent field of plastic surgery, an *approach* to certain difficult problems, which in this case involve the osseous structures of the orbit, and also the adjacent cranium, maxilla and even mandible. In most cases, an osteotomy with repositioning of one or more of these structures, and bone grafting, is carried out. The surgeon performing these procedures must have a thorough background in general surgery (fluid and electrolyte balance, blood replacement, respiratory management), be expert in harvesting bone grafts from various parts of the body, be experienced in methods of nasal, eyelid, lacrimal and other soft tissue reconstruction, and be well versed in managing malocclusion. At a minimum, he must have a neurosurgeon, neuroradiologist, ophthalmologist and orthodontist to aid him in the preoperative planning, the operative procedures themselves, and postoperative rehabilitation. This should not be an occasional surgery for any members of the team, nor should it be undertaken by those who are inexperienced or not fully trained. Ambition alone is no substitute for proper training in craniofacial surgery, and in *all* the areas mentioned above.

Incisions for Exposure, and the Harvesting of Autogenous Bone

The coronal incision is essential for the wide exposure of the orbital region that is required by most craniofacial procedures (Fig. 15.1). It should be begun at least 3–4 cm behind the anterior hairline, and is carried in the avascular plane between the galea and the pericranium to just above the supraorbital rims, where the dissection then goes beneath the pericranium and into the orbit. The frontal nerve and artery, if they pass through a foramen instead of a bony notch, should be preserved by chiseling away the lower portion of the foramen to convert it to a notch. Laterally, the dissection is kept close to the fascia of the temporalis muscle down to and beyond the zygomatic arch. This will spare the temporal branch of the facial nerve. Mannitol is generally given at this point in the procedure, even if a craniotomy is not planned, as it decreases the size of the orbital contents. The medial orbital dissection is carried back beyond the anterior ethmoidal foramen, the superior dissection goes back to the superior orbital fissure, and the lateral dissection sweeps around to the interior orbital fissure. The remainder of the orbital floor dissection can be done through a transconjunctival incision, and dissection of the infraorbital area carried out from this incision and from the coronal incision.

Figure 15.1 The upper half of the facial skeleton is accessible through a coronal incision (*broad-striped area*), the orbital floors and infraorbital region through a conjunctional incision (*striped area*), and the lower half of the facial skeleton can be approached through the mouth (*finely striped area*)—with the result that major craniofacial procedures can be performed without *any* visible facial scars.

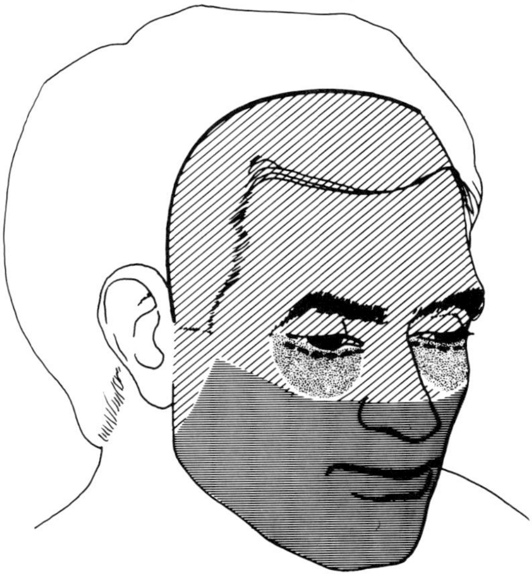

Osteotomies of the orbital floor can easily be performed through the transconjunctival incision, but if bone grafts are going to be placed in the infraorbital region, wiring them into position against the infraorbital rim is very difficult through a transconjunctival incision alone and a short skin incision in a skin crease below the lower lid should be made as well.

Autogenous bone is generally taken from one or more of four areas: ilium, rib, tibia, and skull. Iliac bone, beyond the age of 9 or 10, is ideal bone for grafting, since it has a high proportion of cancellous bone. The lips of the iliac crest are split and reflected, with muscle and periosteum attached, and the ilium beneath this, which has large amounts of cancellous bone, is harvested (Fig. 15.2). Bone grafts are best tailored to the size that will be required before removal from the ilium. Further cancellous bone is removed with a currette, and the preserved lips of the crest are wired together and to the remaining stable anterior superior spine.[9]

Ribs can be removed at any age, and if they are taken subperiosteally, considerable regeneration can be expected to occur in children. Generally a 5-cm incision over the right sixth rib is sufficient to allow harvest to three ribs 12–15 cm in length in an adult, providing 80 cm or more of split rib. If three ribs are taken, two should be taken above and one below a rib lift in place to prevent flailing of the chest.

Another good source of purely cancellous bone is the anterior tibia, just below the medial tibial tuberosity. A trapdoor of cortex is lifted up attached by periosteum superiorly, and cancellous bone removed with a currette. The trapdoor is then wired back into place, and immediate weight bearing is permitted.

In children, if a concomitant craniotomy is planned, strips of skull can be taken as graft material and reossification will quickly occur. Bone paste resulting from the drilling of burr holes for the craniotomy should be kept moist and preserved, and the outer table of the skull can yield large amounts of this type of "bone pate" in an adult.[10]

CRANIOFACIAL PROCEDURES

Craniofacial Stenosis

The craniofacial stenoses (CFS), or the Crouzon and Apert deformities, are transmitted as autosomal dominants. Because of an underlying lack of growth potential of cranial and cranial

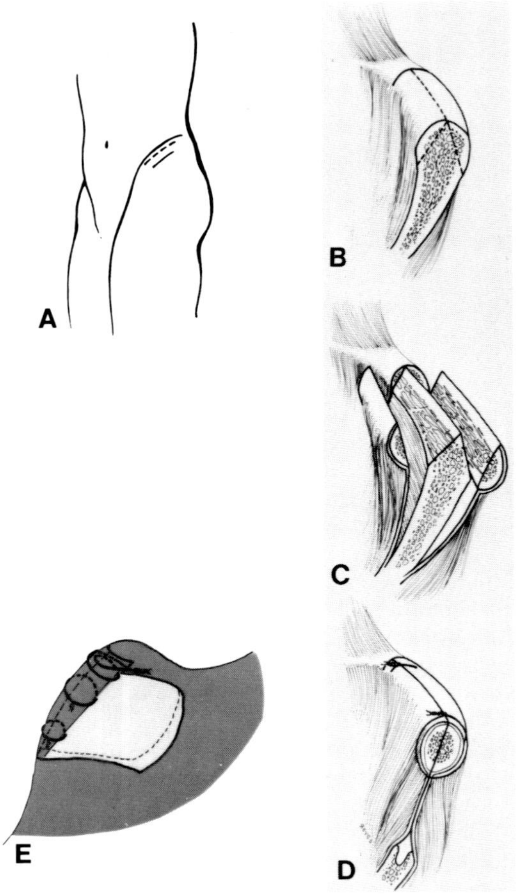

Figure 15.2 Method of harvesting iliac bone which preserves the contour of the iliac crest and provides stability for immediate postoperative ambulation. (*A*) The skin incision (*solid line*) is placed below the incision into the iliac bone (*dotted line*). (*B–D*) The lips of the iliac crest are reflected laterally, with periosteum and muscular attachments undisturbed. (*E*), All the bone beneath the reflected lips is available for harvest (to lower extent of the *dotted line*), and the lips are then wired to one another and to the intact anterior superior spine. (Reproduced with permission from S. A. Wolfe and H. K. Hawamoto: *Journal of Bone and Joint Surgery*, *60A*:411, 1978.[9])

base sutures (reason unknown), cranial deformity (oxycephaly, brachycephaly, turrencephaly) and/or maxillary underdevelopment (exorbitism, nasopharyngeal atresia, retromaxillism) occur. Patients with Apert's syndrome in addition have syndactyly of the hands and feet, more pronounced lateral canthal dystopia with an antimongoloid slant of the palpebral fissures, bregmatic furrows, thicker, oilier skin, and a more chaotic dental malocclusion with an anterior open bite. The palatal mucosa may be thickened and laden with a mucopolysaccharide material. The two syndromes should be viewed as a spectrum, since the cranial deformity can occur without the maxillary deformity, or vice versa, and there are some patients who appear to have Crouzon's deformity and who show slight webbing of fingers or toes.

Initial treatment should be neurosurgical, and should be carried out as soon as the condition is recognized. A thorough strip craniectomy (Fig. 15.3) of the coronal sutures can prevent a good deal of the cranial deformity, as well as the development of intracranial hypertension which may lead to mental retardation and even blindness. There is now evidence that if the craniectomy is carried intracranially, across the cranial base and the roof of the orbits, and anteriorly to the inferior orbital fissures, this release of the cranial base sutures will also prevent a considerable portion of the facial deformity.[11]

Even after this interceptive treatment, however, and in cases seen at later ages, there may be the need to advance the entire maxilla by a Le Fort III osteotomy (Fig. 15.4). This simultaneously corrects the exorbitism, the nasopharyngeal atresia, and the retromaxillism. Onlay bone grafting of the supraorbital and infraorbital areas and zygomatic arches, and a

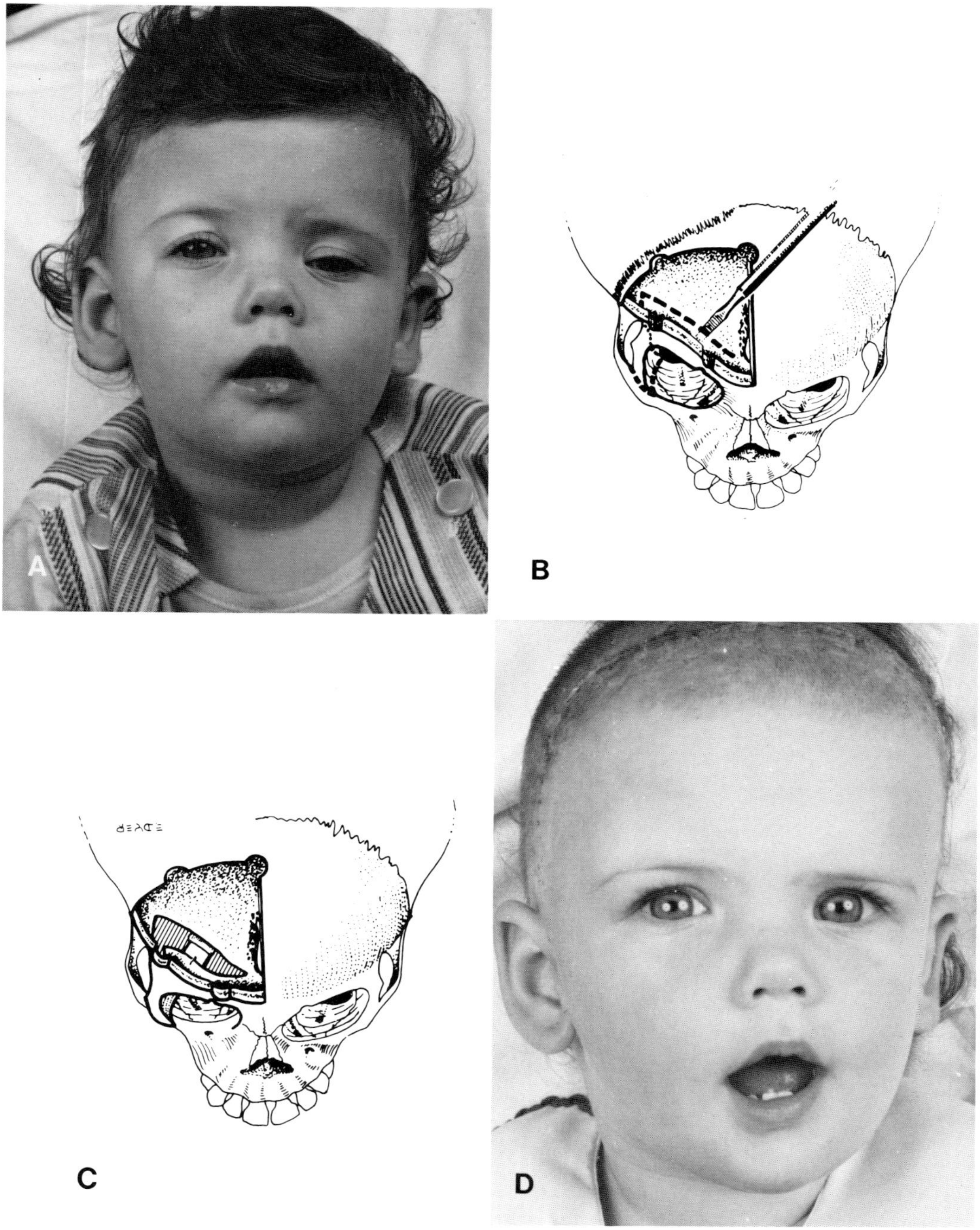

Figure 15.3 (*A*) One-year-old child with plagiocephaly due to right hemicoronal synostosis. Note the revision of the right frontal region and superior orbital rim. (*B*, *C*) Advancement of the right superior orbital rim and lateral orbital wall, with a small bone strut placed in the defect in the orbital roof to maintain the advancement. Silastic cap at lower end is to prevent bony union. The frontal bone is then attached to the repositioned superior orbital rim. (*D*) Same patient, 2 weeks after right hemicoronal strip craniectomy carried to the inferior orbital fissure and across the roof of the orbit, with advancement of the superolateral orbital rim and repositioning of the right frontal bone segment.

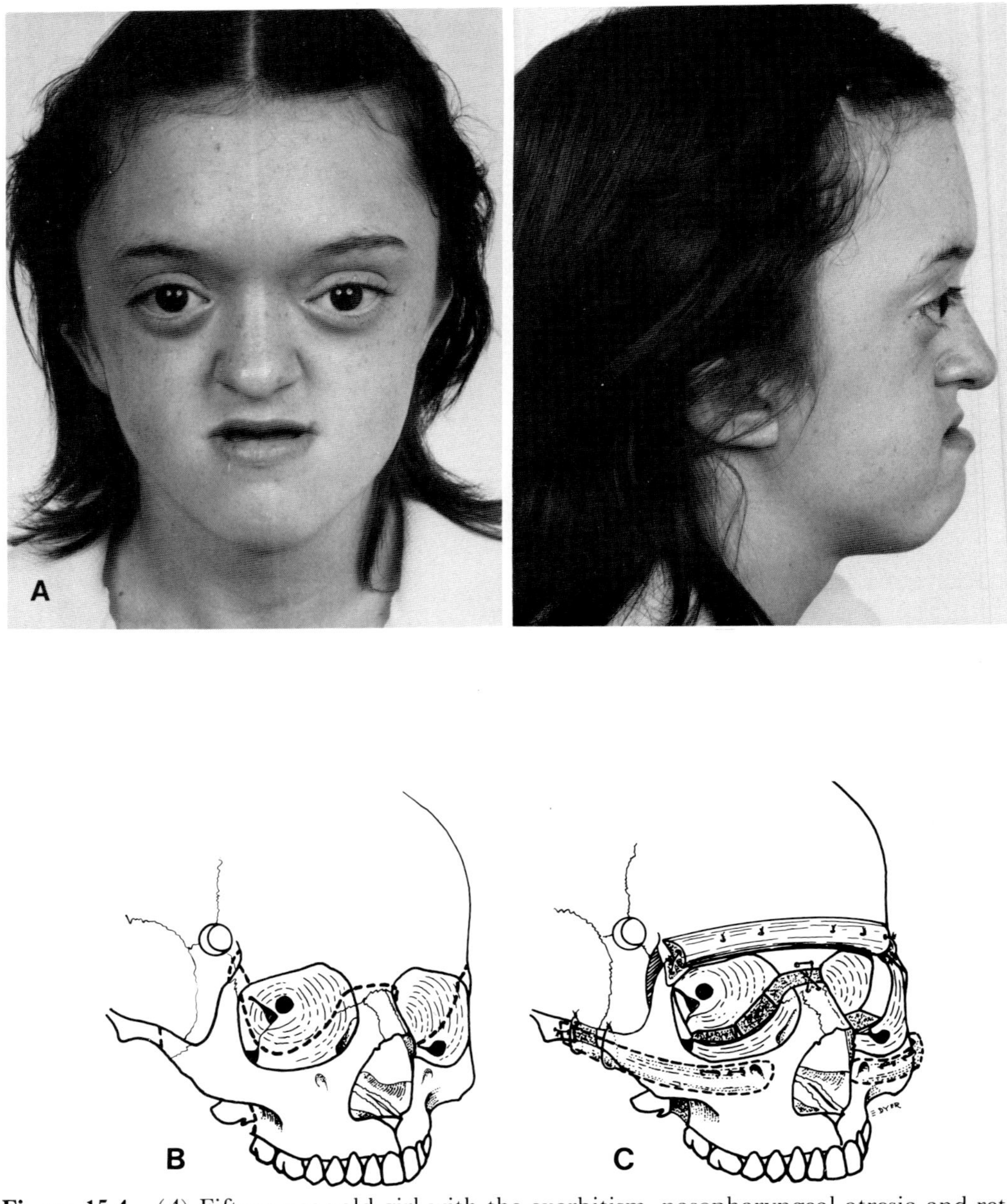

Figure 15.4 (*A*) Fifteen-year-old girl with the exorbitism, nasopharyngeal atresia and retromaxillism characteristic of Crouzon's disease. (*B*) Markings for the "semi-open skull" Le Fort III osteotomy (after Tessier). Note the burr hole to protect the frontal lobe during the cut for the vertical frontal spur. (*C*) After advancement of the midface with osteosyntheses and bone are grafts in place. Nine points of support of the advanced midface shown here.

genioplasty are often carried out at the same time (Fig. 15.5). Burr holes are made above the "vertical frontal spur" (designed to provide autocontention[12]) to protect the frontal lobes from damage during the osteotomy, and the nasofrontal cuts are made in a "keel-shaped" fashion to avoid damage to the cribriform plate. After the maxilla has been freed from the skull and advanced into its new position (determined both by the correction of the exorbitism and the

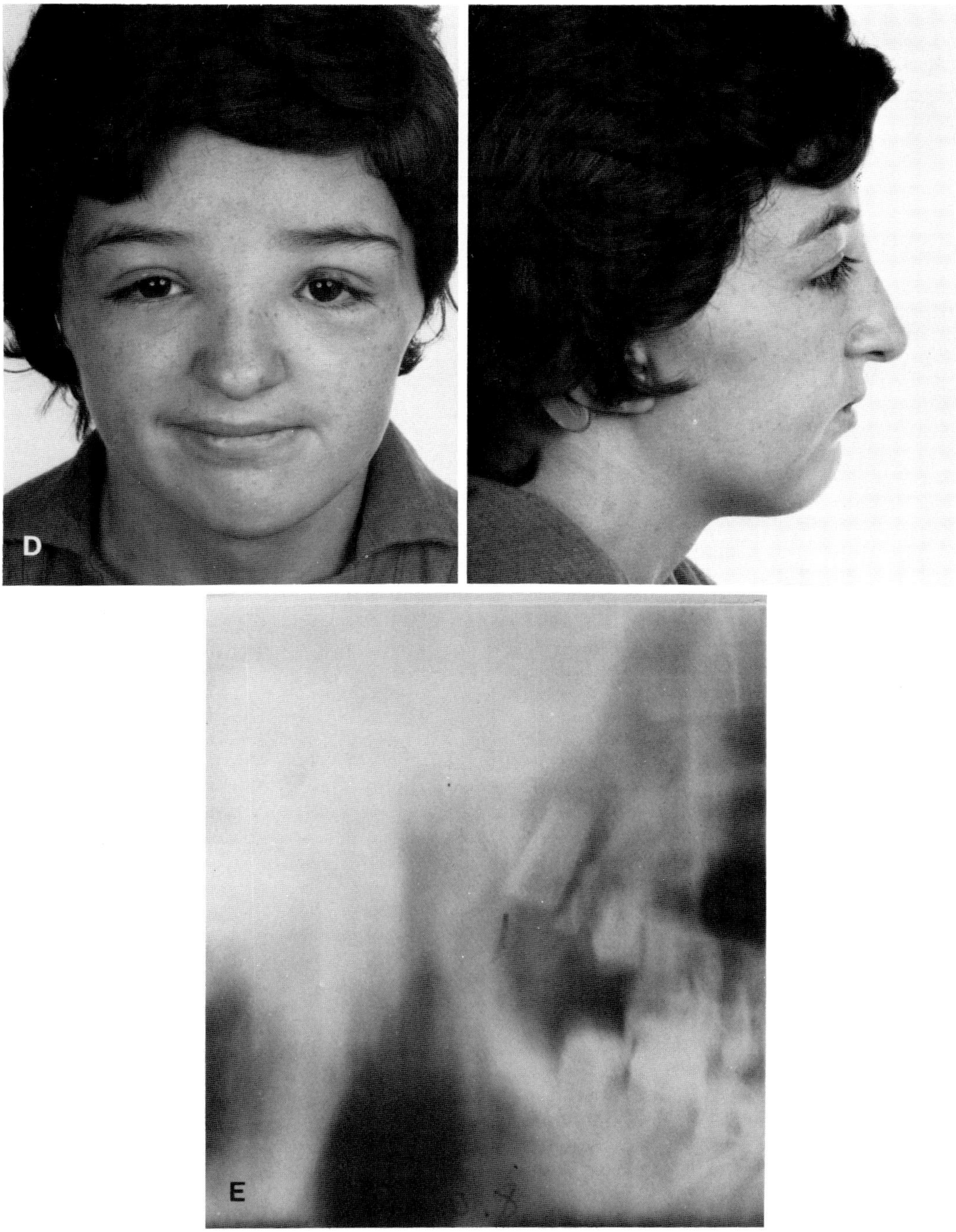

Figure 15.4 (*D*) Same patient 2 weeks after the procedure shown in (*B*) and (*C*). There have been small lower eyelid incisions in addition to the conjunctional incisions to allow wiring split rib grafts to the infraorbital rims. (*E*) Tomogram of the bone graft is the pterygomaxillary space. (Reproduced with permission from S. A. Wolfe: *Journal of Maxillofacial Surgery*, *5*:249, 1977.)

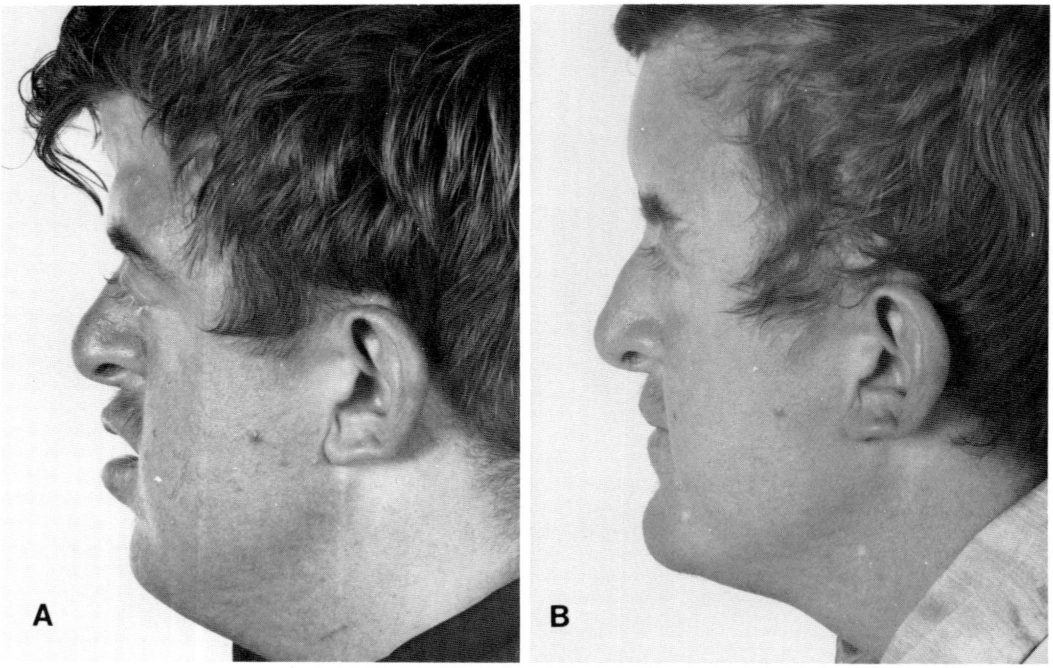

Figure 15.5 (*A*) Patient with Apert's syndrome preoperatively. (*B*) After Le Fort III osteotomy, genioplasty, and onlay bone grafting of forehead. (Reproduced with permission from S. A. Wolfe: *Annals of Plastic Surgery*, *1*:146, 1978.[10])

malocclusion), it is maintained in its new position by nine bone grafts and osteosyntheses (zygomatic arch,2; frontal spur,2; nasofraontal,1; pterygomaxillary,2; zygomatic arch-infraorbital split rib,2; see Fig. 15.4C). The final reconstruction is often stable enough that intermaxillary fixation can be avoided altogether, or begun a week or more after the surgery.

The extent of the exorbitism and retromaxillism may differ, and these cases can be treated by simultaneous Le Fort I and III osteotomies, permitting differential movement of the upper and lower portions of the maxilla.

The ideal age for carrying out a Le Fort III osteotomy has not been established, and must depend on the individual patient and the severity of the deformity. By the age of 4, most of orbital growth has taken place,[13] and the exorbitism can be corrected at this age without fear of return. However, there has been no evidence of growth of the maxilla in cases which have been treated by Le Fort III osteotomy at or before this age,[14, 15] so that with further growth of the mandible, which will continue well into the teens, the class 3 malocclusion will return with progressive severity. These patients will then need to undergo Le Fort I osteotomy to correct the malocclusion. Thus, it is the opinion of this author that patients can undergo Le Fort III osteotomy, if required for functional reasons (severe exorbitism or nasopharyngeal atresia), at 4–6 years of age, fully expecting that they will require another procedure (a Le Fort I osteotomy) at around 15. If severe exorbitism requires treatment at a younger age than this, an advancement of the orbital roof can be carried out (Fig. 15.6). For moderate to mild cases, I feel that it is reasonable to wait until around age 14, when the deformity can be corrected completely with one single operation. This does not dismiss the psychological effects of the facial deformity on the child and his parents, but with proper counseling it can be minimized. The surgeon should not lose sight of the fact that a second major operation is also a very traumatic psychological event. Such a waiting period has been observed for years for young patients undergoing rhinoplasty.

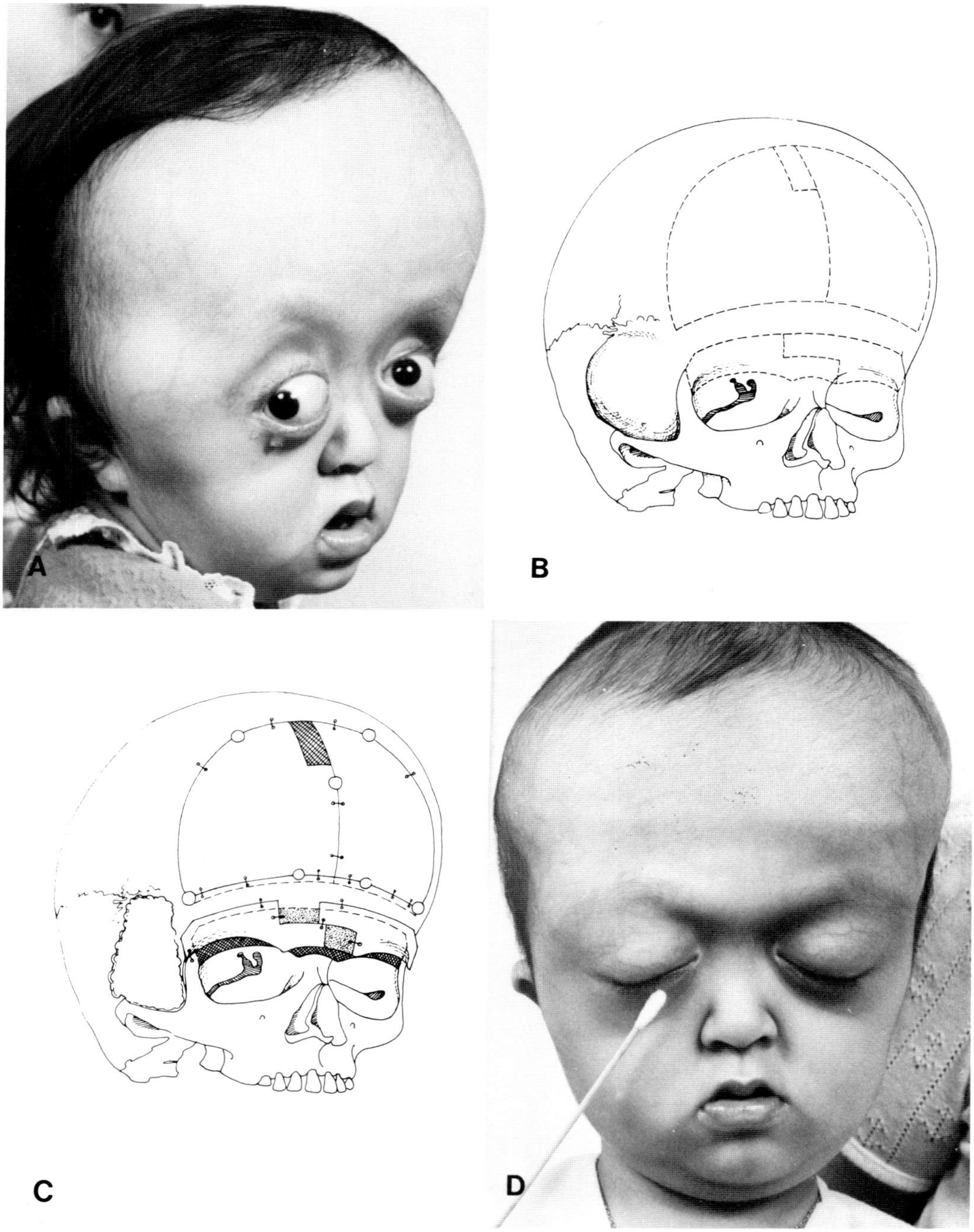

Figure 15.6 (*A*) Two-year-old child with severe exorbitism who could not achieve palpebral occlusion preoperatively. (*B*) Marking of osteotomy for advancement of orbital roof. (*C*) After expansion of orbital roof in the sagittal, horizontal, and vertical planes. Also, reduction of the cranial vault and use of skull as a graft source (*stippled areas*). (*D*) One month postoperatively the child can easily close her eyes. The visible edge of the "frontal bandeau" smoothed out with bone remodeling. A Le Fort III osteotomy will be needed in patient at a later age. (Reproduced with permission from S. A. Wolfe: *Journal of Maxillofacial Surgery*, *5*:249, 1977.)

Telorbitism

Telorbitism (orbital hypertelorism) is an abnormally great distance between the bony orbits, as measured between the dacryons[16] (the point of fusion of the lacrimal, maxillary and frontal bones, located just above the lacrimal fossa). As mentioned in Chapter 14, this is not a primary condition, but is always secondary to craniostenosis, a facial cleft, encephalocoele, or other disorder interfering with the developmental rapprochement of the orbits. Telorbitism should not be confused with telecanthus, which is an increased separation of the medial canthi with the underlying bony structures in normal position.

In distinction to CFD, orbital hypertelorism can be corrected at a much earlier age (Fig. 15.7). Since most of orbital growth, as noted, is complete by age 4, surgery can be carried out at this age, or even earlier in severe cases. Since the ocular globe functions as a determining agent for the growth of the bony structures surrounding it, the bony orbits can thus be repositioned before growth is complete. However, excellent results can be also achieved in adults (Fig. 15.8).

In cases where the transverse width of the cribriform plate is relatively normal (Fig. 15.9*A*), this central section should be spared, thereby preserving olfaction (Converse[17]). If the vertical level of the cribriform plate is normal, an infrabasalar procedure can be carried out without the need for a craniotomy. Even with preservation of the central segment, however, a nasal bone graft is generally necessary (Fig. 15.9*B*), since most of these patients have small, underdeveloped noses. There is no tendency for change in the position of the orbits if proper mobilization was carried out at the time of surgery (Fig. 15.10). Occasionally secondary procedures are required to tighten slackened canthopexies or add to nasal bone grafts which do not keep up with the rest of facial growth. These same techniques can be applied to the correction of orbital dystopia, where only one orbit requires repositioning (generally in the vertical plane), and portions of the orbital walls can be moved to expand small, underdeveloped orbits (microphthalmia) or even normal ones (thyroid exophthalmos).[18]

Plagiocephaly

Plagiocephaly results from hemicoronal synostosis, and the attendent deformity can range from a slight flattening of the frontal base on the affected side, to a severe distortion of the entire cranial base and an orbit which lies superior, lateral and posterior to its expected position. This "expected position" is sometimes quite difficult, since the opposite orbit and nasal structures can be abnormally positioned as well. The interincisive space is the best indication of the midline. Treatment should be carried out as soon as the diagnosis is established (Fig. 15.11), so that the growth-directing influence of the adjacent brain and eye can be used to minimize the deformity. Besides the coronal sutures, the frontosphenoidal and frontoethmoidal sutures can be involved as well (causing the orbital deformity), and the strip craniectomy should be carried intracranially across the orbital roof, and inferiorly to the inferior orbital fissure.

Hemifacial Microsomia

Hemifacial microsomia (previously called the first and second branchial arch syndrome) is a condition which Poswillo[19] has now reproduced in an animal model by causing an occlusion of the stapedial artery early in embryonic development, and the deformity can range from a minor anomaly of the ear or shortness of the mandibular ramus on the affected side, to a severe malformation (or lack of formation) of an entire half of the face, involving the

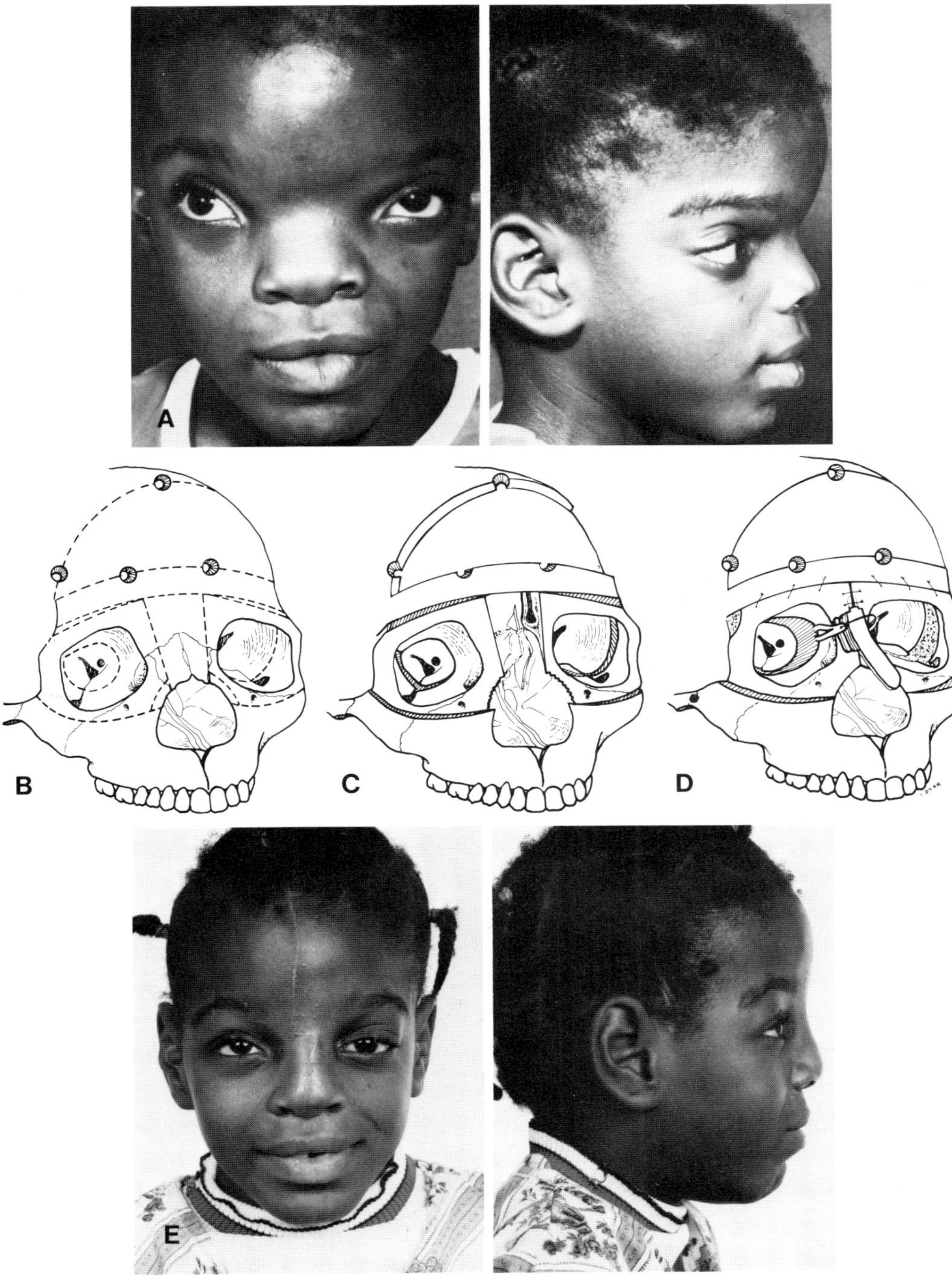

Figure 15.7 (*A*) Six-year-old child with telorbitism. Note the shortness of the nose and the divergent strabismus. (*B*) Markings for correction of telorbitism by rapprochment of the "effective orbits" and central ethmoidal resection. (*C*) After resection of the central frontoethmoidal segment and osteotomies to allow orbital mobilization. (*D*) After approximation of the "effective orbits." Note that the position of the optic foramen does not change. The orbits undergo "rotation" since the distance they must move is greater superiorly than inferiorly. The sagittal projection of the orbits should be at or behind the frontal bandeau to prevent enophthalmos. (*E*) Same patient after reduction of the interorbital distance from 44 to 21 mm. She also has had extraocular muscle surgery to attain orthophoria.

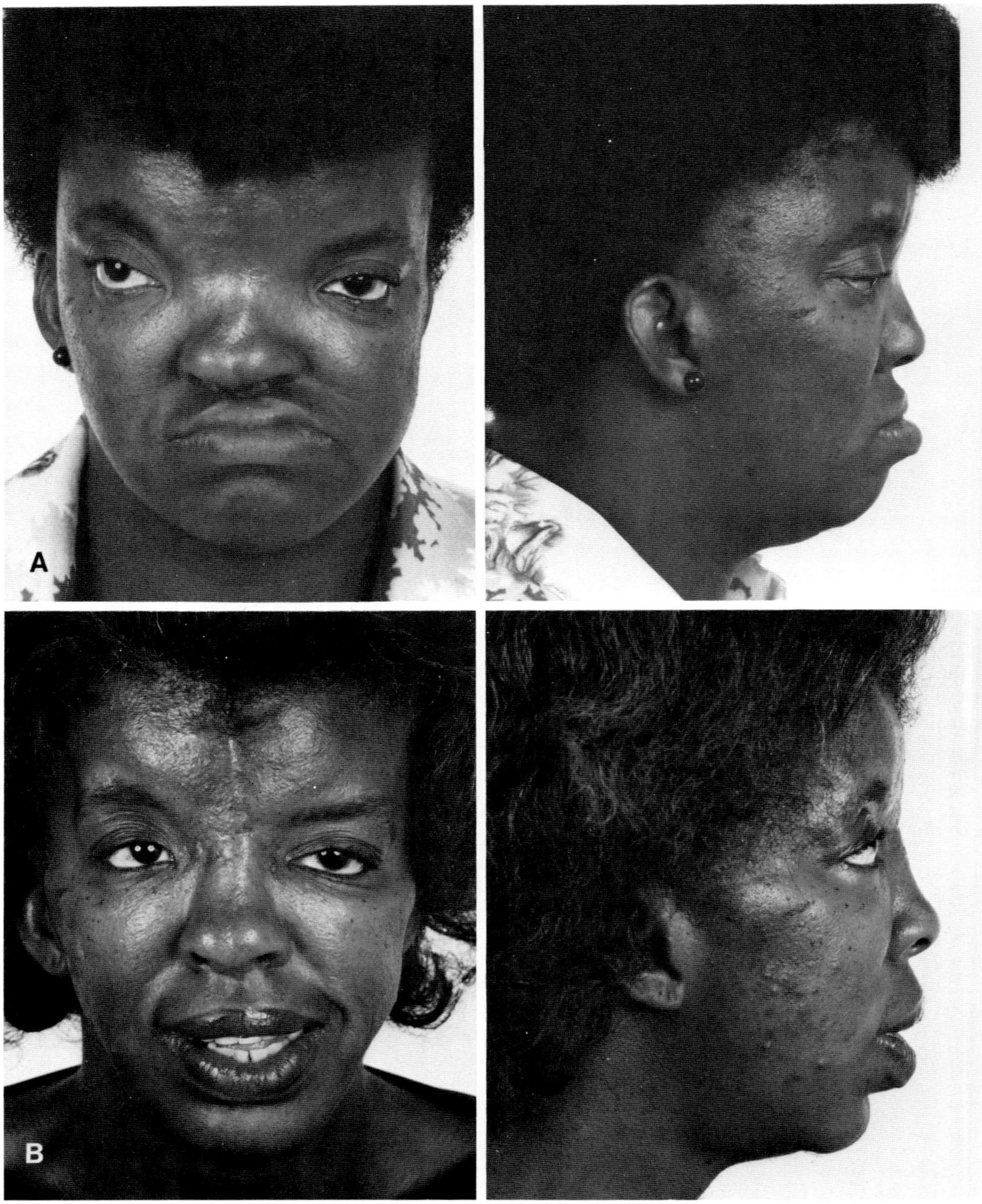

Figure 15.8 Patient before (*A*) and after (*B*) the procedure described in Figure 15.7, *B–D*. An intraoral sagittal split osteotomy and genioplasty were performed at a first stage for the class III occlusional relationship. Note the improvement in the exotropia postoperatively without extraocular muscle surgery.

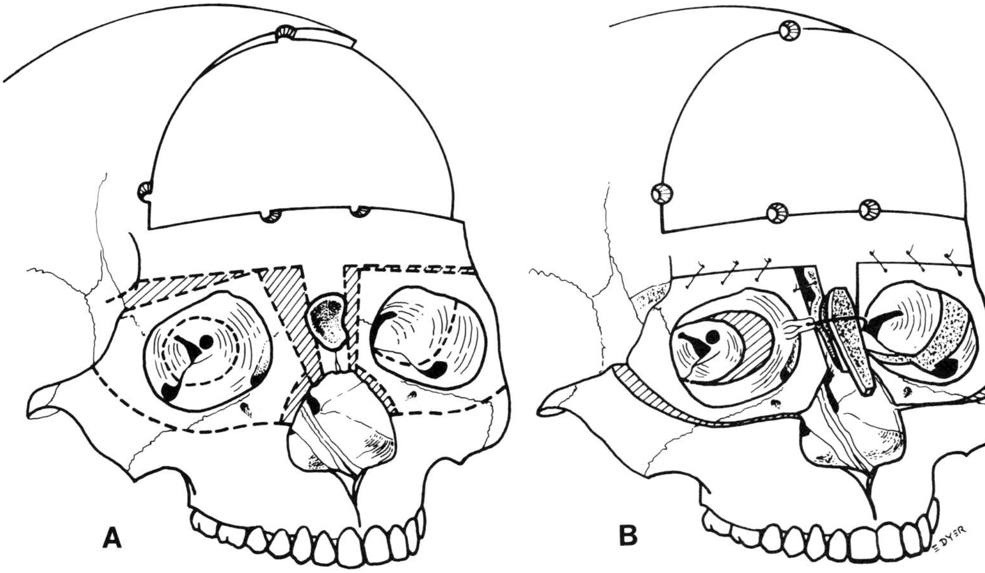

Figure 15.9 (*A*) Preservation of the central frontoethmoidal segment is possible if the anatomy of the cribriform plate is normal (Converse). (*B*) After paramedian (asymmetic) ethmoidal resections with preservation of olfaction. A nasal bone graft is still generally required.

orbit, maxilla, mandible, cranial base and temporal bone of the affected side. The term hemifacial microsomia is not ideal, since the condition can occasionally be bilateral, and Ross[20] has therefore suggested the term of lateral facial dysplasia. The condition is sporadic, and there is no tendency to pass it on to offspring. Mild forms can be treated by ear reconstruction or onlay bone grafting to the mandible through an intraoral approach, and these procedures can be carried out at age 5 to 6. The apparent severity of the condition increases with growth. Most severe cases will have an upward tilt of the occlusal plane on the affected side, and these patients will require a procedure to bring the occlusal plane to horizontal. In cases in which maxillary growth is already complete, age 14 or older, this is accomplished by a Le Fort I osteotomy, and downward and forward rotation of the maxilla on the affected side, using the maxillary tuberosity of the normal side as pivot point (Fig. 15.12). In more severe cases, the maxilla on the normal side will need to be raised as the blighted maxilla is lowered,[21] which requires removal of bone on the normal side. Here the interincisive space will be the pivot point. Bilateral osteotomies of the mandibular rami are carried out at the same time so that the mandible can follow the maxilla into its new position. An intraoral sagittal split is performed on the normal side, and on the affected ramus if it is well enough developed. If not, an extraoral oblique or L-shaped osteotomy with interposition of a bone graft will need to be done on the affected side. In the most severe forms (Fig. 15.13), the glenoid fossa is absent, and the first stage should be to construct a glenoid fossa and zygomatic arch, followed at a second stage by rotation of the maxilla to the horizontal plane, an intraoral sagittal split of the normal ramus, and rib graft (with a cap of costal cartilage to serve as condyle) to construct the missing ascending ramus. When soft tissue is quite deficient, lining and cover must be brought in before the bone construction is done, which is an exception to the general rule of first the hard tissue, then the soft.

In severe cases which are seen at an early age, an osteotomy of the ramus of the affected side with a bone graft can be carried out without a maxillary procedure. The open bite thus

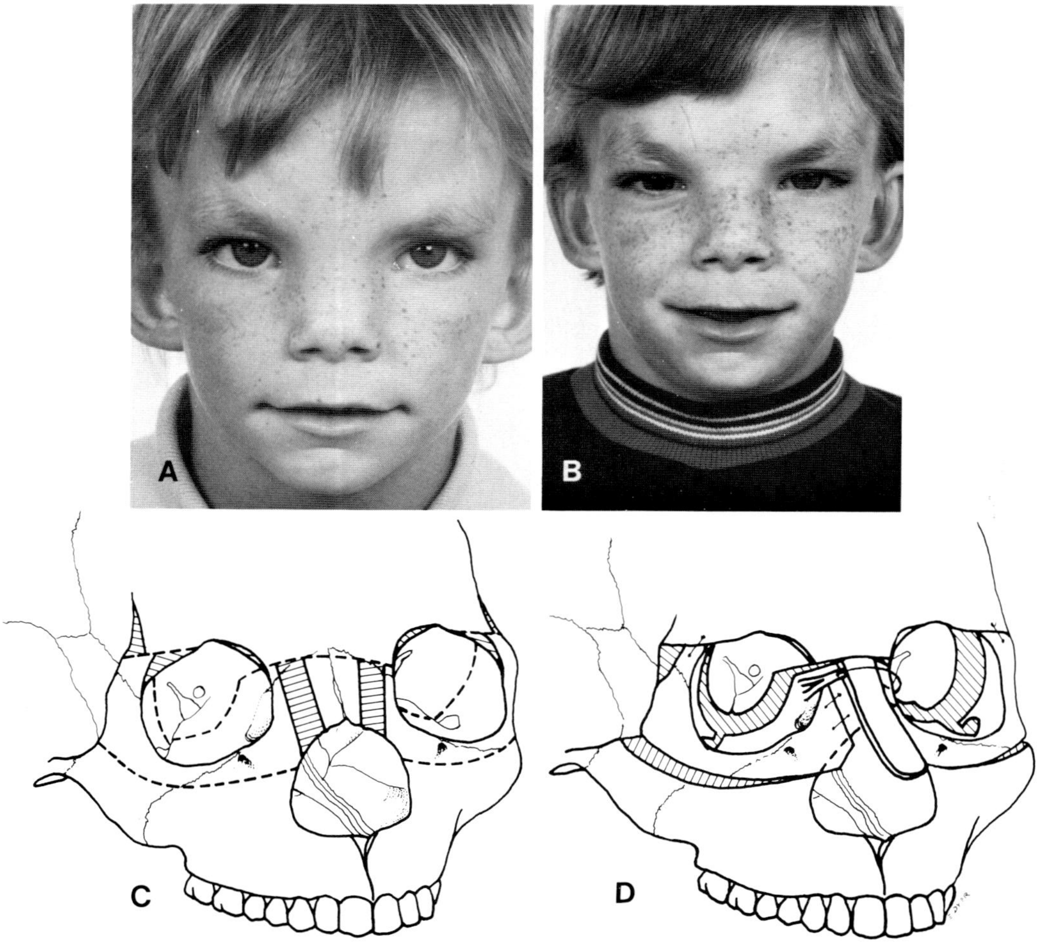

Figure 15.10 Six-year-old patient before (*A*) and 1 year after (*B*) infrabasilar extracranial osteotomies with preservation of olfaction. (Bilateral ostoplasties also performed.) The straight midline incision seems to be less obtrusive than the previously employed frontonasal Z-plasty. The nasal and frontal incisions are required because of the excess skin in this region. (*C*, *D*) Extracranial infrabasilar osteotomies for correction of lesser degrees of telorbitism (with preservation of olfaction).

Figure 15.11 (*A*) Two-year-old patient with telorbitism and plagiocephaly. (*B*) Markings for the osteotomies—considerably more complex than usual due to the sagittal as well as transverse dystopia of the left orbit. (*C*) After resections and osteotomies. The left orbit was displaced approximately twice as far as the right orbit. Note the rotation to the right, reshaping and repositioning of the frontal bandeau. (*D*) View from above of the frontal bandeau. Note the widely separated cribriform plates and bifid crista galli which prevented preservation of olfaction. (*E*) After rotation, reshaping and repositioning of the frontal bandeau. Both the left orbit and frontal bone segment will be attached to this repositioned frontal bandeau. (*F*) Final position of both orbits, the frontal bandeau, and the repositioned frontal bone segments. (*G*) The patient 1 month after surgery. Correction of the esotropia is to be performed about 6 months postoperatively.

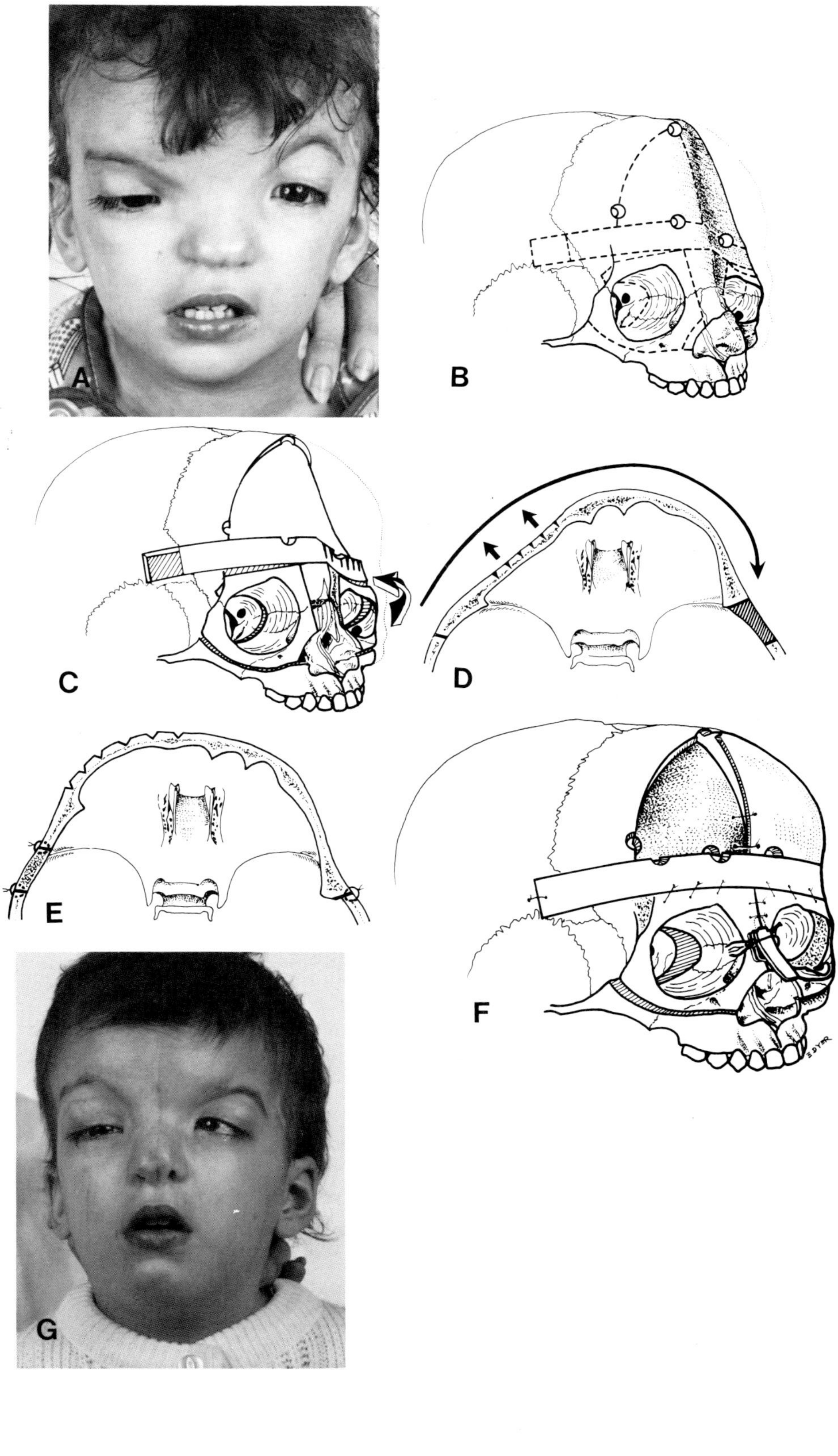
A
B
C
D
E
F
G

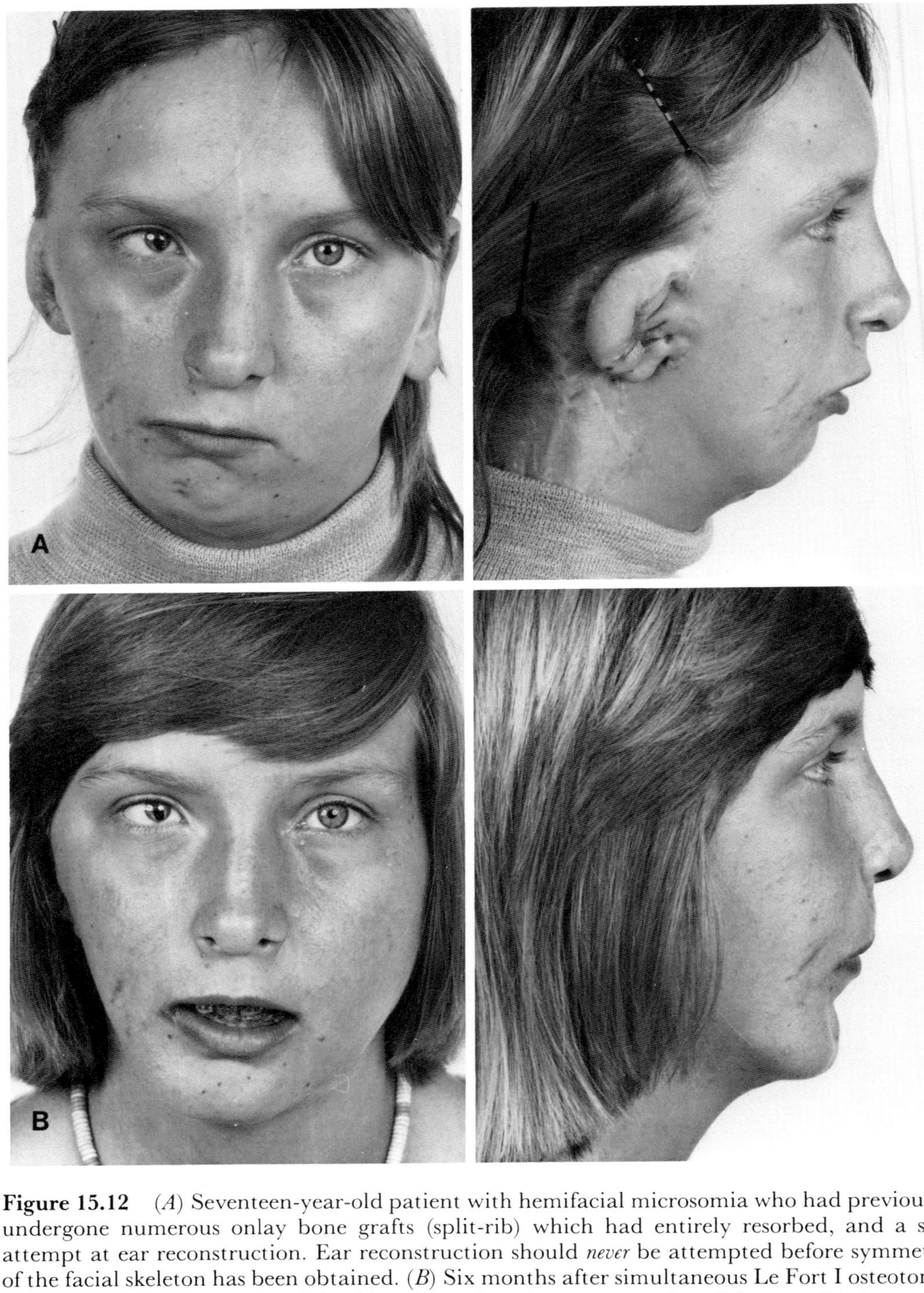

Figure 15.12 (*A*) Seventeen-year-old patient with hemifacial microsomia who had previously undergone numerous onlay bone grafts (split-rib) which had entirely resorbed, and a sad attempt at ear reconstruction. Ear reconstruction should *never* be attempted before symmetry of the facial skeleton has been obtained. (*B*) Six months after simultaneous Le Fort I osteotomy to lower the maxilla on the right side, bilateral sagittal osteotomies of the mandibular rami, and an advancement genioplasty. A fat dermal graft to the right cheek is planned.

created between maxilla and mandible is then maintained by a bite block, which is then gradually decreased in size by the orthodontist, allowing the maxilla to descent to the now horizontal occlusal plane of the mandible. This must be done before the final growth spurt of the maxilla, between 10 and 12, and probably not before age 6 (fixation of appliances to deciduous teeth is difficult). Whether or not the maxilla has the potential for growth is a debated point, but *anything* that can be obtained by growth is preferable to obtaining it by surgery, and may lessen the final amount of maxillary movement required. This treatment should be carefully coordinated with the orthodontist. Harvold[22] has shown that in moderate cases an "activating" appliance which brings about increased use of the existing musculature of the affected side can stimulate growth. Of course, if bone and soft tissue are entirely absent, such orthodontic endeavors will be futile.

Final treatment will consist of addition of further small amounts of soft tissue (fat dermal grafts), removal of skin tags, closure of the macrostomia on the affected side, and possibly, when all else is in perfect order, an ear reconstruction. Efforts at ear reconstruction should not be undertaken until the facial skeleton and soft tissue are symmetrical. If an ear is present, with an ear canal which is low in position, the entire ear can be raised to a proper position on a superior pedicle, bringing the ear canal out beneath and behind the ear lobe to allow for drainage. In my opinion there is no use for silicone, or other alloplastic materials, either by injection or implantation, and these cases should be cared for by a surgeon who can reposition the facial skeleton and carry out bone and soft tissue reconstruction using autogenous tissues. This is one of the most difficult conditions to correct, since one is trying to obtain symmetry with a "normal" side which may be actually overdeveloped.

Treacher-Collins-Franceschetti Syndrome

The Treacher-Collins-Franceschetti syndrome is transmitted as a Mendelian dominant, and is felt to arise from a lack of migration of neural crest ectoderm destined for bone and soft tissue structures in the malar region. The deformity, unlike cases of "bilateral hemifacial microsomia" is symmetrical, and there is often agenesis of the malar bone and zygomatic arch, with a fusion of the temporal, pterygoid and masseter musculature. As one dissects downward along the surface of the temporal muscle in search of a remnant of zygomatic arch, one can arrive directly on the mandibular coronoid process. There is downward overgrowth of the frontal portion of the lateral orbital wall, which, with a bone deficiency of the lateral orbital floor and lateral canthal dystopia, gives a pronounced antimongoloid inclination to the orbits and palpebral fissures. There is a lateral coloboma, and cilia are often deficient medial to it. A beaklike nose and underdeveloped mandible, with a variable amount of ear deformity, complete the picture.

Treatment for severe forms must be carried out in stages, since there is a large deficit of bone, and there is a limit to the amount of bone graft that can be expected to "take" at any one time (Tessier[23] calls this the "critical mass" and feels that a bone graft may not exceed 1 cm in more than two of its dimensions). The staged reconstruction can be begun at age 5 or 6, with construction of a zygomatic arch/malar complex, and correction of the orbit by removal of the overhanging frontal bone and filling in of the inferolateral orbital floor defect with bone grafts. Colobomas of the lower lids and the lateral canthal dystopia are corrected[21](Fig. 15.14).

Mandibular advancement, if required, and augmentation of the chin by bone graft or sliding horizontal osteotomy and rhinoplasty are delayed until around age 15.

Other Orbital Applications of Craniofacial Surgery

The procedures mentioned above were developed after a wide experience in the treatment of orbital and maxillary trauma, and the new principles which have been established can now

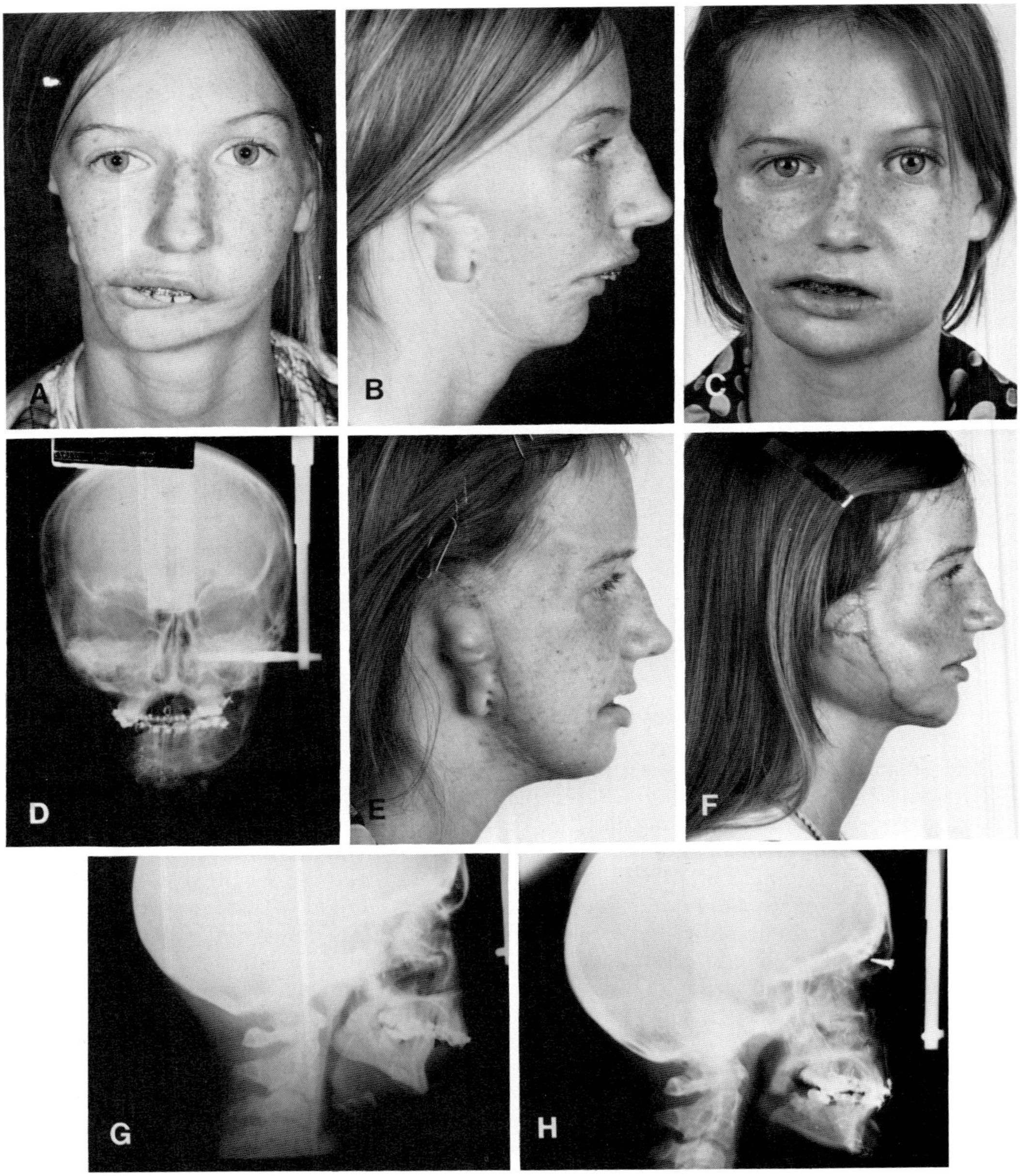

Figure 15.13 Reconstructive saga of a 15-year-old girl with severe hemifacial microsomia. She had previously undergone a metatarsal transplant and insertion of a Silastic prosthesis, both of which had failed due to infection. Preoperative frontal (*A*) and lateral (*B*) view. (*C*) After creation of glenoid fossa (first stage operation) and simultaneous rotational Le Fort I osteotomy, saggital split of left ramus, rib graft with cartilage cap for right ramus (visible on x-ray (*D*) and bone graft to chin (second-stage operation). (*E*) After stage 1 and 2 (see above). An ear reconstruction at this stage and in this position would be a disaster. (*F*) After removal of cartilage remnants of the ear, and insertion of a deepithelialized tube pedicle flap (from abdomen) (stage 3). A small fat dermal graft will eventually be placed in the residual depression in the right malar region. (*G*) Cephalometric x-ray taken after stage 1 (glenoid fossa and zygomatic arch construction). (*H*) X-ray after stage 2. The screw in the frontal sinus (Kufner) permits additional skeletal support of the maxilla, in addition to the usual circumzygomatic suspension.

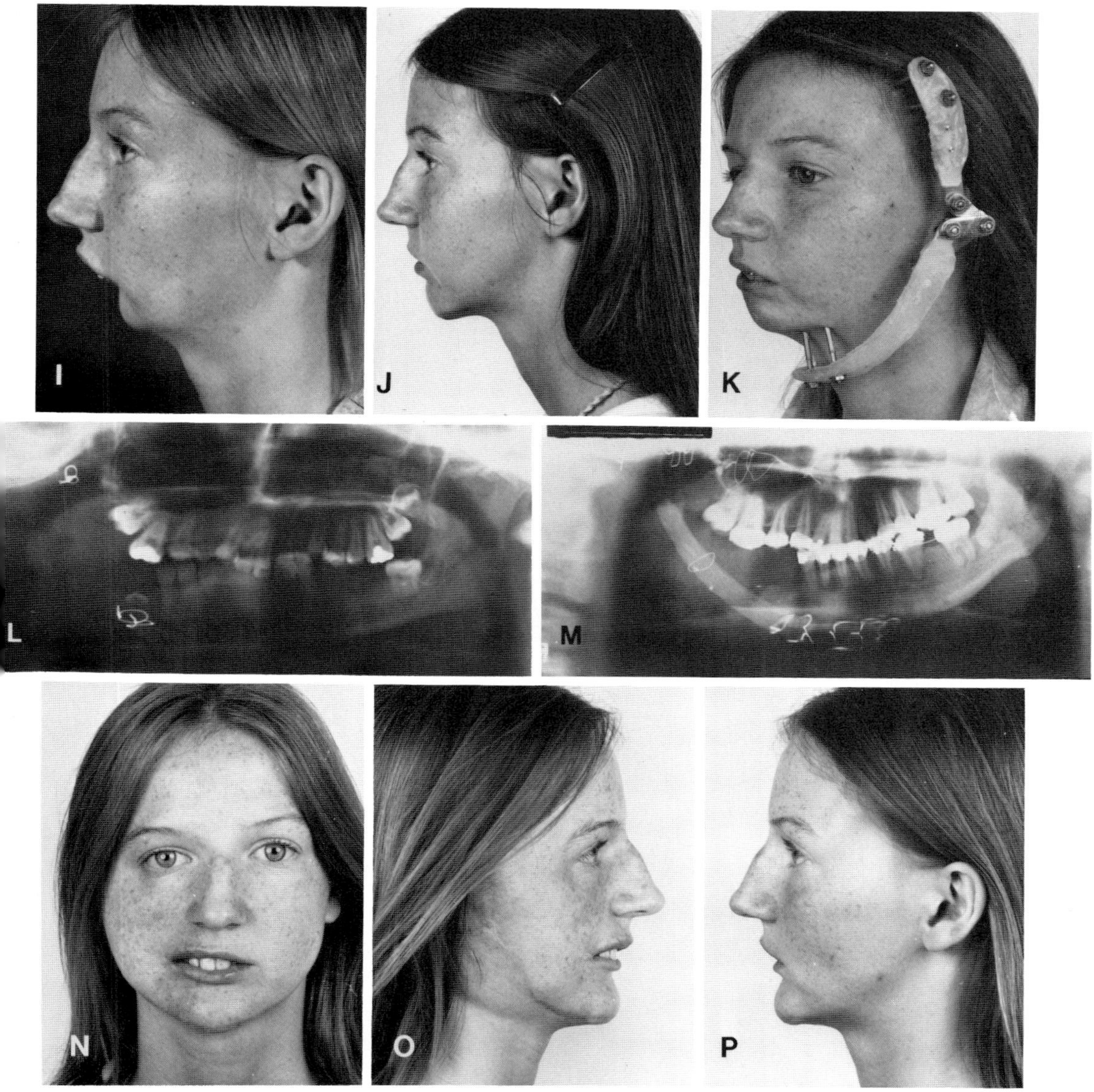

Figure 15.13 (*I*) Properative left profile. (*J*) After stages 1, 2 and 3. (*K*) Articulated biphasic external fixation appliance used during stage 2 to permit mouth opening in the proper plane, but prevent severe initial stress on the right mandibular construction (*L*).

be reapplied to these traumatic conditions. In severe Le Fort I, II and III fractures in the past, even with careful reapproximation of the parts and the use of extracranial traction with a halo device, there was a considerable incidence of postoperative relapse and development of a "dish-pan" face. The pterygoid plates are generally shattered in these cases, so there is no posterior buttress for the midface to rest upon, and consideration should be given to the use of primary bone grafting, along the maxillary fracture lines, in the pterygomaxillary region, in the orbital floor, and in the nose. The grafted bone will provide more material for a firm osteosynthesis, and may aid in preventing the late enophthalmos which after the contraction of the ocular muscles and soft tissues is difficult to correct. A medial canthopexy led into a

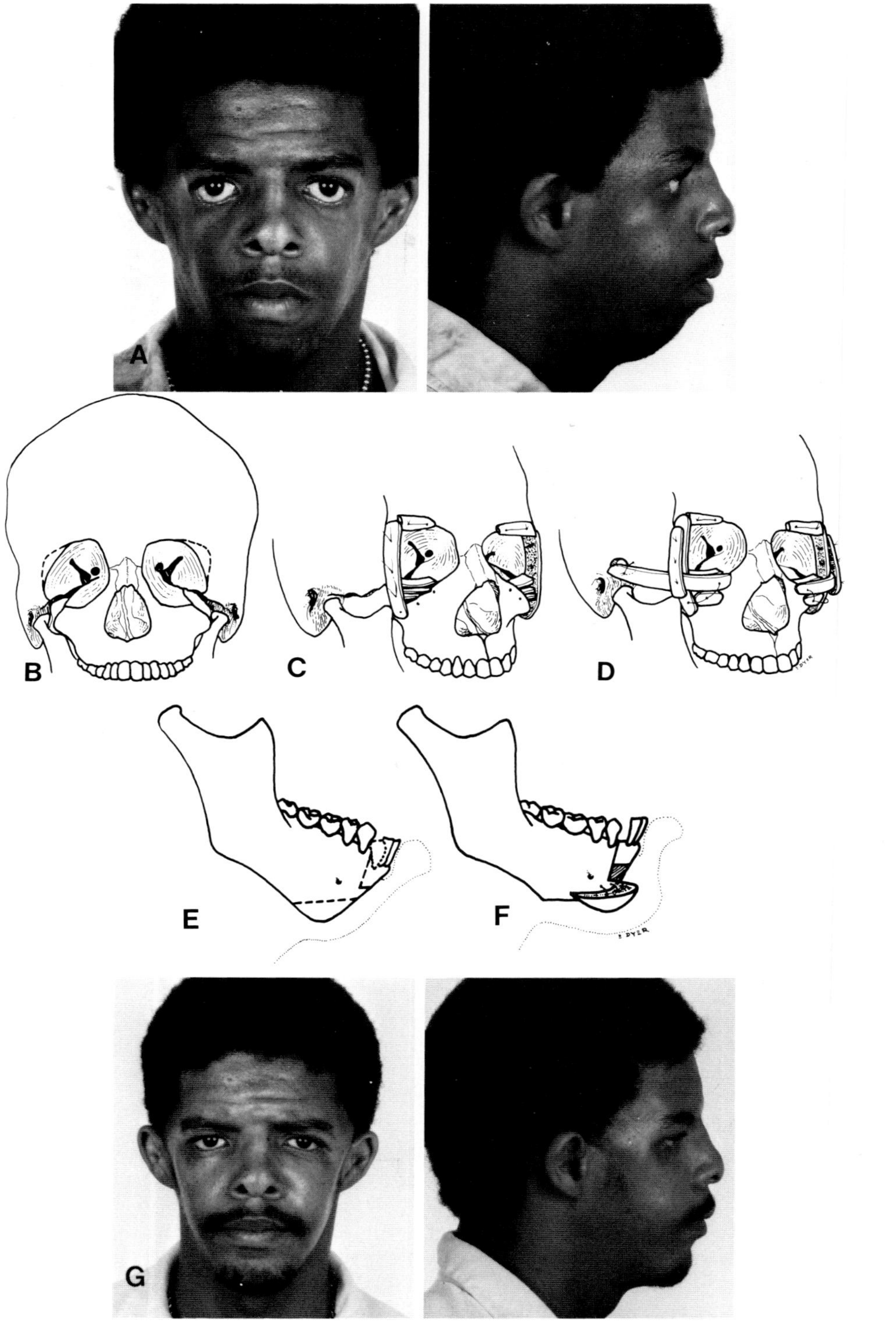
A
B
C
D
E
F
G

solid, stable bone graft will do better than one going into shattered, comminuted nasal bone fragments.

In elective procedures in the orbit, the craniofacial surgeon can provide much better exposure and working conditions for the ophthalmologist who is going to perform intraperiorbital procedures deep in the orbit. Through a coronal incision (Fig. 15.15), the lateral wall of the orbit can be removed to give excellent exposure, and then replaced at the end of the procedure. With neurosurgical participation, the orbital roof can be similarly removed, giving exposure of even the optic foramen. And working with the neurosurgeon, cranial and orbital roof defects can be restored primarily with the use of autogenous bone grafts.

In patients with exorbitism, as mentioned above, treatment is aimed at expanding their underdeveloped orbital volumes to house the normal orbital contents.[24] Patients who have had hyperthyroidism may have persistent exophthalmos after the medical or surgical control of their thyroid disease, and since little can be done to decrease orbital contents, treatment must consist of orbital expansion. Mild cases can be treated by lowering of the orbital floors through a lower eyelid incision with removal of as much orbital fat as possible, which will give 2–3 mm improvement in the exophthalmos reading (the distance between the most posterior point of the lateral orbital rim and the anterior surface of the cornea, generally 16 mm or less). Moderate cases can be treated with orbital floor lowering (Fig. 15.16) plus a valgus step osteotomy of the lateral orbital wall. Severe cases can be treated with a Le Fort III osteotomy to advance the orbital cone in a sagittal direction, plus a Le Fort I osteomy to allow for posterior movement of the lower half of the maxilla to maintain dental occlusion.[21]

Blepharophimosis

Blepharophimosis is a Mendelian dominant condition which has ptosis, shortness of upper eyelid structures, telecanthus, a floating lateral canthus, and hypertrichiasis of the eyebrows (Fig. 15.17). It is also now recognized that there is a deformity of the orbit as well, with orbital height being greater than orbital width (the contrary is normal), and a lateral orbital wall which is thicker than normal, and slants back almost parallel to the medial orbital wall instead of at a 45° angle to it.[23] Correction of the orbital anomaly should be part of the treatment of the condition, which also includes a medial canthopexy, correction of epicanthal folds, a lateral canthopexy and possibly canthotomy, and treatment of the ptosis by levator shortening or suspension to the frontalis muscle.

Figure 15.14 (*A*) Twenty-year-old patient with Treacher-Collins-Franceschetti syndrome. (*B*) The overhang of frontal bone in the superolateral orbital rim is removed. Note the enlarged inferior orbital fissures which are "open to the skin" (a form of facial clefting). (*C*) Revision of the orbital framework with split rib grafts (lateral orbital rim) and cancellous iliac bone (inferolateral orbital floor defects) (after Tessier). (*D*) Further split rib used to construct a zygomatic arch. A burr hole in the temporal region allows solid contention of the graft to the skull. A coronoidectomy should be performed at this time from above if there is limitation of mouth opening due to contact with the zygomatic arch construction. (*E*) The procedure used to correct the open bite and chin deformity—a superior displacement of the anterior mandibular alveolar segment (Köle) with a stabilizing bone graft and an advancement and superior transposition of the interior border of the mandibular symphysis (*F*). (*G*) The patient 3 months after the procedures described in *B–E*.

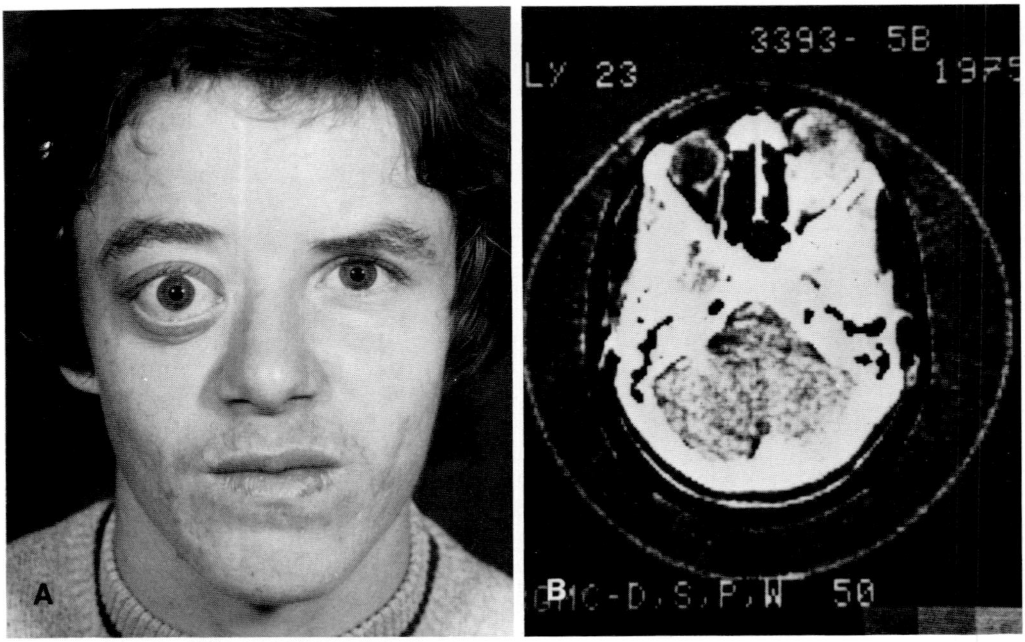

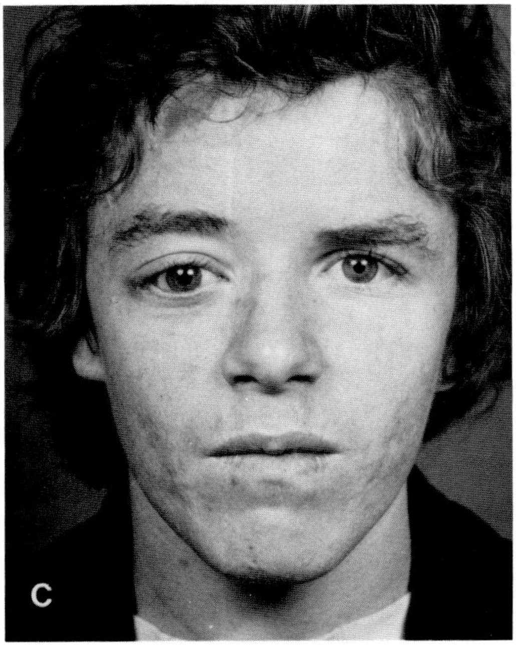

Figure 15.15 (*A*) Nineteen-year-old patient with slowly progressive unilateral exophthalmos who had had a previous exploration of the anterior orbit by an ophthalmologist, with negative findings. (*B*) Computerized axial tomogram demonstrating an abnormal mass in the posterior portion of the right orbit. (*C*) After a coronal incision and removal of the lateral orbital wall by the craniofacial surgeon, the ophthalmologist had excellent exposure of the posterior orbit and could remove a tumor (hamartoma) which completely encircled the optic nerve, without affecting vision or ocular motility. If further exposure is required for such procedures, the neurosurgeon can join the team and the orbital roof can be removed (and of course replaced). (Reproduced with the permission from S. A. Wolfe: *Journal of Maxillofacial Surgery, 5:* 249, 1977.)

Romberg's Syndrome

Romberg's syndrome is a condition which generally arises during the first decade of life, and involves different areas of the face. The etiology is not known, but since it involves both bone and soft tissue in "watershed" areas, it is felt to be on the basis of developmental vascular inadequacy. Treatment, once the condition has "burned out" and been quiescent for a few

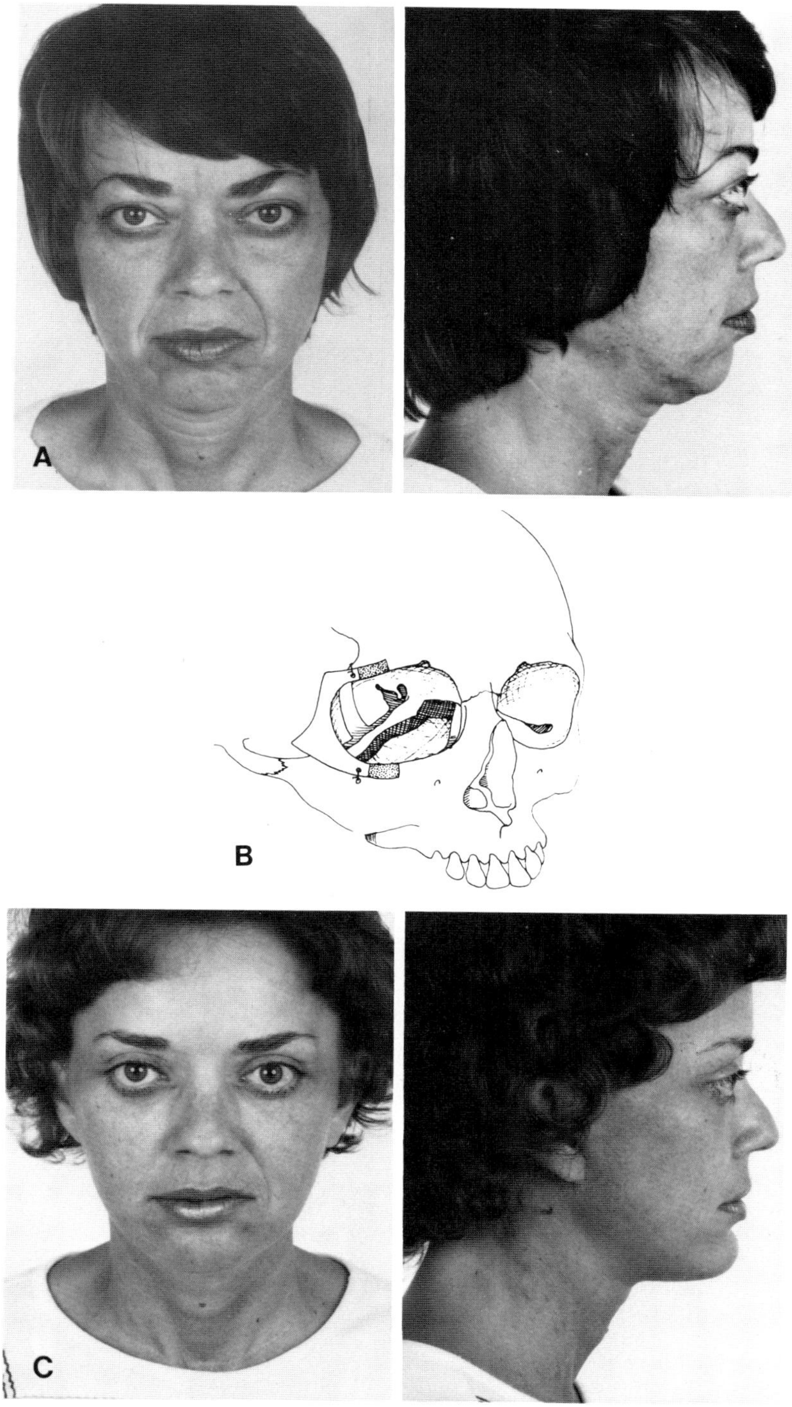

Figure 15.16 (*A*) Forty-year-old patient who had hyperthyroidism (now medically controlled), before orbital expansion. The exophthalmos is best appreciated on the lateral view. (*B*) Tessier's method of orbital expansion which impacts the medial orbital wall, lowers the orbital floor, and produces a valgus movement of the lateral orbital wall. An increase of up to 50% in the capacity of the orbit can be achieved with this procedure.[24] (*C*) Same patient several months following orbital expansion by the method shown in *B*. She is shown several weeks following meloplasty and chin advancement.

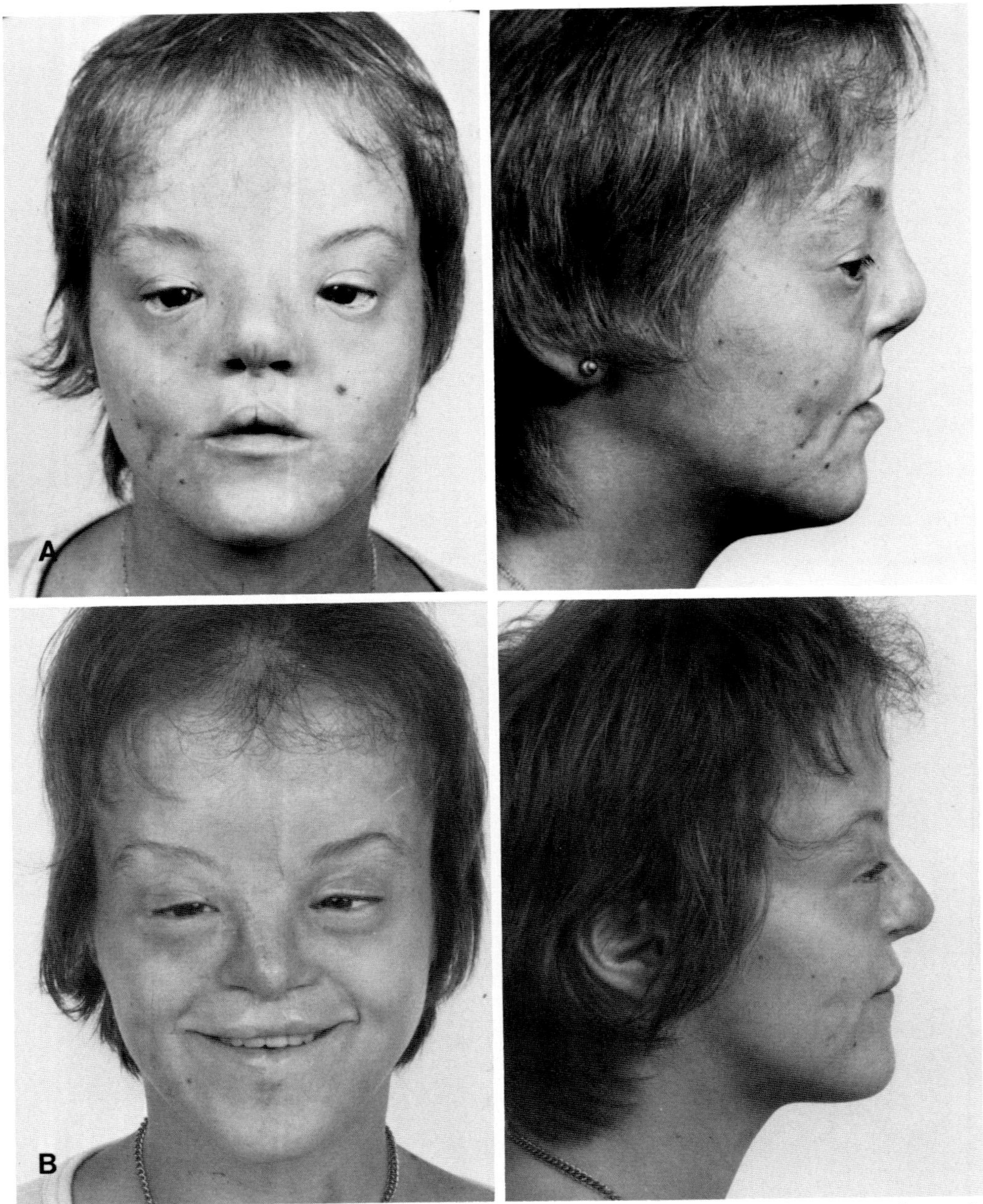

Figure 15.17 (*A*) Patient with telorbitism, a no. 0 facial cleft (see Chapter 14), and a palpebral and orbital anomaly (ptosis, palpebral shortness, telecanthus and an orbit with a greater vertical than transverse dimension) *resembling* blepharophimosis; this was not hereditary, and this is not true blepharophimosis. (*B*) After correction of the telorbitism (as in Fig. 15.7, *B–D*) and revision of the orbits so that the transverse dimension was greater than the vertical dimension. The medial canthopexies and lateral canthorrhaphies lengthened the palpebral fissures. An Abbé flap was performed for the lip. Great care had to be taken here to avoid injury to the temporal branch of the facial nerve which inverates the frontalis muscle, since this patient had no levator function and relied entirely on a frontalis sling for eye opening.

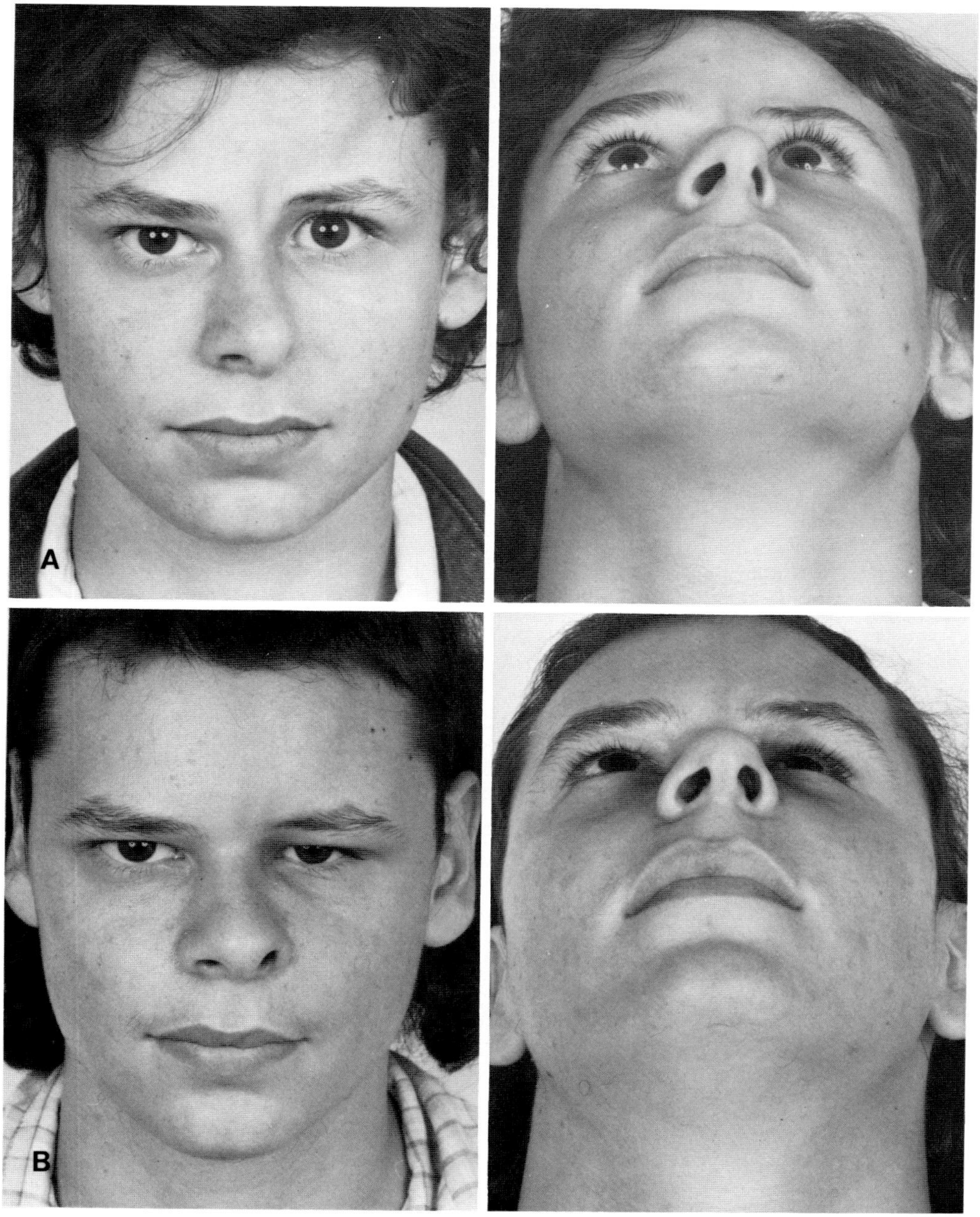

Figure 15.18 (*A*) Eighteen-year-old patient with Romberg's disease which has involved bone and soft tissue in the left frontal and supraorbital regions. (*B*) After an iliac bone graft to the left frontal region, superior orbital rim and orbital roof with coverage by a large pericranial flap. The patient had fusion preoperatively and, as anticipated, experienced diplopia for several months postoperatively.

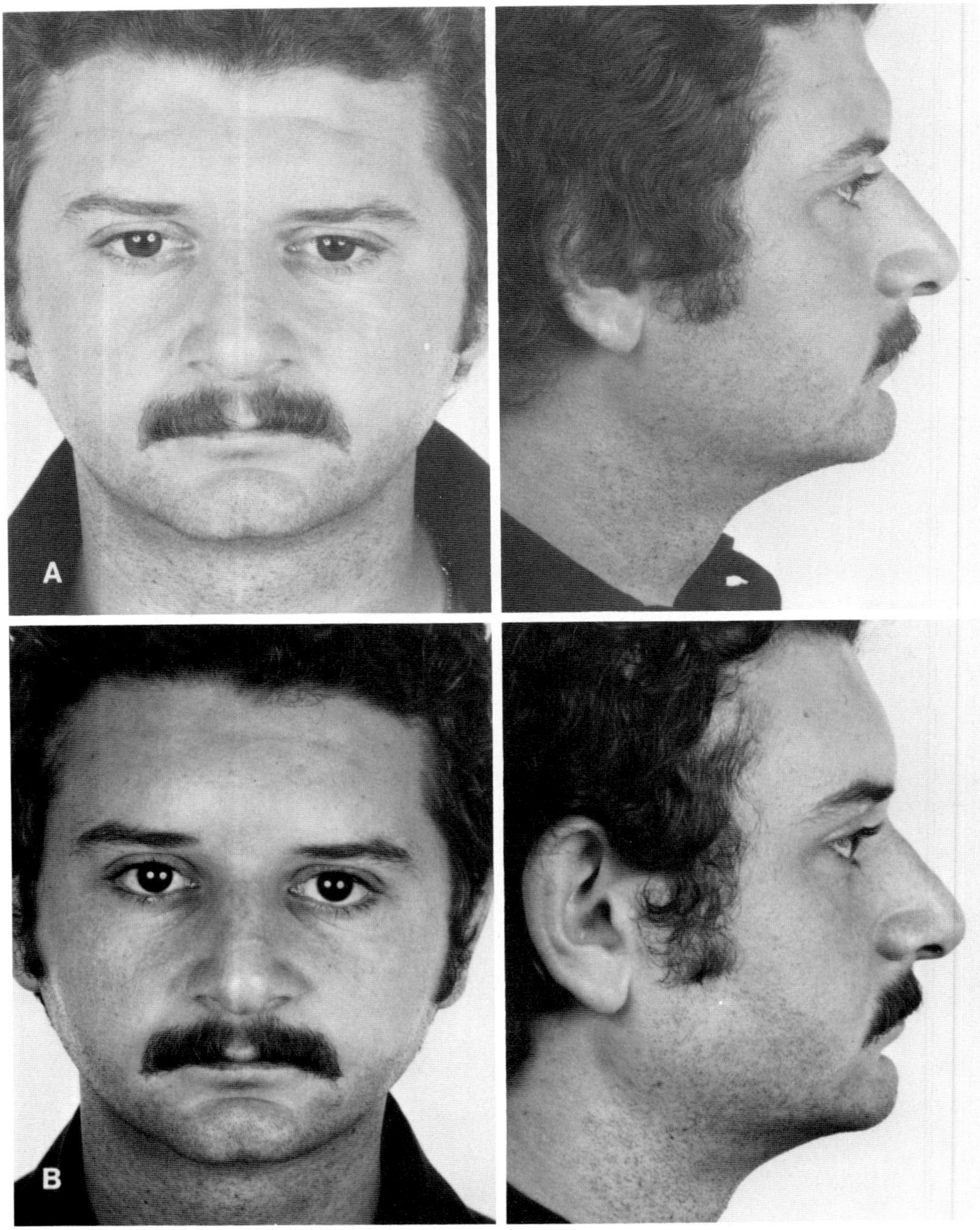

Figure 15.19 (*A*) Young man who was disturbed by the appearance of his forehead. (*B*) Postoperative result—after burring down of the supraorbital ridge and resection of portions of galea and frontalis muscle through a coronal incision (local anesthesia).

years, should consist of replacement of the missing tissue: bone grafts for missing bone (Fig. 15.18), and muscle or pericranial flaps or fat-dermal grafts for deficient soft tissue. In the area of *cosmetic surgery* (Fig. 15.19), the applications of craniofacial surgery are relatively unexplored. The coronal incision is now used without hesitation for the correction of forehead deformities, and orbital expansion is now being performed for esthetic as well as functional reasons.

The distinction between "aesthetic" and "reconstructive" surgery we feel is an artificial one, since all "functional" surgery must bear aesthetic considerations in mind, and all aesthetic surgery must consider function.

References

1. Wassmund, M.: *Lehrbuch der praktischen Chirurgie des Mundes und der Kiefer,* Bd. 1, 260, 282, Hermann Meusser, Berlin, 1935.
2. Schuchardt, K.: Ein Beitrag zur chirurgischen Kieferorthopädie unter Berücksichtigung ihrer Bedeutung für die Behandlung angeborener und erworberen Kieferdeformitäten bei Soldaten. *Dtsch. Zahn. Mund. Kieferheilk., 9:*73, 1942.
3. Gillies, H. D., and Harrison, S. H.: Operative correction by osteotomy of recessed maxillary malar compound in a case of oxycephaly. *Br. J. Plast. Surg., 3:* 123, 1950.
4. Obwegeser, H. L.: Surgical correction of small or retrodisplaced maxillae. *Plast. Reconstr. Surg., 43:*351, 1969.
5. Trauner, R., and Obwegeser, H. L.: The surgical correction of mandibular prognathism and retrognathia with consideration of genioplasty. *Oral Surg., 10:*677, 1957.
6. Tessier, P., et al.: Osteotomies cranio-naso-orbito-faciales, hypertelorisme. *Ann. Chir. Plast., 12:*103, 1967.
7. Tessier, P.: Osteotomies totales de la face. *Ann. Chir. Plast., 12:*273, 1967.
8. Gillies, H., and Millard, D. R., Jr.: *The Principles and Art of Plastic Surgery,* p. 51, Little Brown, Boston, 1957.
9. Wolfe, S. A., and Kawamoto, H. K.: Harvesting iliac bone. *J. Bone Joint Surg., 60A:*411, 1978.
10. Wolfe, S. A.: The utility of pericranial flaps. *Ann. Plast. Surg., 1:*146, 1978.
11. Hoffman, H. L., and Mohr, G.: Lateral canthal advancement of the supraorbital margin. *J. Neurosurg., 45:*376, 1976.
12. Tessier, P., Callahan, A., Mustarde, J., and Salyer, K. (Eds.): *Symposium on Plastic Surgery in the Orbital Region,* p. 283, C. V. Mosby, St. Louis, 1976.
13. Tessier, P., and Delaire, J.: Considerations sur le development de l'orbite; ses incidences sur la croissance faciale. *Rev. Stomatol., 63:*27, 1964.
14. Adduss, H.: Personal communication, 1977.
15. Freihofer, H. P., Jr.: Results of osteotomies of the facial skeleton in adolescence. *J. Maxillofac. Surg., 5:* 267, 1977.
16. Tessier, P.: Orbital hypertelorism; 1. Successive surgical attempts, materials and methods, causes and mechanisms. *Scand. J. Plast. Surg., 6:*135, 1972.
17. Converse, J. J., et al.: Ocular hypertelorism and pseudohypertelorism. *Adv. Surg. Treat. Plast. Reconstr. Surg., 45:*1, 1970.
18. Tessier, P.: Les exophthalmies. Expansion chirurgicale de l'orbite. *Ann. Chir. Plast., 14:*207, 1969.
19. Poswillo, D. E.: The pathogenesis of the first and second branchial arch syndrome. *Oral Surg., 35:*302, 1973.
20. Ross, R. B.: Lateral facial dysplasia (first and second brachial arch syndrome, hemifacial microsomia, in *Birth Defects: Original Article Series, Vol. XI,* No. 7, pp. 51–59. National Foundation-March of Dimes, White Plains, New York, 1976.
21. Rougier, J., Tessier, P., Hervouet, F., Woillez, M., Lekieffre, M., and Derome, P.: *Plastic Surgery of the Orbit and Eyelids* (translated by S. A. Wolfe). Masson, New York, 1978.
22. Harvald, E. P.: New treatment principles for mandibular malformations, in *Transactions of the Third International Orthodontic Congress,* pp. 148–154, C. V. Mosby, St. Louis, 1975.
23. Tessier, P.: Personal communication, 1975.

CHAPTER 16

Microvascular Methods of Reconstruction

Rollin K. Daniel, M.D., F.R.C.S.(C)

The demands of reconstructive surgery in the head and neck region are unique in plastic surgery for many reasons. First, the results are immediately visible to the patient and to society thus demanding as perfect a result as possible. This challenge is particularly arduous as the defect often represents only a portion of the face allowing comparison to the remaining normal structures. Second, several different types of tissue may be required for reconstruction of a single defect including skin, subcutaneous padding, muscle, bone, and oral mucosa. Third, local tissues may be compromised by radiation therapy or previous surgery thus restricting alternatives and mandating tissues from a distance. Fourth, primary reconstruction at or immediately following tumor extirpation is often necessary rather than prolonged multiple procedures. Due to these restrictions, microsurgery with its direct transfer to tissue from a distance is increasingly being considered as a solution to difficult problems in head and neck reconstruction.

MICROSURGERY

Microsurgery may be strictly defined as surgery performed under the magnification of an operating microscope. The first microsurgeons were otolaryngologists who employed the operating microscope for middle ear surgery in 1921. Ophthamologists initiated ophthalmic microsurgery in the 1950s. Each of these disciplines has developed operative techniques which are predominantly restricted to their own surgical specialties. It was only with the advent of microvascular and microneural techniques that microsurgery was liberated from sensory organ surgery thus permitting a new discipline to emerge—reconstructive microsurgery. The latter may be defined "as the functional restoration of tissue utilizing microsurgical techniques." The practitioners of this art were initially plastic surgeons who achieved clinical success in replantation of amputated parts and free tissue transfers, plus neurosurgeons who attempted cerebral revascularization. Recently, hand surgeons, orthopaedic surgeons and urologists have adapted many of these procedures for use in their own specialties after acquiring proficiency with these basic techniques.

Microsurgery demands sophisticated operating microscopes with variable zoom magnification and focusing. In the head and neck region, flexibility is of primary importance as is the availability of an assistant trained in microsurgical techniques. Selection of microinstruments and microsutures are determined by the specific microsurgical operation rather than the body region. Of critical importance is the need to achieve proficiency in the microsurgical teaching laboratory prior to clinical implementation. Basic exercises for acquiring fundamental skills in microvascular and microneural techniques have been published elsewhere.

Specific microvascular surgical techniques are required for anastomosis of arteries and veins 2 mm or less in diameter utilizing multiple methods including end-to-end, end-to-side, and interposition vein grafts. In addition, microsurgical repair of peripheral nerves is often necessary due to the small size and significant branches of the nerves as well as the difficulty of fascicular nerve grafts.

MICROVASCULAR SURGERY

Microvascular techniques are required for replantation of amputated parts or revascularization of tissue transferred from a distance.

Replantation Surgery

The vast majority of amputated parts in the head and neck region involve the scalp and associated parts including the ears or forehead. Successful replantation requires the following: (1) retrieval and cooling of the amputated part in normal ice as soon as possible, (2) control of hemorrhage and resuscitation of the patient, (3) transferal of the patient to the center specializing in replantation surgery, (4) assessment of the technical feasibility of replantation, (5) meticulous debridement of the amputated part, (6) multiple microvascular anastomoses frequently requiring insertion of numerous vein grafts, and (7) dedicated postoperative management. With this regime, it is often possible to achieve successful replantation despite severe avulsion injury following varied etiological agents (industrial machinery, automobile accidents or dog bites). Thus far, replanation with microvascular anastomoses of avulsed ears and facial parts has not been reported, but evaluation by an experienced reconstructive surgeon is always recommended.

Free Tissue Transfers

A free tissue transfer may be defined as the physical movement of tissue from one point of the body to another with revascularization, usually requiring microvascular anastomoses. It is comprised of three basic steps: (1) evaluation of recipient vessels, (2) isolation of donor tissue, and (3) vascular anastomoses. The recipient vessels must include a healthy recipient artery with a strong perfusion pressure and one or more draining veins. In the head and neck region, the recipient artery is often palpable and the recipient vein visible; unfortuantely, the former may be damaged by radiation therapy and the latter may be resected during tumor ablation. Thus multiple vessels must be available and the donor tissue must be able to survive on a reduced and reoriented blood supply following isolation on only those vessels which will be anastomosed at the recipient site. Each tissue of the body tolerates ischemia to a variable extent with muscle and gastrointestinal tissue withstanding deprivation to a minimal degree. Vascular anastomoses of vessels 2 mm and below is required with significant vessel size discrepancy being a frequent occurrence. Early recognition and definitive treatment of vascular

Table 16.1
Free Tissue Transfers

A. SINGLE TISSUE TRANSFERS
  1. Free flap transfer
    a) Free skin flap
    b) Free myocutaneous flap
  2. Free bone transfer
  3. Free muscle transfer
  4. Free nerve transfer
  5. Free intestinal transfer

B. COMPOUND TISSUE TRANSFERS
  1. Free osteocutaneous flap transfer
  2. Free musculocutaneous flap transfer
  3. Free neurovascular flap transfer
  4. Free toe transfer

complications is required thus potentially compounding an already difficult postoperative period.

The complexity of free tissue transfers, including a prolonged operative time and a multiteam approach, is justified by the superior results which can be acheived in primary reconstruction. No longer is it necessary to switch an intraoral defect to the forehead to achieve adequate oral lining nor to accept an oral cripple as the inevitable result of a close-range shotgun blast to the face. This transformation in reconstruction of the head and neck region is due to recent advances in free tissue transfers and will be discussed in depth (Table 16.1).

FREE SKIN FLAPS

Originally, tube pedicle flaps were employed in staged reconstruction of the head and neck region but these multistage transfers proved too time consuming thus leading to "jump" flaps and local flaps. A major advance was the perfection of regional arterial flaps. However, the forehead flap produced significant donor site morbidity and the deltopectoral flap often obligates a dependent phanyngostome and multiple stages. Thus, the free flap is attractive for head and neck repair as it allows unlimited flap tissue, transferred in one stage from an inconspicuous donor site with definitive insertion.

Free skin flaps have now been utilized to restore external skin, scalp coverage, oral lining, subcutaneous bulk, and various combinations. They have been employed to cover open wounds following trauma, tumor resection, and radiation as well as to correct closed wounds due to scar contracture, congenital anomalies (Rhomberg's disease, craniofacial defects), and so forth. The two most commonly employed free flaps are the free groin flap and the free dorsalis pedis flap. Each possesses distinct advantages when transferred to the head and neck region which are summarized in Table 16.2.

FREE GROIN FLAP

The free groin flap is a regional flap which straddles the expected course of the superficial circumflex iliac artery (SCIA) supplied by either the SCIA or superficial inferior epigastric artery (SIEA) with venous drainage through either the superficial inferior epigastric vein (SIEV) or the venae comitantes of the SCIA.

The essential anatomical landmarks are marked: public tubercle, anterior superior iliac spine, and femoral pulse. The axis of the free groin flap is a line drawn from the lowest possible

Table 16.2
Free Skin Flap Donor Site

	Groin Flap	Dorsalis Pedis Flap
SKIN FLAP		
Size	30 × 20 cm	10 × 10 cm
Thickness	2–3 cm (minimum)	0.5–1.0 cm
Donor site	Primary closure	Skin graft
BLOOD VESSEL		
Artery	Superior circumflex iliac (1.0–3.0 mm)	Dorsalis pedis (2.0–4.0 mm)
Vein		
Superficial	Superficial inferior epigastric (2.0–4.0 mm)	Greater saphenous (2.0–5.0 mm)
Deep	Paired venae comitantes (1.0 mm)	Paired venae comitantes (1.0 mm)
OPTIONS		
Bone	Iliac crest (10 × 2 × 6 cm)	Second metatarsal
Nerve	No	Superficial peroneal
MORBIDITY	Minimal	Significant

origin of the SCIA through the anterior superior iliac spine to the inferior angle of the scapula. The flap axis is *not* outlined parallel to the inguinal ligament, but rather on a more inferior to superior oblique line. A pattern of the defect is then placed on the flap axis with allowance to assure overlap of the donor and recipient vessels. The medial border of the flap can be placed as far medially as 15 cm from the femoral artery, but in the vast majority of cases, it is placed within 3–4 cm of the femoral pulse. When the borders of the flap have been completely outlined, one can do a controlled inferior lateral to superior medial dissection. The inferior lateral border is incised with reflection of the sartorius muscle fascia which allows visualization of the SCIA on the undersurface of the fascia. The femoral artery is then identified and the dissection continues along the top and medial sides of the femoral artery. This precludes possible transection of the SCIA while allowing identification of the artery at its origin prior to commitment to flap elevation. With this approach, it is possible to identify the vessel origin on the femoral artery or the other possible parenteral vessels which occurs in 17% of dissections. Once the supplying artery (SCIA or SIEA) is identified one can complete the more superior medial dissection with isolation of the SIEV and the possible entrance of the SCIV. The venae comitantes of the SCIA are identified as they pass underneath the femoral artery to reach the femoral vein. One now has complete control of the vascular pedicle to the free groin flap allowing total isolation of the flap from lateral to medial with absolute assurance of the vascular pedicle. If the leg has been draped completely free primary closure of the donor site can be accomplished without great difficulty.

The flap possesses numerous advantages including the following: (1) proven clinical reliability, (2) vast size (30 × 20 cm), (3) multiple arteriovenous systems, (4) inconspicuous donor site, and (5) optional inclusion of bone. Its disadvantages are few, but significant, especially in the head and neck region: (1) excessive thickness, (2) poor color match, and (3) a relatively short vascular stalk. The free groin flap is favored when large areas of skin are required or with a compound osteocutaneous flap following comando resection. Due to its bulkiness, the flap has limited intraoral application unless an extensive resection has been done.

FREE FOOT FLAP

The free foot flap straddles the dorsalis pedis artery, extending on either side for 5 cm and from the proximal web-space to the extensor retinacular ligament. Following outline of the flap, the distal half is incised on the medial and lateral margins followed by elevation in a distal to proximal direction. The flap is elevated from its inferior medial border up to the extensor hallicis longus tendon. Attention is then directed to the lateral border which is elevated up to the tendon of the extensor digitorum brevis muscle to the great toe must be transected at its insertion and also as it emerges from under the extensor digitorum longus. Following this transection it is possible to elevate the flap with the surgeon sitting distally and elevating the flap with the scissors pointed into the tarsal bone. Essentially the vascular stalk is reflected off the bones into the flap. Once the flap is completely elevated the vascular stalk can be further dissected by dividing the extensor retinacular ligament and then continued into the lower leg. The donor site is covered with a thick skin graft (Fig. 16.1).

The flap advantages are numerous including: (1) large diameter supplying arteries and veins (2.0–4.0 mm), (2) a long vascular stalk (8 cm or longer, (3) extreme thinness, (4) potential reinnervation through the superficial peroneal nerve, and (5) acceptable size (10 × 10 cm). However, its disadvantages are formidable: (1) a *difficult* dissection even for the experienced surgeon, (2) restricted size with minimal expansion on delay, and (3) significant donor site morbidity. The free dorsal foot flap is favored for small to moderate size intraoral defects where its thinness permits contoured closure with passage of its long vascular stalk into the suprahyoid region. For completeness, it is necessary to mention the free deltopectoral flap and the free intercostal flap although these flaps have not been routinely utilized in the head and neck region.

THE ROLE OF FREE FLAPS IN HEAD AND NECK RECONSTRUCTION

Free flap transfers to the head and neck were initially done to correct burn scar contracture and subsequently for reconstruction following tumor resection. The essential advantage was their application in areas above the zygomatic arch which could be reached only with great difficulty utilizing a deltopectoral flap or staged jump flap. Following this success, multiple surgeons began to review the possible utilization of free groin flaps in the oral cavity with the initial reports of Kaplan and Finseth leading to a negative conclusion due to failure secondary to infection. However, clinical success by Fujino and Panje mitigated this negativism and subsequently confirmation by Leeb, Daniel and Acland has proven the value of free flap transfers to the oral cavity concurrent with tumor resection. One of the major difficulties in a free flap transfer following tumor resection is identification of recipient vessels. Although virtually any branch of the external carotid artery is available, ranging from the supraclavicular to the lingual facial vessels, recipient veins are often compromised. Leeb has shown that the majority of anterior mandibular resections require a standard radical neck resection on the side of dominant involvement and a suprahyoid dissection on the contralateral side with the latter offering numerous recipient vessels. Due to its long vascular pedicle, the free dorsalis foot flap can be inset in the oral cavity and its vascular pedicle easily passed into the suprahyoid dissection. This maneuver allows utilization of the external maxillary vessels, both artery and vein. The second major difficulty complicating free tissue transfers is the effect of radiation on the recipient vessels as well as possible secondary radiation damage to the transferred flap.

The author has successfully utilized previously irradiated vessels (5000 rads) without encountering significant vessel wall hypertrophy or reduced blood flow. However, the absence of pathological damage may be related to the time period following radiation (6–18 months) and vessel diameter (1.5 mm). At the present time, previous radiation therapy has not been a significant factor causing loss of free flaps nor has secondary radiation therapy (2000 rads) compromised a successful free flap transfer. The possibility of radiation damage must be considered, but not as a contraindication for transfer.

As shown by Acland, a high success rate (93%, 13/14) free flap transfers to the oral cavity can be achieved and thus obviate the need for additional deformity or dependent fistulas. At

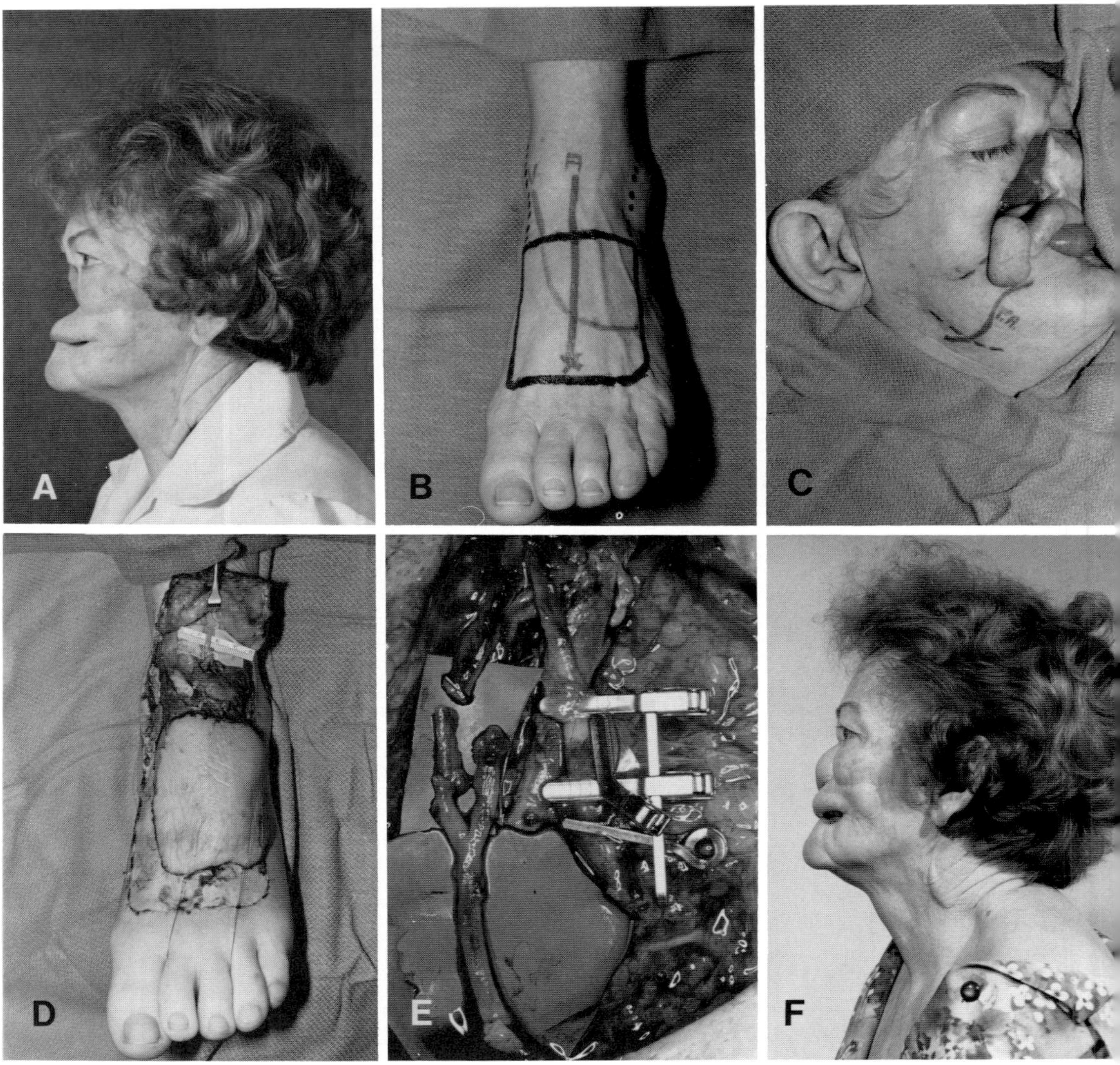

Figure 16.1 Total nasal reconstruction in a 55-year-old woman with previous irradiation and 9 flap reconstructions ravaged by multiple recurrent basal cell carcinoma. (*A*) Complete absence of the nose and its bony base. (*B*) Outline of the dorsal foot flap on the dorsalis pedis artery (*Line A*). (*C*) The nasal-maxillary defect with remnants of previous tube pedicle flaps. (*D*) The foot flap, which was previously elevated and lined with a split-thickness skin graft is isolated on its vascular pedicle. (*E*) Completion of the arterial anastomosis (*A*) and insertion of a Y-shape vein graft (*VG*) in the venous system. (*F*) The patient 3 months postoperatively.

the present time, it would appear that free flap transfers for oral cavity reconstruction are equal to conventional techniques both in their overall success rate and their absence of dependent fistulas or additional cosmetic deformity.

Free Bone Transfers

For decades, bone grafts have been used in facial reconstruction with variable results due to secondary extrusion from infection or absorption due to avascularity of the recipient bed. This problem achieves complex proportions following mandibular resection and/or radiation therapy. Recent advances in microsurgery have attempted to solve this problem with the vascularized bone graft whose essential intrinsic blood supply is restored by microvascular anastomoses to recipient vessels. Thus, the vascularized bone graft is independent of the recipient bed regardless of previous radiation therapy. Three bones have been employed in head and neck reconstruction: rib, iliac crest and metatarsals. Each donor site differs significantly in its blood supply and clinical application.

RIB

The rib is a malleable, curve bone where a nutrient artery arises from the posterior intercostal artery. Its isolation onto the intercostal artery and vein requires a thoracotomy with disarticulation at the costovertebral junction. The rib can be employed as an isolated bone for simple mandibular replacement or incorporated into a compound osteocutaneous flap. Its advantages include the following: (1) a long curved bone, (2) a long neurovascular stalk, (3) minimal donor site morbidity, and (4) option inclusion of skin, muscle, and/or sensory innervation. Its disadvantages are numerous: (1) attempts to force curvature will result in fracture or compression of the medullary blood supply, (2) a deep difficult dissection, and (3) unproven clinical applicability and viability. At the present time, free rib transfers would appear most valuable for compound central segment defects where soft tissue coverage and bony stability is required.

ILIAC CREST

The iliac crest is largely a cancellous bone which can be incorporated into a free groin flap. The periosteal blood supply via the SCIA is retained by incorporation of a thick muscle cuff. The advantages of the free osteocutaneous groin flap are the following: (1) the iliac crest can be shaped to fit mandibular, maxillary or zygomatic defects by appropriate osteotomies, rather than extensive bending; (2) donor site morbidity is minimal; (3) a large amount of associated skin coverage can be provided; and (4) the operative technique represents an extension of the proven free groin flap rather than an entirely new procedure. Its principal disadvantage is that the blood supply is marginal at best and long term viability has *not* been proven. Currently, the free osteocutaneous groin flap is valuable for reconstruction of compound defects of the mandibular body and ascending ramus with associated soft tissue loss (Fig. 16.2).

METATARSAL

The second metatarsal can be incorporated into a free dorsal foot flap. The nutrient blood supply to the metatarsal bone is from the plantar metatarsal arteries rather than the dorsalis pedis artery which nourishes the overlying flap. However, the numerous interconnecting branches probably ensure adequate perfusion thus maintaining viability of the bone. The principal advantage of this osteocutaneous flap is the malleability of the dorsal foot flap and

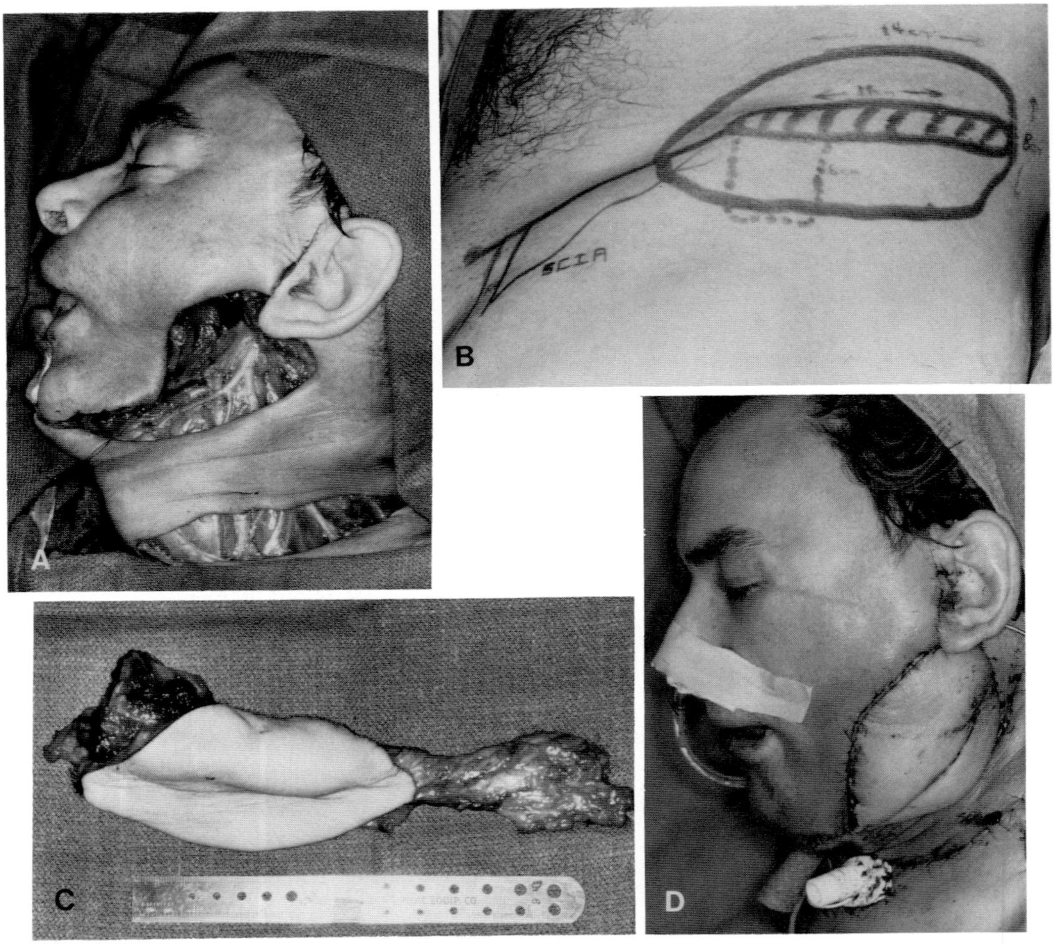

Figure 16.2 A 55-year-old man following extensive resection of a T_4NoMo retromolar squamous cell carcinoma which recurred despite previous surgery and radiation therapy (6500 rads). (*A*) Skin defect following pteryoid dissection plus commando resection. (*B*) Outline of a free osteocutaneous groin flap (14 × 8 cm) incorporating a portion of the iliac crest (11 × 6 cm) which will be isolated on a 14-cm long vascular stalk. (*C*) The free osteocutaneous groin flap. (*D*) The patient following primary reconstruction of the mandible and overlying skin with a free tissue transfer.

the rigidity of the second metatarsal, especially in reconstruction of anterior segmental defects of the mandible or total nasal replacement.

Free Intestinal Transfers

Free intestinal transfers were utilized for replacement of the cervical esophagus as early as 1961 with early proponents being Hiebert, Roberts and Nakayama. These transfers, performed in the premicrovascular surgical era, represented a dramatic solution for an apparently hopeless situation. However, the subsequent introduction of the deltopectoral flap, which permitted two-stage hypopharyngeal-cervical esophogeal reconstruction, appeared to be a simpler and more expedient technique. Recent perfection of microvascular techniques, as applied to clinical free tissue transfers and a realization of the limitation of esophageal reconstruction with skin flaps has led to a reawakening of interest in free intestinal transfers. At the present time, one may transfer segments of jejunum or colon for esophageal replacement following extensive resection or failure of conventional techniques.

As emphasized by Nakayama and May, the critical step in a successful free intestinal transfer is selection of the optimal operative sequence with emphasis on proven intestinal viability prior to completion of the bowel anastomoses. In irradiated patients, it would appear prudent to do a two-stage procedure consisting of free intestinal transfer with controlled fistulas at either end followed several months later by hypopharyngeal and esophageal hookup.

The proximal segment of jejunum distal to the ligament of Treitz is usually isolated on the large marginal arteries which arise from the superior mesenteric artery. A portion of the right colon can be harvested on the colonic vascular branches. Selection of intestinal segment is influenced by numerous factors including the following: (1) availability which is determined greatly by previous operations, (2) bacterial contamination, (3) donor site morbidity, and (4) resistance to ischemia. Both the jejunum and the colon have their purposes. The majority of diameter discrepancies between donor and recipient vessels can be accommodated by variable anastomotic techniques thus providing a higher margin of safety. Recent reports by May and Acland emphasize the value of this procedure in difficult cases of esophageal reconstruction. Whether free intestinal transfers will ultimately replace conventional bowel pedicles of colon, which are frequently plagued by catastrophic complications, must await additional experience.

Free Muscle Transfers

Free muscle transfers to the head and neck region have been utilized for correction of facial paralysis. The basic hypothesis is that, following prolonged denervation, the facial muscles will become irreversibly fibrotic requiring replacement with healthy functioning muscles from a distance.

Rather than accepting the partial viability and random reinnervation of Thompson's free muscle grafts, microsurgeons have attempted the direct transfer of muscle with preservation of normal function via microneurovascular anastomoses. Tamai's initial experimental confirmation of this technique has been confirmed clinically by Chen, Harii, Ikuta and others. However, the essential problem remains selection of an appropriate recipient nerve. Obviously, any remaining facial nerve branch is the first choice with a cross-facial nerve graft from the normal side being preferable to trigeminal or hypoglossal nerves. Harii had documented progressive reinnervation beginning at 3 months with maximum contractibility achieved at 8 months and an associated 50% decrease in bulk.

GRACILIS MUSCLE

The gracilis muscle originates from the pelvis and pubic arch, passes superficially down the medial surface of the thigh to insert on the tibia. Its dominant nutrient artery and its vanae comitantes enter the muscle in its proximal third. They originate most commonly from the profunda femoris or medial circumflex femoral artery. The main motor nerve is a branch from the obturator nerve and can be easily identified with a nerve stimulator. The gracilis muscle is extremely bulky (33 cm long, 8 cm wide, 5 cm thick) thus allowing mass action replacement. The muscle is fixed proximally to the temporal fascia, split distally, and inserted into the upper and lower lips. The principal disadvantage of the gracilis muscle is its excessive bulk and excessive contractility.

EXTENSOR DIGITORUM BREVIS

Thompson employed the extensor digitorum brevis from the foot as a donor site for nonvascularized muscle grafts. The extensor digitorum brevis originates from the calcaneus and sends its tendons to the medial four toes. Its blood supply is from the lateral tarsal artery, a branch of the dorsalis pedis artery, while the neural innervation is from the deep peroneal nerve. The origin of this muscle can be inserted into the zygomatic arch and the tendons inserted into the paralyzed portion of the face. Although contractility is minimum, it is superior to a static fascial sling. In the final analysis, the value of free muscle transfers for facial reanimation is far from proven and they represent a salvage procedure at best.

Free Omental Transfer

The omentum has long been transferred beyond the peritoneal cavity to revascularize ischemic areas and to recover critical structures. Despite multiple methods of lengthening its essential blood supply, its dependence on continuity with the peritoneal cavity results in possible bowel strangulation and adhesion formation thereby limiting its application. Thus recent introduction of microvascular anastomoses permits transfer of omentum to distant sites with immediate revascularization. McLean and Buncke were the first to investigate the application of this technique and emphasized several pertinent points: (1) a rich blood supply from large diameter vessels, (2) malleability and availability, and (3) minimum morbidity. The omentum is harvested on a vascular stalk incorporating either the right or the left gastroepiploic vessels with the former being the larger. The omentum is then transferred to the exposed skull or other sites to provide a vascularized bed which can then be covered with split thickness skin grafts. The principal application of the omentum is in areas of poor blood supply where few recipient vessels are available or correction of curved contour deformities such as the skull and/or subcutaneous defects. The value of the omentum in head and neck reconstruction has decreased following perfection of free skin flap transfers particularly the free deltopectoral flap for coverage of skull and the deepithelialized groin flap for reconstruction of subcutaneous defects associated with Romberg's disease.

References

1. Ch'en C. W.: *Zhonghua Yixue Zazhi No. 8:*530, 1975 (published in Chinese).
2. Daniel, R. K., and May, J. W.: Free flaps: an overview. *Clin. Orthop.*, May 1978.
3. Daniel, R. K., and Swartz, B.: Advances in microsurgery, in *Advances in Surgery, Vol. XI*, edited by C. A. Robb, Yearbook, Chicago, 1977.
4. Daniel, R. K., and Tyalor, G. I.: Distant transfer of an island flap by microvascular anastomoses. *Plast. Reconstr. Surg., 52:*111, 1973.
5. Daniel, R. K., and Terzis, J. K.: *Reconstructive Microsurgery*, Little Brown, Boston, 1977.
6. Daniel, R. K., Terzis, J., and Midgley, R. D.: Restoration of sensation to an anaesthetic hand by a free neurovascular flap from the foot. *Plast. Reconstr. Surg., 57:*275, 1976.
7. Harii, K., Ohmori, K., and Torii, S.: Free gracilis muscle transplantation, with microneurovascular anastomoses for the treatment of facial paralysis. *Plast. Reconstr. Surg., 57:*133, 1976.
8. Hiebert, C. A., and Cummings, G. O., Jr.: Successful replacement of the cervical esophagus by transplantation and revascularization of free graft of gastric antrum. *Ann. Surg., 154:*103, 1961.
9. Ikuta, Y.: Autotransplant of omentum to cover large denudation of the scalp. *Plast. Reconstr. Surg., 55:*490, 1975.
10. Ikuta, Y.: Free muscle transfer, in *Reconstructive Microsurgery*, edited by R. K. Daniel, and J. Terzis, Little Brown, Boston, 1977.
11. May, J. W., and Bunting, P. D.: Free jejunal transfer for irradiated esophageal reconstruction, in *Reconstructive Microsurgery*, edited by R. K. Daniel, and J. Terzis, Little Brown, Boston, 1977.
12. McCraw, J. B., and Furlow, L. T.: The dorsalis pedis arterialized flap. *Plast. Reconstr. Surg., 55:*177, 1975.
13. McLean, D. H., and Buncke, H. J.: Autotransplant of omentum to a large scalp defect, with microsurgical revascularization. *Plast. Reconstr. Surg., 49:*268, 1972.

14. Miller, G. D. H., Anstee, E. J., and Snell, J. A.: Successful replantation of an avulsed scalp by microvascular anastomoses. *Plast. Reconstr. Surg.*, *58:*133, 1976.
15. Nakayama, K., Yamamoto, K., Makino, H., Odaka, M., Ohwada, M., and Takahashi, H.: Experience with free autografts of the bowel with new venous anastomosis apparatus. *Surgery*, *55:*706, 1964.
16. Östrup, L. T., and Fredrickson, J. M.: Distant transfer of a free, living bone graft by microvascular anastomosis. *Plast. Reconstr. Surg.*, *54:*274, 1974.
17. Östrup, L. T., and Fredrickson, J. M.: Reconstruction of mandibular defects after radiation, using a free, living bone graft transferred by microvascular anastomoses. *Plast. Reconstr. Surg.*, *55:*563, 1975.
18. Roberts, R. E., and Douglas, F. M.: Replacement of the cervical esophagus and hypopharynx by a revascularized free jejunal autograft. *N. Engl. J. Med.*, *264:* 342, 1961.
19. Serafin, D., et al.: A rib-containing free flap to reconstruct mandibular defects. *Br. J. Plast. Surg.*, *30:* 263, 1977.
20. Spira, M., Daniel, R. K., and Agris, J.: Successful replantation of an avulsed scalp with regrowth of hair. *Plast. Reconstr. Surg.*, *62:*447, 1978.
21. Tamai, S., Komatsu, S., Sakamoto, H., Sano, S., Sasauchi, N., Harii, Y., Tatsumi, Y., and Okuda, H.: Free muscle transplants in dogs with microsurgical neurovascular anastomoses. *Plast. Reconstr. Surg.*, *46:* 219, 1970.
22. Taylor, G. I., and Daniel, R. K.: The anatomy of several free flap donor sites. *Plast. Reconstr. Surg.*, *56:* 243, 1975.
23. Taylor, G. I., Miller, G. D. H., and Ham, F. J.: The free vascularized bone graft: a clinical extension of microvascular techniques. *Plast. Reconstr. Surg.*, *55:* 533, 1975.
24. Taylor, G. I., and Watson, N.: One-stage repair of compound leg defects with free, revascularized flaps of groin and iliac crest. *Plast. Reconstr. Surg.*, *61:*491, 1978.
25. Thompson, N. Treatment of facial paralysis by free skeletal muscle grafts, in *Fifth International Congress of Plastic and Reconstructive Surgery*, Butterworth, London; 1971.
26. Weiland, A. W., and Daniel, R. K.: Free vascularized bone grafts for reconstruction of segmental bone defects. *J. Bone Joint Surg.*, in press.

Index